The Garbage Collector

Root Canals, Disease and
what the dental profession
refuses to acknowledge

ROBERT GAMMAL BDS., FACNEM(dent)

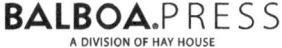
BALBOA.PRESS
A DIVISION OF HAY HOUSE

Balboa Press books may be ordered through booksellers or by contacting:

Balboa Press
A Division of Hay House
1663 Liberty Drive
Bloomington, IN 47403
www.balboapress.com.au
AU TFN: 1 800 844 925 (Toll Free inside Australia)
AU Local: (02) 8310 7086 (+61 2 8310 7086 from outside Australia)

Interior Image Credit: Robert Gammal

Print information available on the last page.

ISBN: 978-1-9822-9515-8 (sc)
ISBN: 978-1-9822-9516-5 (e)

Balboa Press rev. date: 06/24/2022

Contents

The acquisition of a new truth is like the acquisition
of a new sense, which renders a man capable
of perceiving and recognizing
a large number of phenomena that are
invisible and hidden from another,
as they were from him originally.

—Liebig, in *Chemische Briefe*, as quoted often by Dr Weston Price

Foreword

Dr Mike Godfrey, MB, BS

It has been fortunate over the years that there have always been a few who refuse to walk away from the truth. I have known Robert Gamal for forty years and consider him to be one of those few. Predictably, just as with those earlier pioneers, there was opposition and ridicule followed by ad hominem attack. However, Robert remained true to his principles, and this book reveals the reasons.

Robert does not call a spade a spade. He quite justifiably calls it a *bloody* spade. The reader will feel Robert's pain and frustration as he details the impeccable but rejected research of one hundred years ago, when the leading American researcher Western Price collaborated with Drs Rosenow, Billings, Mayo and other luminaries demonstrating how dental procedures could result in serious chronic illnesses. Thirty years ago, in Hal Huggins's home, I saw Price's metal trunk with his accumulated root canal research papers in a black hard back 2 volumes 1100-page book. Inside the book's cover I read the dedication to his son. Before he knew better, Weston Price, as a leading dentist, had performed a root canal on his son, who subsequently died, and Price then realized the cause of his son's death.

I graduated in 1963, but like Robert, I had to wait twenty years before I became aware of possible underlying reasons why my patients were remaining ill. The moment was at a medical conference in California when a research dentist, Hal Huggins, told us to look at teeth. A few months later, I flew to Colorado to spend a week at Hal's clinic, little realizing how it would change my medical practice. I had more hugs from happy patients in the last ten years of my practice than the first forty.

Problems occur in both medical and dental professions, as Robert shows, where standard investigations cannot reveal the real cause. I also had to become reasonably proficient in electrodermal testing (EDT or EAV) with minimal available training. A couple of anecdotal examples could suffice here. Melanie was a twenty-year-old lass with a two-year history of non-stop left earache for which she was on three medications, including morphine. She had consulted ENT and neurological specialists, including an oral surgeon, to no avail. The latter's rooms were right below mine. With EDT, I identified the likely cause as an impacted left upper wisdom tooth (back molar) that, according to acupuncture meridians, was also on the inner ear. I took her downstairs and asked the surgeon to do a standard nerve block (as per Neural Therapy). Fifteen minutes later, he came running up shouting that the earache had gone. I told him to extract the tooth. Three months later, Melanie came back with her mother to thank me. Her mother then revealed that her daughter had been scheduled for nerve ablation as a desperate final solution.

Another example was an elderly lady with a permanent unpleasant head pain described as like a very tight bathing cap. It started after a Maryland bridge had been placed on two titanium implants some months before. As galvanic testing confirmed a very high current between the bridge and the implants, I informed her that either the bridge had to be unscrewed or she would continue to suffer. She eventually went back to the oral surgeon, and the nerve pain disappeared the instant the bridge was detached. How rapidly does pain stop when you let go of an electric fence? Unfortunately, outside of Europe, there is now even less training available in these additional modalities.

Last century, I somewhat naively thought that my mercury toxicity diagnoses from dental amalgam in patients suffering from chronic symptoms would be welcomed by my fellow GPs. However, with written support from a couple of European professors, both being past-presidents of their Oncology Societies, I successfully kept the Medical Council disciplinary boards off my back for forty years prior to retirement. My main concern with mercury was the proven association with dementia. In 1968, there was an average of sixteen amalgam fillings in the mouths of twenty-one-year-olds thanks to the post WW2 socialized school nurses being trained to "fill the valleys" where the natural grooves in all posterior teeth were drilled and filled to prevent them getting decay. This practice only stopped only in 1976. However, that cohort had become the middle-aged and elderly, with a remaining amalgam load greatly exceeding the WHO safer upper limit of eight fillings. My warnings in the 1990s were apparently disregarded, and we are now seeing an increasing epidemic of early-onset dementia.

Ironically, both medical and dental resistance to accepting the mercury factor could be due in part to one of the amalgam manufacturers listed adverse effects besides irrational anger, being resistance to criticism. A perfect example to this was Adolf Hitler who refused to listen to his generals' advice to quit whilst ahead. WW2 could have ended in 1943, but Hitler had numerous amalgams, along with two gold bridges and crowns, which would have guaranteed a continuous flood of mercury to his by then demented brain.

Weston Price led the way with his famous tome *Nutrition and Physical Degeneration*. Ralph Steinman then confirmed this theory in the 1960s and 1970s, with his primary research proving that the direction and volume of the normally retrograde dentinal fluid was hormonally controlled and negatively influenced by raised sugar levels in the blood. Thus, dental decay was nutritional and not a fluoride deficiency disease. Notably, both the Aboriginal and the Maori populations drinking fluoride-deficient rain and river waters, had no dental decay before adopting foods based on white flour and sugar.

Robert's position on fluoride is fully justified and well supported by science. One of the less known effects of fluoride is musculo-skeletal fluorosis, which presents as diffuse painful joints and is often misdiagnosed and treated as arthritis. Many middle-aged people are long-term tea drinkers with several cups per day. Notably, there can be more fluoride in a teabag than in one litre of fluoridated water. This is then exacerbated by fluoridated toothpaste. A seventy-nine-year-old lady consulted me for an opinion when she was on the waiting list for her second hip replacement, having also had both knees done. She admitted to drinking six cups of Bell's tea per day since her teens and used Colgate toothpaste twice a day. Both her urine and blood fluoride levels were elevated. but after changing to herbal teas and toothpaste, her "arthritis" pains decreased so much that she went on a cruise instead of having surgery. The *New Zealand Medical Journal* published the case in 2018. Notably, arthritis and related hip and knee replacements are annually costing health departments several billions of dollars. Additionally, fluoride blocks iodine uptake, with resulting obesity, diabetes, and breast inflammatory diseases.

It is still a tragedy that proper nutrition is not taught at medical or dental schools, but health is not profitable. Indeed, one could cynically state that the human carcass is unique by only having a commercial value when diseased

Robert's very well-referenced book ought to be read by all who, as Huggins succinctly put it, are interested in their health.

Acknowledgements

Many thanks to Myra, Tesa and Ysabel, who had to deal with me during my mad hatter phase and survived it. I thank you for your love, the constant support, and many debates.

Thanks to my parents, who worked so hard to put me through dentistry and taught me how to be in the world.

Thanks to my friend Myrop Moyne, for the initial edit, who laughed as she told me that what I had written was not English.

Thanks to my dear friend Suzi Alesandra for her painstaking work to correct my terrible grammar.

Thanks to the many dentists and doctors and other less-acknowledged health care practitioners that I had the pleasure of working with and who guided me to greater knowledge.

And, finally, thanks to all the patients who taught me the realities of what is printed here.

A Note from a Colleague

My life changed forever early in the 1990s when Robert Gammal tapped me on the shoulder and invited me to a dental meeting at which he was debating another dentist. The topic—mercury.

Following that meeting, Robert invited me to attend a lecture being given by Prof Fritz Lorscheider. Upon hearing the real science about mercury toxicity and realizing what I was subjecting my patients to and how my education at Sydney University was basically a sham, my dental education began anew. Meeting the giants of dental and medical research, namely Fritz Lorscheider, Professor Boyd Haley, Dr Murry Vimy, Dr Jerry Bouquot, Dr Chris Hussar, Dr Wes Shankland, and the master clinician of them all, Dr Hal Huggins, meant that I never practised dentistry as I had been taught again. Amazingly, I was now receiving thank-you cards and letters from patients who were so very grateful for their new-found health. For the uninitiated, the secret to regaining defective health is to *first* address your dental condition with a biological dentist, and not by a dentist who calls himself or herself "holistic." The rubbish Robert and I were taught at dental school was appalling. Our "professors" should have known the current science at the time yet chose to ignore it and pursue their and the profit-centred dental dogmas that prevailed at that time and ignore the true science.

The Garbage Collector will pique the interest of both the dentally informed and the person struggling to recover his or her health in the aftermath of toxic dental interventions. Robert uncovers and lays bare the politics, scientific cover-ups, and money-driven "science" of past and current-day dentistry. You will love the read and knowledge provided. Enjoy.

Dr Andrew Taylor BDS

Some Terminology

Alice's Adventures in Wonderland gave us many insights into the world as seen by Lewis Carroll. One of those is conveyed through the character of the Mad Hatter. At the time the book was written, the hatters of the society used mercuric nitrate to cure the felt was used to make hats for presidents and nobility. The exposure to mercury caused them to go quite mad, hence the phrase "Mad as a Hatter".

"Quecksilber" is the German word for "quicksilver" or **"mercury"**. When amalgam was first introduced to the world in 1812, the German and Swedish dentists who used this new wonder material were called "Quecksilber dentists" or "Quacks"—thus the origin of the word. All current dental associations were formed by the dentists who wanted to use mercury amalgam. All current dental associations today were originally formed by the Quacks.

Biography

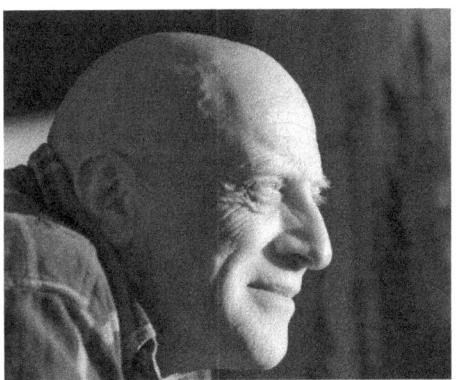

My graduation from Sydney University in 1974 set the stage of an amazing journey. I worked as a dentist for about forty years in Australia, England, and Nepal, with both Nepali and Tibetan people. It was a truly magical experience. I retired in 2014 and have not looked back.

For the first thirteen years, I did everything that I was taught to the best of my abilities. I did thousands of root canals, advised all pregnant women to take fluoride tablets, and of course poured mercury amalgam into as many people as I could. I did this in good conscience, as it was what I had learnt form great professors. I thought that I was doing everyone a great service. I can only apologize to the people I hurt in this period. I poisoned my friends and family. I poisoned every patient that came near me. I poisoned myself with mercury and a couple of root canals. I am not grateful to the people who taught me how to do this.

Then came a period of new knowledge and new experiences. I met great teachers who were able to show me how these "treatments" that I performed in good faith could be doing more harm than good. These teachers took many forms. Dr Horst Poehlman, a German medical physician in Adelaide, introduced me to ways of thinking about the body that none in Australia had done. I was fortunate to study with Dr Hal Huggins in Colorado, and I then continued a long, continuous learning relationship with him. These people opened a world of knowledge and introduced me to many other great teachers.

I spent the next twenty-seven years doing the opposite and watching the most amazing healings in many of my patients. I took out amalgam fillings, removed dead root-canalled teeth, and banned fluoride from my practice. I worked in areas with and without water fluoridation. By this stage, it was no surprise that the children I saw with the best teeth and best health were drinking tank rainwater. The worst teeth were in kids in fluoridated areas.

In 1994 I worked with a small group of doctors and dentists to set up the Australian Society of Oral Medicine and Toxicology. This was the first time that the dental establishment in Australia was faced with scientific proof that what they were advocating was in fact making people sick. As a group we brought information into the public and dental sphere about the dangers of mercury amalgam and root canal procedures. We held international conferences in Sydney, Melbourne, and Brisbane with great attendance.

I also decided that the messages had to get out further to the public, so I made a couple of documentaries: *Quecksilber—The Strange Story of Dental Amalgam*, in 2004, and *Rooted* in 2006. They are available on YouTube.

By 1994 I had completely changed my approach to dentistry. The treatments were no longer based on what the dental association and professors were advocating but instead were based in published science. As strange as this may sound, the teaching of dentistry at universities throughout Australia is still based in dogma that maintains a status quo of vested interests. It is not scientific, nor is it health enhancing.

My best teachers were the patients. Their stories still amaze me even in my retirement.

Forty years of working as a dentist has provided me a wealth of experience. I cannot sit back and let this knowledge pass with me. I hope that this book will be a way of passing some of this knowledge on to others, which I hope will be of benefit and bring to the world a greater understanding and better treatments. I hope that some dentists will read this information, question it all by reading the references, and then change the way they practise.

I always told the patients who came to me for treatment that I was good at taking out the rubbish but the healing had to come from inside the patient. I just take out the rubbish, and you do the healing. I am much more of a garbage collector than a healer.

I hope the information in this book will benefit you and your loved ones.

Informed Consent

This is what informed consent could look like:

> The Root Canal Procedure I am about to perform on your tooth is impossible to do well, because each of the basic premises is impossible to achieve. It will leave you with a dead, gangrenous, infected toxin factory buried in your jaw, just a few centimetres from your brain. It will cost you about $6,000, after a crown has been fitted as well.
>
> All materials used in this procedure are at best toxic and at worst carcinogenic. Some are used only for minutes, some for months, and the root filling itself will stay in your tooth forever. All will spread from your tooth to the rest of your body.
>
> The bacteria that remain, and the toxins they produce, will also escape from the tooth and spread throughout your body. The bacteria may find other organs that suit their life cycle and cause infection in that part of your body.
>
> The decaying, dead tissue that remains in your tooth will continue to release gangrenous gases, which will also leave the tooth and enter the rest of your body.

These gases are highly carcinogenic. They are similar in action and structure to the mustard gas used in the First World War.

Such a tooth will continue to release toxic substances into your body, which will travel throughout your body. These substances may affect every organ in your body, especially heart, kidneys, reproductive system, and thyroid gland. It will have a deleterious effect on your whole immune system.

These toxins have been related to the development of cancer, cardiac failure, neurological diseases, including Multiple Sclerosis, weight loss, and Trigeminal Neuralgia and a host of other ill-defined conditions.

Please sign this form if you wish to proceed. _____

Introduction

A number of appendices to this book are published on my website at www.realdentalinfo.com

Modern dentistry, as it is taught and usually practised, is one of the single greatest causes of systemic diseases, from rashes to headaches to cancer. Mercury from amalgam and the fluoride in our water supplies are supported by the practice of Root Canal Procedures. Together, this holy trinity of unchallengeable dogmas form the basis of many degenerative diseases.

The desire to help people was the main driving force for me to enter the dental world. In my retirement, I am now able to offer some of the knowledge and insights I picked up along the way. It's been an amazing journey of discovery, and I have been fortunate to have had great teachers who pushed me in directions of truth. They have been earlier researchers, dentists, doctors, massage therapists, naturopaths, chiropractors, spiritual healers, Tibetan shaman and less-credentialed great thinkers. My greatest teachers, however, have been the patients who came to see me. Each one had a different story to tell, and each one showed me another aspect of how to approach health. Almost all treated dentistry as only one of several modalities that they worked with to improve their health.

I have never made a promise to any patient that I could cure their disease. I strongly recommend that you treat the information that follows in the same way. Yes, this is a sort of medical disclaimer, but it is also a reality. There are many causes of disease, and dentistry is but one of them.

If the disease state is progressed, then you may need to approach your healing with other modalities, as well as getting rid of the cause.

Challenging the status quo in any field is always difficult. When Dr Semmelweis introduced the concept of washing hands after handling cadavers in hospitals to reduce cross-infection in the late 1800s, he was ridiculed and ostracized. Many readers will take this information to their own dentist for comment, which will usually be along the lines of the accepted paradigm. I know that some individual dentists, who have done root canals all of their careers, will become angry for my "advocacy of returning dentistry to the dark ages of extractions and gummy smiles."

I make no apology for discrediting the people and organizations who teach that keeping dead teeth in your head is good for you. None of this information is new. It's been available for 150 years. This information has also been suppressed and denigrated for just as long. It is not outdated, though, as the dental teachers would have us believe. It is in fact, supported by the very latest research from the twenty-first century, and much of that is published in the dental journals themselves. I am merely adding another volume to those already published by other greater minds. Mine is just another scream in the medical wilderness.

The information presented here is not readily available to either dentists or patients.

With this knowledge, you are at least armed to make decisions about your dental treatments. By the time you get through this book, you will know more about how dead teeth can affect your health than 99 per cent of dentists worldwide. You will also be more discerning about finding a dentist who is trained enough to help you.

It's time for a new paradigm in both medicine and dentistry, if we are to reach health and a great life. Doctors need to get into the mouth and learn what dentistry is doing. There is no pill that can fix the disasters that dentistry creates. Dentists need to get out of the mouth and their molar-mechanic mentality and learn enough medicine to understand what their treatments are doing to their patients. It's time for all of us to gain a greater understanding about medical principles that are not dictated by industry and drug companies.

Dr Meinig, a seriously well credentialed endodontist and the author of *Root Canal Cover Up*, broke his silence after reading the research from Dr Weston Price: "Millions of people are ill and suffering from degenerative diseases that the medical profession is at a loss in the cause and treatment, while the degenerative disease problem continues to bankrupt our people and country. These two extremely alarming issues and the root canal research sheds upon them, persuaded me to blow the whistle and alert the public to Price's substantial findings, which could help the public tremendously."

A Hope

My hope is that the teachers of dentistry will take heed and show responsibility for what they are teaching. If the teachers don't get it, then it is to be hoped that many other humans will get it and will learn enough to make changes in their own lives. It seems that I have screamed for too many years with too many of my colleagues, and still the status quo is just as firmly entrenched as it was in the 1970s. Too many have suffered unnecessarily because of the teachings of modern dentistry. Our society is far less healthy than it was in the 1970s, and part of this can be directly related to what every dentist does every day to make a living. Our cancer rates are approaching one in two. Autism rates have increased exponentially and are currently running at one in forty. IQs have dropped across the board. Mercury is still a huge part of our existence, and our environment is more polluted than any of us thought possible. Millions of root canals are done every year with absolutely no understanding of the systemic disease they cause. We all need to learn too much too quickly.

Geoffrey Robertson, QC, has been one of my intellectual heroes for a long time, and I can only wish that my command of the language was as brilliant as his. For those who have not read Geoffrey Robertson's work, I strongly recommend it, simply for the pure pleasure of reading really bloody good English. A quote from *Rather His Own Man* inspires many of the concepts I hope will carry through this book:

> "I recite the story of the headmistress who sent all her new teachers this letter:
>
> Dear Teacher
>
> I'm a survivor of a concentration camp. My eyes saw what no man should witness, gas chambers built by learned engineers, children poisoned by educated physicians, infants killed by trained nurses, women and babies shot and burnt by high school and college graduates. So, I'm suspicious of education. My request is to help your students become human. Your efforts must never produce learned monsters, skilled psychopaths, educated morons. Reading, writing, arithmetic are important only if they serve to make our children more human."

1

The Dedication to Ignorance

● ●

The story of how a "cast of millions" become
entrenched inside the structure of teeth
and end up causing the largest number of
diseases ever traced to a single source.

—Dr. George Meinig

My father used to tell me to believe nothing of what I heard and only
half of what I saw. When I went to university to learn how to be a
dentist, I promptly forgot his warnings and believed everything I was
told. Needless to say, I graduated and became a dentist. Sometime in
my thirties, I stopped being a dentist and started to become Robert. It
was about the same time that I was introduced to very different ways
of looking at and approaching disease, connecting cause and effect
between the physical, mental, and spiritual states. From then on, I
was very blessed to be led along a path by many great teachers who
were all able to shine some clarity on the connections between these
three states of being. This new knowledge gave me a greater depth of
understanding and was supported by such a vast array of published
science that I had to sit up and take notice. Suddenly I had new tools
with which to see my patients and present treatment models that
would benefit their health instead of ruining it. This new approach was
opposite to my previous training. Everything that I had done to my

1

patients till then, which included family and friends, was all based on the officially sanctioned training. I had to make a choice to either keep following the traditional methods or relearn all that I had been taught. At that time in the early '90s, all the dentists that were beginning to take on this new information were still under the oppression of the dental associations and what they claimed was correct knowledge. Everyone had to tread carefully for fear of retribution in the forms of fines or deregistration. It was clear from the start that we needed to support our treatments and every bit of written information with serious scientific references. The research that was never spoken of at university was indeed voluminous, published in peer-reviewed journals, and supported by other published scientific research. Much of this material dated back about 150 years and, although denied by the establishment, has been supported by scientific research ever since.

I spent he first thirteen years of my career doing everything that the good professors taught me. I used mercury amalgam, I did thousands of root canals, and I recommended fluoride to all my patients. I believed my professors and deans. I have no idea how much disease I caused in this first stage of my career. I spent the rest of my forty years in dentistry doing the opposite. In this latter period, I saw multiple sclerosis disappear after extracting one dead tooth. I saw suicide notes torn up after extracting one dead tooth. I've witnessed brain tumours disappear after extracting one dead tooth. And it goes on and on. All these dead teeth had had root canals which were done by dentists who I am sure had the best interests of their patients at heart, just as I did. The end results of their state-of-the-art treatments became glaringly obvious. The body can often heal itself very quickly if given the opportunity.

Surely the teachers have a responsibility to keep up to date and adapt their teaching to the latest scientific findings. Considering that dental students will one day be the caretakers of one of the most important parts of the body, I thought that the teachers would take responsibility for teaching what ultimately would always benefit the patient's health and general well-being. They are still teaching the same nonsense today as they did fifty years ago. Every dental school in Australia, and many other parts of the world, are still teaching dental students to implant mercury amalgam fillings into living human beings. They continue to teach the lie that fluoride reduces tooth decay and that poisoning the water supply is beneficial for everyone's health. Of course, they continue to teach dental students how to "save a tooth" with root canal therapy. People are being made sick every day by what dentists are taught to do.

Hopefully this book will give ample evidence and resources to allow the reader to make informed decisions about treatments that may be offered by dentists. I am also hopeful that a few dentists will take the time to check the references and find out that this information is critical if the health of their patients is foremost in their minds and paramount to their practice. There is no shame in not knowing, but it is definitely time for dentistry to take responsibility for the devastating effects that current treatments are having. I understand there will be ferocious criticism of this work, as there has been of me for many years. I know also that this work rests on a vast foundation of scientific evidence as well as clinical evidence that has been published since the 1880s to this very day. I always used to tell my patients that they should not believe a word I say but instead go and read the information for themselves and then make up their own minds. I repeat this to you, the reader. After all, what follows is opposite to what is taught at universities. If you are a dentist who is only now being introduced to these concepts, then I hope that this is just the first of many books and much information that you will be reading. It is a great learning curve, and everyone benefits.

Dentists are trained to only look in the mouth and leave the rest of the body to the doctors. Doctors are trained to *not* look in the mouth. Doctors have no idea what dentistry does or that it could affect the health of their patients. Nor do they realize that their income is directly related to what dentists do every day. Clearly a good reason to not tread on each other's toes.

Although the mouth is a part of the body, this is the one area that medicine does not concern itself with. There are both historical and financial reasons for this, but the net result is that we have a group of mercury-poisoned mad hatters[1] Medicine has abdicated all responsibility for this part of the body. I'm beginning to think these days that medicine has abdicated responsibility for the body as a whole. The drug companies are the only long-term beneficiaries of our failing health. Medicine does not consider dental conditions as causative of anything. Dentistry simply denies that dental treatments could negatively affect the health of the rest of the body. It appears that the tonsillar folds are the Great Dividing Range between the two worlds. So long as the status quo is maintained, they both live in harmony — the patient is the sacrificial lamb.

Medical students do *not* learn about the mouth or teeth. I have met some who don't even know where the jaw joint is. The limit of their oral knowledge really is limited to basic anatomy. They are forced to believe the fallacious protocols of the dental teachers and private trade organizations (PTOs) because that is all that is available to them. I've spoken to many medical specialists over a forty-year career, and very few have a clue about anything that I tell them. I recently spoke to a young doctor who told me that the only thing she learnt about dentistry in medical school was that fluoridation was the greatest public health measure ever. She did not know anything else.

Many chronic degenerative diseases can be linked directly to dental treatments. Doctors, not knowing or understanding this, can only treat symptoms without ever finding a cure. They, like the dentists, have been misled for far too long. They do not know that dead teeth can create cancer or that mercury may be responsible for infertility. They all believe that fluoride in the drinking water stops tooth decay and that it cannot calcify your pineal gland or cause hypothyroidism, osteosarcoma, or heart disease.

Dentistry is *not* the only cause of disease.Its just
the most neglected cause of disease.

The issues related to root canal procedures are particularly difficult for the dental private trade organizations (PTOs) because although they claim that this is the bee's knees among treatments, their own literature contradicts this stance. A quick browse through the references will demonstrate this. The aims of root canal procedures are clearly identified and upheld in the dental journals. These same dental journals also make it astoundingly clear that none of these aims are achievable. This is quite a dilemma for a dentist who, on the one hand, reads that success of this procedure depends on the total elimination of bacteria from the tooth and, on the other hand, that complete sterility of a tooth remains "an elusive goal." The idea that mercury from amalgam is safe and that fluoride stops tooth decay completes the holy trinity of lies that carry a whole profession into wealth and a population into disaster. Belief is just that—it is a universe away from knowing.

As Carl Sagan said, "You can't convince a believer of anything, for their belief is not based on evidence, it's based on a deep seated need to believe."

The Noble Dental Authorities

All dental associations worldwide are Private Trade Organizations. Most specialist dental organizations, such as the endodontic associations, are also private trade organizations. They are not scientific bodies, nor are they government bodies. They are private trade organizations *for profit*. They have their own well-entrenched vested interests. They are answerable only to their shareholders! So long as their share prices continue soaring towards heaven, life is good. Anything which might make those shares drop in value is guarded against and stomped on as fast and hard as possible. Did you really think they are scientific bodies who have a wealth of honesty, integrity, and are backed up by well researched and true information? They do like to sprout off about ethics and things of that nature. Perhaps you think that they are there to look after the well-being of the dental consumer – you, the patient. Perhaps you think that they are looking after the welfare of their membership – the dentists.? Wrong again. If they did look after the welfare of the dentists, they would not allow them to be exposed to the third most toxic substance known to man. Instead, they actively promote the use of mercury amalgam as the best filling material on the planet and go so far as to say that it is unethical for a dentist to remove such amalgam fillings for the benefit of their patients' health. These Private Trade Organizations are merely concerned with the share price, their influence over government, and their association with other Private Trade Organizations, including the medical ones and toothpaste manufacturers. (From now on I will refer to them all as PTOs.)

A World Unto Its Own

The PTOs point to the millions of root canals done each year, to demonstrate their efficacy, their safety, and the supposed scientific research that underscores this procedure. Unfortunately, just because millions of the same procedures are done each year does not make that procedure either safe or effective. Show me references, not anecdotes. The same numbers argument is also used by the PTOs to justify how good mercury amalgams are. These are the same people claiming that a schedule 6 poison - fluoride - is good for our health and that everyone in the population agrees. It has nothing to do with science and everything to do with convincing the greatest number of individuals that numbers matter, which is underscored by our human need to belong.

The dental world calls "saving" a tooth, keeping the tooth in your head and being able to chew on it. They make a lot of fuss about having a "functional bite" and one's teeth being aesthetically pleasing. The average suburban dentist can repeat the mantra word for word, stating that if you lose your tooth, your whole head will cave in, and your ugliness will kill you.

To me, saving a tooth means keeping it alive. This important distinction is the basis of what may be deemed safe or unsafe. In the words of Dr Joseph Issels, who was one of Germany's leading oncologists:

"The over-riding consideration must not be conservation of the tooth but preservation of its vitality. If this is impossible, even the most beautiful crown must not delude us that the lifeless tooth beneath is anything other than a "corpse in a golden coffin," whose decomposition toxins slowly but surely are destroying the organism."[2]

Not only is 'root canal treatment' supposed to be 'safe and effective', but the practice is also supported by a whole specialty of dentistry called "endodontics" and the specialist dentists who carry out this procedure - endodontists. They even have their own specialist organizations like the American Endodontics Society (AES), American Association of Endodontists (AAE) and the Australian Society of Endodontology Inc. (ASE). These groups have their own specialty journals. Some make claims that are almost truthful. Some make claims that putting a carcinogen in your tooth is a good treatment.

These clubs, like all others, have a vested interest in maintaining themselves. Dissent is not tolerated, especially from within the group. Following are two cases in point. One is that of Dr Weston Price, who in the 1920s was the president of the American Dental Association's Research Institute. As soon as he published information contradicting the status quo, he was labelled a misguided fool and has been defamed ever since. The other is that of Dr George Meinig. After being one of the founding members and past president of the American Association of Endodontics, he has become relegated to the level of "moron idiot" who strayed down the wrong path like Dr Price. From being one of the world's most renowned endodontists, he changed his mind and philosophy after reading Dr Price's research. The professors, deans and specialists repeat the story that they are both wrong. Does it mean that we should believe only the people who hold power? They certainly think so. As Richard Feynman said,

"I would rather have questions that can't be answered than answers that can't be questioned."

The root canal procedure is not based in science. It is a religion unto itself but has nothing spiritual or intellectual or intelligent about it. The procedure has enjoyed support equal to religious fervour with little or no opposition since about the 1850s. That this practice is well supported by published science is a myth. These myths are supported by a range of beliefs, which are programmed into every dentist on the planet.

- It's critical to have a good bite!
- Loose a tooth and you will never chew again!
- Missing a tooth is *UGLY!*
- Lose a tooth and your whole face will collapse.
- Losing a tooth will make you unlovable.
- Save that tooth at any cost!
- Root Canalled teeth are not dead!
- Dead teeth do not affect your health.
- Everything a dentist does is beneficial for your well-being.
- Root Canals are Safe and Effective!
- Deans and professors are always right!

One of Australia's leading professors of endodontics, Dr Paul Abbott, wrote in 1996, "… the main concepts, aims and procedures in Endodontics, have changed *little* during the last **300 years** …"[3] (emphasis addd)

What an amazing admission!

Dr Abbott was Professor of Endodontics at the University of Western Australia. He also acted as guest editor of a special supplement of the *Journal of the Australian Dental Association* dedicated to endodontics.[4] The Australian Dental Association seems very appreciative of his efforts, as can be seen from the editor's introduction:

"… New directions in Endodontics are based on the principles of **evidence based practice** with particular emphasis on a **risk/benefit** approach …"

I hope that this impressive collection of papers will be kept as a handy reference in your surgery and I invite you to carefully read and put into practice the suggestions and recommendations provided in these papers" (Professor P. Mark Bartold, editor, *Australian Dental Journal* [my emphasis]).

If dentists really were to follow the editor's advice and "practice the suggestions and recommendations provided in these papers", root canal procedures would no longer exist, and this book would not need to be written.

The "principles of evidence based practice with particular emphasis on a risk/benefit approach" certainly sounds like a wonderful ideal. To make such a statement, Professor Bartold must be assuming that there is a strong foundation of evidence that this procedure is based on. If the professor said it, then all dentists could assume this to be the case.

If this professor had actually read the articles printed in this collection of papers, he would have seen the following statement:

"White et. al.,[5] in a recent evidence-based review of the outcomes of both treatment modalities, noted that if evidence-based principles are applied to the data available for both treatment modalities, few implant or endodontic outcome studies can be classified as being high in the evidence hierarchy."[6]

The "state-of-the-art" dental treatments of root canals and implants suddenly don't have any legs to stand on! There is *no* evidence base on which this procedure can rest. Unfortunately, Professor Bartold's patronizing arrogance is all too common in dental academia.

My version of evidence-based dentistry is watching the outcomes of my treatments against the improvements (or not) in the health of my patients. The treatments, of course, are based on published scientific research.

I was shocked when I first heard of a dentist who was actively removing root-canalled teeth. I had no idea what would prompt any dentist to do such a thing, so I sought him out and asked him why. The answers he gave me were intelligent and supported by so much science that I had to take a step backwards and look for this new information. It was rather uncomfortable, to say the least. Having been on both sides of the fence, I really do understand the dentists who look at my work and call me the one who makes "dental cripples". I can only suggest that they familiarize themselves with the literature and stop making "medical cripples".

We have been consistently lied to for so many years that finding our way into a more truthful reality is both difficult and also very uncomfortable, as we then need to accept that the treatments we so caringly provided to our patients, friends and families may actually be killing them. No dentist or doctor likes to see themselves as causing harm. We can no longer use the reasoning that we are only doing what we have been taught. The murderers in Nuremburg were only following orders. It's just not good enough.

Dead or Just a Little Bit Dead - Call in the Exorcist

Yuval Harari stated, "People rarely appreciate their ignorance, because they lock themselves inside an echo chamber of like-minded friends and self-confirming news-feeds, where their beliefs are constantly reinforced and seldom challenged."[7] Dental professors like to use big words—the bigger the jargon the more godlike the professor. Even if the words make no sense, most dentists will believe these words and repeat them verbatim.

Dentistry does not like to admit that dead tissue remains in a tooth or that a root therapied tooth is in fact dead. Even the Australian Society of Endodontology have stated that "After endodontic treatment the tooth is pulpless, but it is NOT a dead tooth." This is still current as of 2022.

If the tooth is not dead, then it must surely be alive! If it's alive, it would have a great blood supply and live nerve tissue and no infection. They could not find a reference for this statement, so I supply it for them below.

This idea that a dead tooth is not a dead tooth comes from a paper entitled the *'Endodontic Point of View'*, published in 1977 and used as a propaganda piece ever since. The author, Dr Ehrman states, "It is wrong to speak of Root Canal Therapy as a dead tooth; it is more correct to describe such a tooth as nonvital or, better, pulpless. Even though the central blood supply to the tooth has been lost, the tooth itself still retains its connection to the body via the periodontal membrane and the cementum."[8]

The *Oxford English Dictionary* defines "'non-vital" as "Fatal to Life". It defines "Dead" as "No longer alive". "Pulpless" means that the blood supply is gone. If the blood supply to any tissue is taken away, then that tissue dies.

I wonder whether this explanation, that the tooth is still attached to the body by whatever means, could also be applied to a dead brain. This is an example of dead brain being published by a private trade organization which is still attached to its shareholders. Dentists actually believe this stuff. They repeat it verbatim to patients and to my face when confronted with this information. It is always used in the propaganda. The Australian Society of Endodontology repeat it today in 2022 on their website. Root canalled teeth are simply not allowed to be dead. Why? Because if they were, then there would have to be an acceptance that they can become gangrenous, as is the case with all dead tissue unless mummified. This would then affect the whole body, and focal infection would be understood as a reality instead of a theory. Dentistry is the only modality which claims that it is good to keep dead, infected, and gangrenous tissue in the body.

Dead is Dead Is Dead!
Only dentistry believes in a "Little bit Dead"

Save That Tooth at Any Cost

It may seem an enigma that root canal procedures (RCPs) are allowed, let alone protected by just about all medical, dental, and government worlds. There is a never-ending bucket of money to fund the propaganda, as has been the case since the time of Dr Price. According to the American Dental Association and most others, "When endodontic treatment has been completed, a filling or crown (cap) will be necessary. This will restore your tooth to its original shape and function."[9]

According to the 2017 national dental fee survey, the average cost of a root canal without a crown in Australia ranges between $2,000 and $3,400.[10] In Australia, a molar root canal with three canals can cost up to $2,760 without a crown and up to $4,760 with a crown. Save that tooth at any cost! Amen.

In 2019 in Australia, the *conservative estimated* costs are as follows:

•	root canal procedure	$2,500
•	posts and pins	$400
•	core buildup	$500
•	new crown	$2,000
•	total cost	$5,400

On finder.com.au/root-canal-therapy, it is stated that a root canal treatment will cost between $2,000 and $3,500. My estimate is very conservative. They also make an incredible statement. It is incredible for its honesty: "It's also worth pointing out that re-treatment could cost up to one-third more than first-time root canal treatment, so keep this in mind when budgeting for the cost of the procedure."

Thus, retreatment could cost $7,200 (making the total cost $12,600)

But why would you need to retreat the tooth with another root canal? The simple answer is that about 30 per cent of all root canals fail, even when done by a 'really good endodontist'.[11] That's right. This site is actually acknowledging the horrendous failure rate of this "treatment".

The Australian Dental Association also acknowledged this high failure rate in 1996:

> "Endodontic re-treatment is a relatively common procedure, particularly amongst specialist endodontists. Some endodontists estimate that up to two-thirds of their referrals are for endodontic re-treatment ... A large proportion of the re-treatment cases are for cases originally treated less than two years prior to the need for re-treatment."

> "... previous root canal filling should be removed so that the root canal system can be re-cleaned, shaped and disinfected through the use of irrigating solutions and inter-appointment anti-bacterial medicaments prior to the placement of a new root canal filling."[12] (my emphasis)

Special Note

In 2007, the same author, Dr Paul Abbott, admitted that all of the aims of root canal procedures are unattainable and that there is little in the way of an evidence base to support the procedure at all. Therefore, removing the old filling, cleaning the canals again, and putting the same useless antibacterial mess in the tooth, as well as an attempt at sealing it up at the end, is an elegant way of providing a regular and large income for the dentist. It does nothing positive for the patient. You cannot improve on bad by doing bad again. About 33 per cent of all root therapies done by specialists will fail.

Dr Price, in 1920, pointed out that 17 per cent% of all root fillings done by endodontists will be overfilled. This alone counts as a failure! Specialist endodontists rely on redoing the procedure for 66 per cent of his or her income. They are happy to take your money and believe that doing the same thing over and over will produce a different result. In other words, if the first hit-and-miss approach doesn't work, you'll be advised to have a second go at the very same hit-and-miss approach.

Do the same thing over and over again but expect a different result? This is the thinking of a fool. Don't be a fool and pay again and again to have this abuse foisted on you. Remember that the only dental measure of success or failure of a root canal is gauged by local symptoms. If systemic effects were included, we would see a failure rate closer to 100 per cent.

Any medical treatment with a 30 per cent failure rate would no longer be available. Very few patients are warned of this potential crappy result and the crappy amount of extra money they will spend for the privilege of having this crappy "treatment" redone. No one talks about the failure rate of the tooth that has had two or three or more attempts at being retreated. By this stage, patients are usually advised to have the tooth out and an implant put in.

The American Association of Endodontists in 2017 stated that 25 million endodontic procedures were performed annually in the United States.[13] We should all be impressed by this very big number! If, for the sake of simplicity and generosity, we were to estimate the cost of a root canal procedure and restoration to only be about $5,000, then simple maths means that root canal procedures are a $125 billion industry in the USA. If dentists paid only 30 per cent of their earnings in tax, this would represent a $37 billion income for the government. Now ask yourself whether an endodontist or a government would want to shut down such a good earner? This is still petty cash compared to the cost of medications to treat the diseases caused by this procedure.

Don't Bite the Hand That Feeds You

For a dentist, it's far more profitable to refer the patient to an endodontist to do the actual root canal procedure than to waste valuable time which could be used to make the crown and a much greater profit. The specialist is dependent on the GP dentist for referral and thus for their income. When 60 per cent of an endodontist's workload is redoing old, failed root canals, there is a guaranteed money stream. The specialist will, of course, be friendly and polite to the hand that feeds him or her while maintaining their lofty position within the trade.

The GP dentist can rely on the endodontist to send the patient back after the root canal is done, with clear instructions that the tooth is now very fragile (because a big, dirty hole has been drilled in the centre of it). To save it now, after spending so much pain, money, and time, the patient will need to have a crown placed over the tooth *immediately*. Anyone who has attended an endodontist's rooms will know the truth of this statement. The patients would come back screaming for me to fit them in that day or the next. There was panic if they had to wait any longer. They could not wait to spend more of their hard-earned money to "save" the tooth. The GP dentist can sit back and do crown and bridge work from morning till close and make a stack more money than by extracting the tooth or doing the root canal themselves. When the "root treatment" fails, this can be blamed on the endodontist, who will then drill a big, dirty hole through the porcelain or gold crown on the dead tooth and charge the patient a second time to redo the "treatment". Of course, the damaged crown will need to be replaced at the patient's cost. After all, it is your tooth that is dead, and if you would have brushed them as a kid, you would not be in this situation. And on it goes. Perhaps it is because your immune system is already compromised that the infection in your tooth is not improving. Either way, it is *ALLLLLL your* fault! Getting the picture? Everyone is a winner except the patient.

For endodontists to accept the information in this book means they are out of business, out of income and, worst of all, out of prestige membership in their club. The same applies to the specialist children's dentists who still put Formaldehyde or Ferric Sulphate in baby teeth and then cover them with nickel-releasing stainless steel crowns.

How do any of these people justify being the cause of such a wide variety of diseases without ever taking responsibility for their so-called treatments? Sadly, it is the patient's health which suffers due to the ignorance (or worse) of these so-called health care providers. They do not read the published science, not even when it's written in their own journals by their own professors! They don't even read the warnings published by the manufacturers about the poisons that they implant into your teeth.

Most of you reading this will have to make difficult decisions. Do you believe what you read here, and in many other similar volumes, and have your dead toxin factory removed, or do you believe your army of dentists who are telling you it is all in your head and your disease has nothing to do with them and that I have been deregistered and discredited?

So, I will answer this right now. Yes, I am not registered. Several years after retiring from dentistry, I chose not to waste the money any more on renewing my dental registration. Thus, I used to work as a dentist until retiring and now am no longer registered. It's as simple as that. As for being discredited—well, that's nothing new. I have been a bit of a thorn in their sides for a while now, but I have yet to see this discrediting put in writing! Become informed by reading the references and other material mentioned in this book. The only way I know to verify what is written here is to read the references. Perhaps I am just a mad old dentist with some ulterior motive. Don't believe me. Read the information and become informed. That is the only way to become empowered to make your own decisions about your health.

Helen's Story—In Her Own Words

Helen was a patient who had a root canal in her left lateral incisor. (Second from the front.) The diagnosis of a brain tumour sent her on a search'

"It first started when I was fourteen years old. I had an abscess which was on the roof of my mouth, so I went to the dentist and he found that it had killed one of my front teeth, so he recommended that I have a root canal therapy done. I started taking antibiotics to treat the abscess and I had the Root Canal Therapy done and everything seemed to be fine for a while.

I was 19 and my period stopped. So I went to the doctor and he said "Don't worry – it will be OK and these kinds of things happen. It went on for six months and they still said it was OK and then said, "we might do a blood test." So, we did a blood test – it came back and it showed that I had really high prolactin levels - which is a hormone that the pituitary gland produces. So, they said "we are going to do a CT scan and MRI scan just to check the pituitary and see how it is. I had both of those scans done and they came back and showed that I had a pituitary tumour. The tumour was about 12 mm, which sounds quite small but in comparison to the pituitary gland which is only 1 cm itself. So, it was actually a MACRO PROLACTINOMA is what it is called - SO that was a bit scary …

Then I came to see you and I had the root canal pulled out and three months later I had another blood test – and the blood test showed NORMAL. We were very shocked but decided not to get too excited yet till we get the results of the other scans back. I had another MRI scan which was three months after having the tooth pulled, and I got the results back and they said there was no tumour there. It's a healthy pituitary gland. There was no other explanation to say that the tumour had disappeared other than having my tooth pulled. My periods returned a few months later after having the scan done. And my blood tests are normal still.

> I went back up to my doctor and he was also shocked. He didn't ask me why, what's happened. He said "Oh that's strange" – he didn't want to know really … so that was a bit sad I thought.
>
> I could have had surgery; they could have taken out the whole gland. I would have had to have been on hormone replacement tablets for the rest of my life. I could have had to be on a drug called Dostinix, which has horrible side effects, like depression and nausea every day – for the rest of my life …"

Three years later, there was still no sign of any pituitary tumour. The only dental treatment this young lady ever had was the root therapy of the upper lateral incisor. None of her other teeth even had a filling. The only treatment she had for the tumour was the removal of the one dead tooth! I make the point that I did not cure her cancer. She did it all by herself. All I did was remove the cause, which gave her body the ability to heal itself. That's all.

The Greater Cost–Professor Patrick Stortebecker

As mentioned, the cost of doing a root canal procedure should also be measured by the cost of the diseases they cause. As will be mentioned several times in this book, dentistry is *not* the only cause of chronic degenerative diseases, but it is one of the most overlooked and ignored causes. You will see later the relationships to cancers, multiple sclerosis, cardiac disease, and a vast range of other conditions. Professor Patrick Stortebecker was professor of Neural Surgery at Karolinska Institute in Sweden. He describes this with reference to a report on the Joint Commission on Neurology from *1975*.

> "Disorders of the nervous system are a leading cause of chronic disease and disability in the United States today. It is conservatively estimated that well over 12

18

million people suffer from one or another of these neurologic conditions.

The social and economic consequences to the individual and the community are enormous. The annual direct cost for the care of only three of the disorders of the nervous system -- EPILEPSY, MULTIPLE SCLEROSIS, and STROKE -- has been estimated by the Department of Health, Education, and Welfare at more than 3 billion dollars, while their indirect cost, from loss to the gross national product and loss to federal taxes, is about ten times higher and totals an additional 30 billion dollars. Added to this national burden is the personal tragedy these disorders bring, which is hardly measurable in monetary terms."[14]

As His Holiness the Dalai Lama stated, "We must attempt the impossible. I am convinced that if we continue to follow a social model that is entirely conditioned by money and power, and that takes so little account of true values such as love and altruism, future generations may have to face far worse problems and endure even more terrible forms of suffering."

2

History, Demons, and Heroes

· ·

... I believe with all my heart that humanity
needs rescuing, not from a willful aggressor
but from an incorrect interpretation, which
has furnished wrong fundamentals for
diagnosis, prognosis and treatment.

A new truth is a new sense, for with it,
we can see things that we could not see
before and things that cannot be seen by
those who do not have that new truth.

—Dr Weston Price, 1925

The Golden Age

The period from 1880 till about 1940 was a golden period for science
and the arts. Some of the most amazing people lived through this
period and gave us the incredibly rich tapestry of today's knowledge.
Great names include artists like Henri Matisse, Wassily Kandinsky,
Pablo Picasso, and Marc Chagall. This was the time when Einstein
developed the theory of relativity and the splitting of the atom. This

is the time when George Gurdjieff brought ancient knowledge from Tibet and the Indus Valley back to the West. Great composers like Debussy and Shostakovich, Stravinsky and Bernstein, filled the world with their music. It was a period of great exploration and discovery. It was the period of the First and Second World Wars and the Great Depression. The great golden age was also one of great suffering. It is upon this stage that some of the most important discoveries were made in relation to health and dental conditions. The contrasts were staggering. In this period, Dr Royal Rife found a way to cure cancer, and the atomic bomb was let loose on the world. Fluoride was introduced as a saviour for mankind even though it was well known to cause cancer. This was also the time when the American dental association began to be influential in their pursuit of "saving teeth" at any cost and using their new-found magazine (journal) as the sounding board. In 1923, Dr Price published his research. By 1925, he had become a great embarrassment to the dental world. This was made public in the famous 1925 debate with Dr Buckley.

The First World War left many scars and much personal destruction. Some people, though, benefited greatly during this period. It was a period when many things happened which set the stage for our current medical and dental systems. This was also the beginning of the demise of traditional medicine as had been practised for hundreds of years with great results.

By 1900, John D. Rockefeller had made a great part of his fortune and owned about 90 per cent of America's oil reserves. Already there were products being made from petroleum, such as Bakelite. It was soon discovered that petroleum could be used to make certain drugs and even the little capsules to put them in. This prompted Rockefeller to do a few things. In 1923, he and some other businessmen founded the American Society for the Control of Cancer (not "the Cure"). He also funded and set up the General Education Board (GEB). He further donated millions of dollars to almost every major medical school in America. This was done with the condition that the medical schools all started to teach a curriculum set by Rockefeller. Almost overnight, these schools were teaching the same course to medical students, based on the use of drugs that could be patented. There were many medical schools at the time that were teaching the long understood traditional medicine of herbs and homeopathic treatments. These schools were shut down or changed their curricula. The teachers and practitioners that refused to give up their tried and tested remedies were simply demonized. Some were run out of town, and some accidentally died. There was simply no room for anything that competed with potential patents. All treatments that worked and had a scientific foundation were no longer allowed. This is the reason that chiropractic treatments were demonized. Mercury and dead teeth, however, were allowed. They did, after all, make people sick. This is the medical model that today is regarded as state of the art.

Dr Weston Price (1870–1948)

[Special Note: The use of rabbits and other animals was common in medical experiments of the time. I am not condoning this practice but simply reporting on the experiments.]

The greatest hero in this story is Dr Weston Price. At the turn of the twentieth century, he was the head of the American Dental Association's Research Institute and was heading a team of some of the most brilliant minds in the dental world of America. His research was dedicated to exploring how dead teeth affected health. His findings were farsighted and compassionate, as were his brilliance and his tenacity to continue while so strongly opposed by the dental establishment at the time. In 1923 he published two major volumes of his research and his findings.

Price's research was mammoth and impeccable. It was conducted over twenty-five years by a dedicated team of scientists, dentists, and doctors under Price's guidance. One of the most amazing feats of research, in my opinion, was that he traced the medical histories of over 1,500 patients back over three generations—without computers. These histories were then correlated against the patients' conditions. He was able to relate these histories to current disease states, X-ray appearance of the dead tooth, many blood parameters, including calcium metabolism, and the patient's "resistance" to infections. These relationships provided a means of knowing whether a patient fell into one of three categories. The first were those with a high resistance to infection (in modern terms, a healthy immune function), the second, those with a susceptibility to lots of diseases (compromised immune system) and the third, those in the middle who start off resistant and gradually lose this resistance as different factors come into play. This was a new concept and really set the stage for what is today considered common knowledge. Immune function is affected by many toxins, diseases, and stress situations. Dentistry is a great contributor to immune dysfunction simply by leaving dead teeth in the mouth and implanting mercury into people's bodies.

Another most important finding that Dr Price was able to demonstrate repeatedly was that organisms and their toxins, derived from the dead teeth, are able to spread throughout the body and cause a wide range of diseases. This finding was also shown by other great researchers, such as Rosenow, Mayo, and Billings. This spread of microorganisms from a "Focus of Infection" (the tooth) causing disease in other parts of the body, is called Focal Infection. To this day, the dental establishment deny the reality of focal infection from a tooth, by calling it a "theory". Current dental schools claim that there are serious flaws in Price's work, but to my knowledge these have never been pointed out. In fact, I didn't get to hear about Dr Price till thirteen years after I left university. Current students are still denied this knowledge. To this day, the dental establishments have never shown one peer-reviewed published scientific paper to demonstrate any support for their position.

Throughout this story, I will be referring constantly to Dr Price's words. In part to demonstrate his correctness in light of current research, as well as to show clearly that the results of this current research have been known and denied for nearly one hundred years. How many millions of people have been killed or made terribly sick by this chilling and obstinate denial? Tell the same lie often enough ...

After Dr Price published his work on root canals, he travelled widely with his wife to just about every remote corner of the world. He studied the African tribal people, Australian aborigines, Pacific Islanders, Eskimos, indigenous Americans, and people living in isolated communities in Wales and Switzerland. He published a monumental work which has today passed its fifty-third publication. "Nutrition and Physical Degeneration" was written in 1939 and demonstrates the importance of ancestral diet in health. He found that all people who had lived on an ancestral diet had healthy and strong bone structures. The dental arches (the bony arch that the teeth sit in) were wide, and there was no crowding of the teeth. Dental decay was present in less than 0.1 per cent of the population.

In contrast to this, just one generation after the introduction of white flour and sugar, the next generation had a dental decay rate that we now consider normal. The dental arches became narrower, and this is the first time that crowding of the teeth became an issue. In men, the pelvis became wider and the shoulders narrower. In women, the shoulders became wider and the pelvis narrower. This, then, was also the beginning of birthing problems for many of these populations. If dental decay rates are increased so dramatically by the consumption of sugar and refined flours, then why are we poisoning our water supplies with fluoride, which has no effect on decay rates *ANYWHERE?*

I have had the good fortune to do some dental work in Nepal with both Nepalese locals and Tibetan refugees. In one particular camp of about fourteen hundred Tibetan people, there were those who had been the original refugees from Tibet, who had eaten only an ancestral diet. The next generation were people in their twenties to thirties. They had both the Tibetan diet and the more westernized Nepali diet, which included sugars and flour. The children of this second generation were the high-contrast group. Their decay and dental crowding were very high. The bone thickness around the teeth was similar to that of Western people—very thin. The previous generations had no crowding and little decay. Bone thickness around the teeth was dramatically different. It was really thick and strong compared to that of Westerners. In fact, their whole bone structure was similar to what Dr Price had reported. Another interesting observation was that the sugar-and-flour generations had lower molars that had the standard two roots, like Westerners' molars. The older generation who ate an ancestral diet had many lower molars with three well-defined roots. The rearmost root (distal root) was often divided into two completely separate roots. Nowhere in my dental training has this been taught. I am so fortunate to have witnessed firsthand some of the findings of Dr Price. Needless to say, the surgical approach I used to take these teeth out had to change quite a bit.

To get an idea of some of the research that happened in the early twentieth century, it is worth looking at some YouTube videos showing the experiments of Dr Pottinger.

One such video may be found at https://www.youtube.com/watch?v=OvQ5F6GCfgI. Additionally, the following is a must-read website:

https://price-pottenger.org/

In one lifetime, Dr Price did the work of ten geniuses. His findings were totally supported by the other geniuses of the time: Mayo, Rosenow, and Billings. His research is still far ahead of its time and still far ahead of modern medicine's and dentistry's criminal denial.

Dr George Meinig (1914–2008)

Dr Meinig was one of the nineteen founding members of the American Association of Endodontics. In 1946, they published the first issue of the *Journal of Endodontics*. In fact, on their website in August 2020 they stated,

"We honor the original and founding members of our Association."[15] George Meinig is still on the list. For many years, he was the president of that association, and thus one of the leading endodontists in America. Incredibly, he did not know of Dr Price's work, even though he was alive for many of the years that Dr Meinig was a specialist in the exact field that should have been teaching about Price's research. Towards the end of his career, he came upon the work of Dr Price, and realized the dangers of his specialty. It was a giant acknowledgement for him to understand the way his many years of treatments had potentially affected his patients. He went on to write a book called *The Root Canal Cover-Up*. He describes root canal procedures as

> "The story of how a 'cast of millions'
> That become entrenched inside the structure of teeth
> And ends up causing the largest number of diseases
> Every traced to a single source"

In an interview on the Laura Lee show, Dr Meinig made some very powerful comments. Here is a brief list of quotations from Dr Meinig:[16]

> ... I practiced some 47 years and in all of that time I never heard about a 25-year research program that was conducted by Dr. Weston Price in the early 1900's and actually before then and it was finally published in 1923. His work was all well documented in two volumes of 1174 pages and in 25 articles that appear in the medical and dental literature.

> ... what he reported and what he found with the tests which involved some 5,000 animals over the 25 year period was root canal distilled teeth, no matter how good they looked, or how free they were from symptoms, always remained infected.

> ... the reason that this is a focal infection is because the infection came from the tooth and travelled from

the tooth to the heart or the kidneys or the lungs or some area of the body and it set up a new infection.

… he had a patient who had kidney trouble and had a root filled tooth. He removed that tooth, put it under the skin of a rabbit, the rabbit got kidney trouble and died within a few days. He took the tooth out of that rabbit, surgically of course, and washed it in soap and water, disinfected it with a disinfectant and put it under the skin of another rabbit and that rabbit got kidney trouble and passed away. He then took that tooth out of that rabbit and put it in another rabbit and he repeated that 30 times.

… Now one of the things that happens with these root filled teeth is that when they are removed it is very often that periodontal membrane that is infected and the surrounding bony socket remains in the jaw and sometimes healing gets rid of that but many times it doesn't. And what happens then is an infection that occurs in the jawbone …

These are huge statements from one of the world's leading proponents of root canals. He not only describes the research that Price, Rosenow, and others did but also demonstrates the bloody-minded ignorance of the dental profession of his time. He worked closely with Dr S. H. Shakman to uncover the historical subterfuge which was created to allow for the development of his endodontic society and dentistry generally. His new-found position about the dangers of root canals did not win him many friends, and he was immediately castigated and spat out by his colleagues and other mad hatters whose income was on the line.

Dr Meinig is a great example of how a person can be dedicated to truth no matter how wrong he was prior to gaining extra knowledge. He dedicated the rest of his life to trying to wake a sleeping profession and a corrupt dental association. His dedication to the well-being of his fellow humans was clear.

Dr Hal Huggins (1937–2014)

The last, but far from least, hero of this story is Dr Hal Huggins. Dr Huggins is personally responsible for bringing Dr Price's writings into current awareness. Great financial and personal expense from Dr Huggins has allowed us all to benefit from this one-hundred-year-old research. He was sent a trunk which was full of Dr Price's original writings. He was smart enough to read and understand the message in the trunk and created a purpose-built concrete bunker to house these volumes. He then paid to have them transcribed. His efforts have been tireless in educating about the dangers of root therapy, even in the face of massive opposition.

Dr Huggins is also the person who took the dental world by the collar and gave it a great big shake in the mid-1970s. He made the world look at the dangers of mercury escaping from dental amalgam. He has authored many books and taught many dentists and cynics that dental amalgam is the most dangerous filling material that could ever be implanted into a living human being. I am lucky to have studied with him in Colorado in 1991 and to have had a long and close relationship with him for years afterward. His insights and knowledge left most professors floundering. His intelligence and wit were matched by his warm humanity and love of people and fun.

There were many researchers in the 1970s and 80s who tried to prove him wrong, firstly about the amount of mercury coming off amalgam fillings and secondly about what this mercury can do to our bodies. They never did prove him wrong. In fact, some of the more honest scientists at the time were horrified that they kept proving him right. They went on to form the International Academy of Oral Medicine and Toxicology.

Dr Huggins is the author of many brilliant books, including *It's All In Your Head*, *The Price of Root Canals*, and *Solving the Multiple Sclerosis Mystery*. He has taught many dentists how to change their dictated work habits for the benefit of their patients. I shall always be indebted to Dr Huggins for teaching me so patiently and graciously. His knowledge and courage are beyond the scope of most mortals. I truly believe that acting on the knowledge that he gave me has saved my life and my sanity.

Dr Huggins was once asked if all root-canalled teeth should be removed. He replied that it was only "for those people who had an interest in their health." This book is for that same group of people. I also hope that some dentists will pick up the information presented here and do their own research to verify it. Only with such verification can we move away from the dogmas of belief and move into knowledge with consequent healing for everyone.

Some Other Clever People

Dr Edward Rosenow (1875–1966) was the medical shining light in a new field of bacteriological research. His research completely supported that of Dr Price. By 1915, Dr. Rosenow was generally regarded in prominent medical circles as the most brilliant of modern scientists. From this already lofty position, he went on to serve as head of experimental bacteriology for the Mayo Foundation for nearly three decades, from 1915 to 1944.[3] His research was supported by the findings of many others, including such prominent people as Dr Charles Mayo (1865–1939), who built the famous Mayo Clinic, and Dr Frank Billings (1854–1932), a president of the American Medical Association who, in a series of lectures in 1915, told the world about the findings that Rosenow's research had uncovered.

All had done laborious research on the effects of microorganisms and their toxic by-products from dead teeth, on a variety of laboratory animal models. Their work was supported by many other research groups around the world that were finding similar results. They all demonstrated over and over how a disease in a human could be replicated in a rabbit or other animals, simply by inoculating the animal with the bacteria from the dead tooth that had been taken from the ailing human. Most of the time, the removal of these foci of infection from the people's mouths was accompanied by either an improvement or complete elimination of their disease. The research was conducted over many years, peer reviewed, and published. Price worked on this for over twenty-five years, and Rosenow for over thirty, and there are many others whose research supported these two great pioneers.

Amongst these geniuses at that time was another doctor named Dr Royal Rife (1888–1971).[17] Refreshingly, he had nothing to do with teeth. He was a brilliant microscopist who built microscopes which allowed light to be passed through quartz crystals on its way to the subject and the eyepiece. By this means, he was able to use specific wavelengths to both demonstrate and affect the viral organisms he found in all cancer tissue which he named BX viruses. "This meant that each organism had a signature frequency at which it vibrated or resonated. Rife further developed this technology by building a frequency instrument which was able to reproduce these MOR's (Mortal Oscillatory Rates) and thus kill the organisms."[18]

He found wavelengths of light which caused the viral particles to explode. As this happened, the cancers were cured. He travelled the world curing cancers. His work was published internationally in the newspapers of the time. This was, of course, unacceptable to the medical establishment, which by this stage was already formulating various chemotherapy concoctions. Ain't *no* profits in light!

Apart from curing cancer, he did something else that to this day has hardly been spoken of. Dr Rife worked closely with another scientist, Dr Kellner, who was an expert in growth mediums. They grew the BX virus in one of these mediums, and by making subtle changes in the formulation of the growth medium, they watched startling changes in the BX virus itself. Gradually the virus changed into many different forms but ended up as a bacteria called *Escherichia Coli* (commonly found in the lower intestine of warm-blooded organisms). By inverting the changes made to the growth medium, they were then able to convert these *E.Coli* bacteria back to a BX virus. This experiment was repeated four hundred times. They demonstrated a principle called Pleomorphism, or Pleomorphic Change (i.e., the ability of an organism to change form [e.g., from aerobic to anaerobic]). (Aerobic organisms need oxygen to live, while anaerobic organisms do *not* need oxygen to live.)

Dr Price also set up a clever experiment to demonstrate pleomorphic change. He had two petri dishes in which he grew two different aerobic organisms. One of the dishes held bacteria, and the other held a fungus which used vast amounts of oxygen. Both petri dishes were joined by a tube and hermetically sealed. As the fungus used up the oxygen, the levels of course changed in both dishes. The aerobic bacteria were gradually deprived of oxygen. Instead of dying, these clever little aerobes changed form and became anaerobes. As the oxygen concentration was gradually reduced, the aerobic organisms changed to anaerobic organisms.

So how does this fit into the story?

The test tubes that Rosenow used were long. In such a culture medium, there was also an oxygen gradient of more oxygen at one end than at the other. When shorter tubes were used, the reliability of the experiments went down. Dentine, which makes up most of a tooth, is a tubular structure. The tubules run from the centre of the tooth to the outside. Each tubule can carry eight bacteria across its diameter. Billions can live in just one of these dentine tubules. Differing oxygen gradients will exist in different parts of the tubule, to allow for a great variety of organisms to inhabit differing depths of dentine. The bacteria that inhabit these dentine tubules can therefore take many and ever-changing forms. They can undergo pleomorphic changes within the dentine tubules. This may be a clue to the extreme virulence of some of these organisms and their ability to cause such a huge variety of disease in the rest of the body.

Focal Infection—Reality or Theory

A Focus of Infection is a source or area in the body that is infected and allows the infecting organisms and their toxins to spread to other parts of the body. If the bacteria find a nice home to live in, they will cause an infection in this new part of the body. This is called Elective Localization. The infection is known as a Focal Infection. All medical teaching is fully cognizant of the reality of infections spreading to remote parts of the body. That is, after all, why antibiotics have been so widely adopted.

The position paper of the American Association of Endodontists in 2014 makes the following claims:

"Decades of research have contradicted Dr. Price's findings since then. In 1951, the Journal of the American Dental Association published a special edition reviewing the scientific literature and shifted the standard of practice back to endodontic treatment for teeth with non-vital pulp in instances where the tooth could be saved. The JADA reviewed Dr. Price's research techniques from the 1920s and noted that they lacked many aspects of modern scientific research, including absence of proper control groups and induction of excessive doses of bacteria."[19]

When Dr Price published his revolutionary findings in 1923, he became the scapegoat of the dental world. At a time when bacteriology was taking its rightful place in medicine, Dr Price was able to show that the current dental practice, which tried to keep dead teeth in the mouth, was contributing to many systemic diseases. What set him apart from the other geniuses who were doing similar research was that he was a dentist rather than a medical person. Dissent from within was not tolerated.

The dental PTOs have systematically condemned the work of Dr Price, under the pretext that it has been proven wrong time and time again by well conducted studies." It is probably the only time you will ever hear Dr Price's name mentioned by these groups. They are so fearful of the concepts and research presented that they use Dr Price as the perfect scapegoat. Denigrating great scientists seems to be the way of these PTOs.

The dental world was only just learning how to attempt root canal procedures and needed the support of the whole industry. These procedures had to be safe. They had to "save" teeth. They were simply not allowed to be infected and nor were they allowed to act as a source of infection. The new information that they could be the cause of so many diseases, including cancer, was far too dangerous to allow. The knowledge that disease was a profitable business model was already well established.

The dental establishment calls focal infection a dangerous concept which was started in 1901 by a man called Hunter, which led to the extraction of millions of teeth that could have been easily saved. They talk about the people who have been incapacitated as dental cripples, whose inability to eat has led to their early demise. These dental organizations, which pretend a scientific basis for their statements, only ever talk about focal infection as a theory, never as definitively demonstrated reality. The use of the word "theory" is nowadays almost always linked with that other word, "conspiracy". All I can suggest is that you take the time to read the references and then you can decide whether it is a theory or a conspiracy. All of Dr Price's research is available to be downloaded from my website, www. realdentalinfo.com.

The integrity of this research, supported by so many of the top scientists of the time, has been arrogantly denied by financially driven private trade organizations and a less-than-competent dental "profession". Dentistry's isolation from medicine has enabled the maintenance of mechanics instead of an understanding that teeth are a part of the body. It created the perfect molar mechanics rather than health practitioners. There is to this day zero responsibility within the dental world for creating anything but a perfect Botox smile. Dentists do learn about how various medical conditions will affect the teeth and the gums. We learn nothing about how our "treatments" can be causing many systemic diseases—I mean *nothing*. Dead, pulpless teeth are not allowed to cause disease. Mercury from amalgam is not allowed to cause mercury poisoning. Systemic diseases caused by our "treatments" are simply impossible.

The knowledge of Focal Infection goes hand in hand with another concept called "Elective Localization," as mentioned earlier. What this means is that the bugs that caused kidney disease in a patient also caused the kidney disease in the experimental rabbits that had these bugs injected into them. Elective localization demonstrates that bacteria have a preferred action on preferred tissues. This makes perfect sense, as any organism will have a preferred home to live in, which allows for a long life and steady ability to eat, grow, and reproduce. When bacteria from a tooth are injected into a rabbit and the rabbit dies of the same disease that the patient had before the focus was removed, serious questions need to be addressed. This caused a major dilemma for dental establishments. If the patient's health improves when the focus is removed, this adds serious weight to the research. When this is demonstrated a few times, it could be a coincidental finding. When researchers like Rosenow, Billings, Mayo, and Price were able to demonstrate this many thousands of times, it became a threat to the very existence of dentistry. "It has long been known that the tendency of organisms to localize depends on a certain extent on virulence, and the virulence of an organism is changed by environment. Rosenow's elaboration has been so extensive, however, as to almost revolutionize former views concerning infection" (William W. Duke, *Oral sepsis in its relationship to Systemic Disease* [St Louis, Missouri: Mosby, 1918],[74]).

As Professor Martin Fischer wrote in his book *Death by Dentistry* in 1949, "Microorganisms seek out the hostelries most comfortable for them."

The evidence is irrefutable, but the dental associations continue to try to discredit it because this would mean the end of root canal procedures. Some of the past leaders of the trade organizations were more honest and concerned for the patients.

Thomas B. Hartzell served as president of the ADA in 1922, a year before Dr Price published, and in an October 1922 article, "TEN YEARS TO LIFE," he addressed some aspects of the problem of oral focal infection: "… in our enthusiasm to save the teeth themselves, we have sometimes lost sight of the greater thought that teeth are only a part of the human mechanism concerned in the digestion and assimilation of food and that they are subject to infectious processes rendering them a menace to the life of the individual even though they are playing their mechanical part in the nutritional process. This oversight I concede to be the greatest error into which our profession has ever fallen."[20]

Oh, how the ADA rhetoric changed so soon after.

A perfect example of a focal infection is bacterial endocarditis. Bacteria from the dead tooth or extraction site enter the bloodstream and find a lovely home in the heart. That is a Focal Infection. Now why is that so difficult for a cardiologist or a dentist to understand? We don't need a flood of bacteria, which happens when a tooth is extracted or any other blood-producing procedure is carried out. All that is needed is a few bacteria to come from the dead tooth to find that new perfect home. Bacteria will, in fact, come from that dead tooth all the time. They will travel through the body, and they will localize in tissue that they find suitable to inhabit. This will happen even if the dead tooth is root-canalled by the best endodontist on the planet. Most medical doctors know that if an infection anywhere in the body is not treated, then there is a good chance it will spread to other tissues in the body. Only dentistry denies this possibility.

In 1840, the *American Textbook of Operative Dentistry* described a focal infection as "a localized or generalized infection caused by the dissemination of organisms or toxic products from a focus of infection."[21]

In 1916, Billings wrote, "A focus of infection may be described as a circumscribed area of tissue infected with pathogenic organisms. Foci may be primary or secondary. Primary foci usually are located in tissues communicating with a mucous or cutaneous surface. Secondary foci are the direct result of infections from other foci through contiguous tissues, or at a distance through the blood stream or lymph channels. Primary foci of infection may be located anywhere in the body."[22]

This is supported by Schuster's words from 1941: "… focal infection implies metastasis from the infected foci, of *bacteria or their toxins*, capable of injuring contiguous or distant tissues."[23]

Even the American Dental Association got in on the act and offered a clear definition of Focal Infection some seventy years ago, in 1951. This is the same year that the American Endodontic Society stated that the American Dental Association proved focal infection to have been discredited.

> "A *Focus of infection*" is a 'circumscribed area, infected with micro-organisms which may or may not, give rise to clinical manifestations."

> "A *Focal Infection*," is 'sepsis arising from a 'Focus of Infection' that initiates a secondary infection in a nearby or distant tissue or organs."

The American Dental Association continued with the following:

> Two mechanisms can produce focal infection: the spread of toxins or toxic products from a remote focus to other tissues by the blood stream.

> If the bacteria pass the barrier (of the abscess wall) three things may happen;

a) they may multiply in the blood setting up an acute or chronic septicemia.

b) they may be carried live to a suitable nidus where they infect the surrounding tissue.

a) they may produce a slow but progressive atrophy with replacement fibrosis in various organs of the body.

The bacteria at the focus may undergo autolysis or dissolution. Some of the products of this dissolution, diffusing into the blood or lymph, may sensitise in an allergic sense, various tissues of the body.

A later diffusion of these products on reaching the sensitized tissue may call forth an **allergic reaction.**

The American Dental Journal in 1951 clearly and emphatically stated, "**The concept of focal infection in relation to systemic disease is firmly established. The origin of many toxic or metastatic diseases may be traced to primary local or focal areas of infection.**"[24]

Strangely, our current dental professors seem to be the only people on earth who now claim that focal infection does not exist. They are also the only people who regard mercury as safe! It seems from where I'm sitting that the principles of focal infection stopped applying in root canal situations roughly at the same time they were forced to accept the fact that it is impossible to sterilize a tooth. This is why focal infection is a theory, just like a conspiracy theory. By continually blurring the lines by calling it a *theory*, there can never be an appreciation of the gravity of this situation.

This concept of focal infection and elective localization was too much to bear for the dental world at the time (as well as now). They looked at the research and feared for their livelihoods. At that time, there was no such field as endodontics, and the discussion was about whether or not to keep pulpless teeth in the mouth, and whether the infection in these teeth was a problem for the rest of the body. They even argued that teeth were infected only if they produced a local reaction in the bone!

They were supported in their quest by another bacteriologist, W. L. Holeman. His mission was to discredit Dr Rosenow's research and, in so doing, that of Dr Price. He did not do any research himself in this area but merely rewrote Rosenow's results to make them look less serious. In a letter to the *Journal of the American Medical Association* in 1927, Holeman wrote, "... the 1916 work of Rosenow does not 'indicate more than a 50% chance for either specific or non-specific strains to cause a given disease condition in the laboratory animals."

The reality was that Rosenow and Price found a 90 per cent likelihood of a certain bug being associated with the specific disease in its human host. When Holeman argued a 50/50 chance of anything, he was really telling the world that the focal infection concept and, especially, elective localization were unimportant. His comments made Focal Infection into a 'theory' rather than a cause of disease. The dental associations were grateful to have someone else arguing on their behalf. Some of the most brilliant and ground-breaking medical research that was ever done was instantly disregarded as a mere theory. That Rosenow continued to research and publish his findings till 1944 made no difference after Holeman's deceptive position was published. It made no difference that the research Rosenow continued to do for another thirty years completely supported his earlier research. It made no difference that the results were duplicated and verified by a host of other researchers. Following are just two examples.

Rhoads and Dick, in 1932, cultured green-forming cocci from all of 209 roentgen-ray-negative pulpless teeth and concluded that "... it seems justifiable to regard all pulpless teeth as probable foci of infection, whether they show apical change in the roentgenograms or not. Certainly that position should be taken in the presence of systemic disease of a type usually associated with focal infection."

Swanson and Van Kirk, in 1936, cultured eighteen hundred extracted pulpless teeth and observed that

> Positive cultures resulted from enough x-ray negative teeth to warrant the statement that absence of x-ray evidence does not guarantee sterility in pulpless teeth.

> … the sterile pulpless tooth under any circumstances may be an extreme rarity.

(Word definition: "X-ray negative" and "X-ray positive" are old terms used to describe the appearance of the tooth on an X-ray. "X-ray negative" means it looks like a healthy tooth in healthy bone. A "X-ray positive" is when there is a big hole in the bone filled with abscessed area that looks like a black hole on the film.)

It is still sadly assumed by modern dentistry that an x-ray negative tooth (one which does not show an abscess at the end of the root) is not infected. In fact, one of the accepted measures of a successful root canal procedure is the change in the x-ray picture of the bone from one which shows an abscess to one that does not. That even seems logical. Unfortunately, this supposition is *not* supported by the published research. Even more unfortunate is the fact that this very supposition is still being recited in all dental schools to this day, as well as by many so-called holistic dentists. Worse still, it means that most people who have a root canal procedure are being misdiagnosed. Dr Price demonstrated this reality, and many other prominent dentists have since published similar findings. Even the Australian Dental Association have agreed with this in their 2007 publication, which will be discussed later in this book.

After Holeman 1927, there appears to be nothing recorded in the literature that speaks against Rosenow's research.[3] No one has published anything that contradicts Rosenow, even though he continued to publish till 1944.

Holeman found great support in the American Dental Association, who were only too happy to try to save face if not survival. Particular individuals continued to quote Holeman and reinforce his grand deception. As S. H. Shakman said, it is possibly the "greatest fraud in medicine that has ever been perpetrated and perpetuated." It has allowed the madness of endodontics to persist. It has prevented the medical world from seeing real causes of disease and treating accordingly. This deception of Holeman is singularly responsible for the deaths and suffering of millions of people. It allowed other prominent and unscrupulous people in the dental field to write textbooks that are used worldwide to this day, still promoting the lie that Holeman created in 1927. One such is the *Textbook of Endodontics* by Louis Grossman, which so many of us have had to study. This and another by the famous root canal proponent John Ingles, provided volumes with which to brainwash dental students. These were the gods of root canal therapy.

"Grossman's textbooks have killed more people around the world than that other famous American export, guns."[3, 25]

In his textbook, Grossman writes,

> "One researcher in 1940 noted 'practically every investigation dealing with the pulpless teeth made prior to 1936 is invalid in the light of recent studies' and that the research of Price and others suffered from technical limitations and questionable interpretations of results."[26]

No reference is given, and blind-faith belief is required and expected. All that is needed to wipe out years of serious research is a "vested interest" textbook! After all, it is only the dental students, in their late teens or early twenties, who will read these textbooks, and they know nothing except what they are taught. Why would anyone bother questioning Grossman or Ingles? Why would any dental student go back and read the earlier research that god just defiled and verify this single comment by Grossman? The amount of time, understanding, and opposing knowledge that is required to demonstrate Grossman's lie is, in itself, years of work. Just because Grossman said it, truth is assumed. Grossman lies, and the dental world believes it. The professors repeat the lies, and the next lot of dentists don't even give it another thought. Blind faith is well defined in dentistry. Blind Faith is the only type of faith there is.

It's worth putting this into the historical perspective of a relatively young and unscientific entity called dentistry. At times, the medical profession did try to at least associate with dentistry but was constantly pushed away. Remember that the people who became the dental faculty started off as apes that came down from the trees and became the "tooth pullers" of the society. As time went on, the noble art of extraction was passed on to the barbers. Have a haircut and have your tooth pulled at the same time. It was a barbaric period with lots of whisky and a few people holding the patient in the chair. They went on to fill holes in teeth with things like molten lead and tin. They rapidly took to filling teeth with mercury amalgam when it was set free on the world in 1812. This was the first time that these "dentists" had an alternative to molten lead or tin. They were ecstatic. It didn't matter that the material expanded wildly and cracked the teeth. It didn't matter that they released vast amounts of mercury, which was already known to be highly toxic.

These molar-mechanic dentists ignored the instruction of their Swedish and American Dental Societies to never implant mercury into their patients. Of course, this new wonder material was not going to go away, and these two societies collapsed and were replaced with new organizations created by the very "dentists" who wanted to use amalgam as a filling material. This was the birth of what are now the American and Swedish Dental Associations. They were built on the backs of mechanics and mercury and had naught to do with health or science. These maniacs wanted to use amalgam, no matter how dangerous mercury was. Two of the world's most popularly used dental alloys for the fabrication of amalgam (i.e., when mixed with equal amounts of mercury and called an amalgam filling) have patents which to this day are owned by the American Dental Association.—US patent 4,018,600, registered in April 1977; and US patent 4,078,921, registered in March 1978. In Germany and Sweden these dentists who used amalgam were called *Quecksilber* dentists. "Quecksilber" is the German word for "quicksilver", or "mercury". They were known as *"Quacks"*. Our current dental associations were, in fact, formed by Quacks. Nothing has changed since then.

These mad hatters also developed ways of filling the canals of front teeth with gold and other less-savoury materials, such as arsenic. A pulpless tooth was merely an empty vessel which could be "treated" and kept (sometimes painlessly) in the mouth for that perfect smile. These two practices of using amalgam and filling root canals were the foundation of what is now called a "dental profession". These molar mechanics were not about to let scientists and medical people get in the way of their incomes and prestigious positions.

To this day, the thinking is the same. Clinical judgement still takes precedence over scientifically demonstrable facts. As with all clinical judgement, it is subject to the colour of the glasses worn by the practitioner. This explains the difference between clinical observation and anecdotal evidence. Anecdotal evidence is what GP dentists like me see in their daily practice, which differs from the status quo. Clinical observation is what the dental specialists see in their practice, which agrees with the status quo. I'm not just playing with words here. These words guide the thinking of most doctors and dentists. They guide and maintain the prestige of the specialists. They tell everyone what is acceptable and draw the proverbial ethical line in the sand that most dentists will never cross.

Grossman arrogantly ridiculed Rosenow's research in 1976: "… to add fuel to the fire, reports from bacteriologic laboratories began to come in that show that infected teeth were a menace to health – the health of *laboratory animals*. It was an emotional period and no cognizance was taken of the fact that the amount of broth cultures injected into the animals was so large that it was no wonder the animal's health was overwhelmed …"

The fact is that the bacteria did electively locate in respective tissues of animals corresponding to diseased tissue of human hosts. Moreover, as early as 1919, Rosenow had published studies using smaller doses, specifically in response to critics of earlier large doses.[3]

Incredibly, these books by Grossman and Ingles are the textbooks from which dentists are still "educated". They are *never* peer reviewed. They are never devoid of bias otherwise, they would not be used by the establishment as textbooks. I cannot see my writing being regarded as a text from which they would teach. Textbooks by their very nature are written to conform to the current status quo and then are used to maintain this position of ignorance and false ideals. It makes no difference whether they have no scientific validity, or that what is written in them makes no sense. It makes no difference that what is taught in these volumes is well known to be unachievable. It makes no difference that the basic premise is false. All that matters is a hard-covered volume that is capable of turning intelligent, open-minded students into well-dressed wealthy morons. Personally, I would not use these texts even as doorstops; what they represent is just too ugly. These two dentists alone have caused more death and suffering than most wars combined.

When I went to Sydney University in 1970 to study dentistry, these were the textbooks that I studied from. (Incredibly, in 2022 they are still being used in classrooms!) At that time, these texts were printed on glossy paper and had hard covers. They were bloody expensive and bloody heavy. I know these texts well, as do all of my colleagues. Considering that Rosenow died in 1966, just four years before my entrance into madness, it is worth noting that the names of Rosenow, Mayo, Billings, Price, and Rife were never mentioned in the five years of brainwashing I received. The concept of focal infection was never mentioned. That teeth could be a source of systemic disease was never mentioned. That there was even a controversy about this was never mentioned. That sterility of the tooth was an unachievable goal was never mentioned. We learnt to do a procedure that has impossible goals and is completely unachievable, and we were instructed to call it a "treatment" or "therapy". A rose by any other name just didn't cut it. Dental students are discouraged from thinking and are given the answers to write in the exams. Professors and deans are untouchable. In a profession dealing with the well-being of other humans, the students will hold the deans and professors in high regard and will know that these gods would never tell lies!

As long as there is a separation between medicine and dentistry, there will always be this reliance on clinical observation rather than science. There will always be an emphasis on mechanical restorations rather than disease and suffering. Remember, dentistry just isn't allowed to cause any disease!

It was clear in the early 1900s that the published science could not be challenged by other published science, as there was none, and thus, to avoid a full frontal attack, the dental associations decided to step sideways by firstly separating further from the medical faculty and by claiming that good clinical observation and judgement took precedence over 'test tube science'. As well, there needed to be an end to Price's publications. It was not enough to just shut down the research institute that Dr Price had headed for twenty-five years, as that would have made him into a martyr. They had to discredit him and his research. Holeman fitted the bill perfectly.

The reliance on clinical judgement instead of scientific research was not an overnight phenomenon. It has been a very long-running and carefully scripted lie that is repeated ad infinitum and to this day is still used to steer dentists away from scientific research. It is repeated in the dental journals as a well-known fact. It is repeated by the PTOs in their newsletters and special publications. It is repeated by the teachers of dentistry, and students are taught to scoff at the idea of focal infection. The same teachers also instruct the students to scoff at anyone who may be badly affected by the fluoride that we are forced to drink. The idea that the medical professions are to be referred to occasionally is the only lip service that doctors are permitted. This has been an orchestrated campaign for over one hundred years. The narrative has not changed.

Of course, this clinical judgement is as biased as the textbooks. This clinical judgement was then, and is now, based solely on mechanical outcomes of their "treatments". If you could eat on the tooth and it looked pretty, then it was a clinically successful "treatment". This "clinical judgement" was made by mad hatters who were themselves poisoned with mercury and were, and still are, genuinely mad. I am not exaggerating or being flippant. The great masters of dentistry were and still are really crazy. That's what mercury poisoning does. It makes no difference whether you have risen to the pompous heights of dean of the faculty; you will still be poisoned by mercury, and you will still be mad—just well paid for the effort.

These holy professors have told us for years that all that matters is what we see in our clinics. All that I now need to look at is the work that I did. I guarantee that every dentist looks at the work they did and can see only magnificence. The tools I have by which to measure my successful clinical treatment will tell me only whether the tooth hurts or not. I have *no* dental tools to show me that a case of brain cancer was caused by a root canal procedure I did two years earlier. (The tools that do tell us this are not well regarded by the TGA, but they do exist.)

Focal infection, although a critical means of producing disease, is only one way that dead teeth can make you sick. This will be discussed in detail later, but it is mentioned here for clarity that focal infection is not the only way that a root-canalled tooth can make you sick. By talking only about an "outdated theory", dentistry can sidestep these other disease-causing mechanisms.

Historically, the attitudes of the dental profession are traceable to the writings of a few special individuals who cast enough doubt on the real research to maintain the continued practice of endodontics. Although based on totally false premises, it remains a powerful driving force of modern dentistry. It is maintained by what these trade organizations regard as ethical.

In America, dentists have been deregistered simply for telling patients that mercury is coming out of their amalgam fillings. Taking out dead teeth that may be causing a disease, is considered unethical. The history of medicine in the last 150 years is one of establishing *organizations that profit from diseases*. These organizations have nothing to do with finding cures or long-term humane treatments, as can be seen in the establishment of a society for the control rather than the cure of cancer. Any disease which can be caused by retaining dead, infected, gangrenous teeth in the mouth will be accompanied by a suitably named organization which promotes and profits from that disease. Billions have been spent on cancer research with no cures over the past ninety odd years. The rate of incidence of multiple sclerosis (MS) is increasing steadily, but the Australian MS Society does not want to hear about a dental relationship, which could save so many lives. Autoimmune disease rates are increasing dramatically, yet we still have lousy poisoned food and lousy poisoned dentistry. Almost every medical specialty is faced with diseases that are caused directly by dentistry.

Setting the Stage

The birth of endodontics did not have a guiding star but did have a few gods. There were many in high places that did care about the continuation and organization of root canal procedures. The supposed reason was that they could save teeth. The same reason persists today. The gods made pronouncements, and all of the dentists were delighted to accept. This did not become a fashionable trend; it became a religion. The religious dogma took the place of rational and objective science. The dogma was published in the magazines and journals of these newly formed dental organizations. We may be forgiven for thinking that it sounds like unsupported, arrogant propaganda. These writings fed the needs of the membership to have their societal status raised to new heights by promoting techniques that added handsomely to their wealth. All they needed to rely on was what they saw before them. God said it, so it must be so!

Some examples from the *Journal of the American Dental Association* illustrate this clearly. For these I am grateful to S. H. Shakman, PhD, for his painstaking research.[3] The pompous attitudes in these quotes are replicated today with the same rhetoric. I have added emphasis to the quotations that follow.

July 1922: *JADA* Vol 9, No 7,

'Radicalism Gone Mad' by the Editor, Otto King

> "During recent years ... altogether too many teeth have been extracted through a distorted point of view as to the significance of focal infection, and the relation of teeth thereto. While the profession needed a stirring up on the role which teeth may play in disease, yet the extreme to which the extraction of teeth has been carried is not creditable to dentistry." "a large element among dentists have been stampeded out of their judgement and ... influenced to extract many teeth which should have been preserved."

In line with the craze for extracting teeth, King asserts that

> the so-called 'surgical removal of teeth' has been carried beyond the bounds of reason ... ***To curette all areas from which teeth have been extracted – even diseased teeth – is a radical procedure which is not justified.***

Not only is the surgical extraction and curettage of bone a justified procedure, but it is absolutely essential if we are to remove all tissue which causes disease and prevents healing. The lack of such curettage is one of the reasons that dry sockets and cavitations form in the bone in the first place. This was already known in the late 1800s!

The history book is being written. The ethical concerns are finding their early strategies. In 2022, a full one hundred years later, the dental boards in Australia and America still consider it unethical to extract teeth surgically if forceps can be used, unethical to remove the periodontal ligament and abscess and to clean the bone, and unethical to suture an extraction site that could just have had gauze over it.

1924 *JADA*: Editorial by C. N. Johnson

> … heaven forbid that this profession of ours should ever arrogate itself an undue importance … the moment that smugness begins to raise its ugly head, hope of advancement is irrevocably lost.
>
> So much for one side of the picture. Now for the obverse side. We are frequently regaled by our detractors, not only from outside, but also from members of our profession …

Johnson dismisses the views of presumably ignorant medical men who have advanced the extraction of pulpless teeth, in contrast to dentists "who had been studying teeth for nearly a century …"

Johnson concludes that "**the one great lesson to be learned from our detractors is to ignore them.**"

Yes, you read it right. The editor of the *JADA* is telling everyone to ignore anybody who criticizes them or their practices or beliefs. Ignore the thousands of well-controlled and well-published scientific studies that demonstrate disease caused by dead teeth. Ignore the world and live in a very tightly controlled closed shop or be castigated! This same attitude is upheld in today's dental organizations.

June 1925: *JADA* Vol12, No 6, Editorial by C. N. Johnson

> I freely, frankly and humbly admit that I am not a research worker in a pathologic laboratory, but I have had somewhat extended clinical experience … and I am thoroughly convinced that, in our present prejudice against pulpless teeth, we have gone far astray, and I hereby make the strongest possible plea for a return to **conservatism and sanity** … my present prediction is that we shall arrive at the truth more surely by **careful clinical observation** and study than through the medium **of laboratory research** …

To limit our understanding to clinical observation only and dismiss the research means to look at the procedures we have done and admire the great outcome. It really does depend on the colour of the glasses we wear. There is only one group of people in the world who dismiss the concept of focal infection and they are dentists.

June 1925: *JADA* Vol12, No 6, "Fads and their Effects," ADA President C. N. Johnson

The broad-scale extraction of pulpally involved teeth was described as a "fad" like some other stupid fads of the time.

> … the so called 'New Departure Creed' (advocating the use of Gutta Percha instead of gold foil) … in the late seventies and early eighties (1870s &1880s) … created a real furore in the profession … this fad of plastics threatened to sweep gold foil from our list of filling materials.

September 1928: *JADA* Vol 15, No 9, by Editor C. N. Johnson

> The question of the pulpless tooth is still with us, but is much nearer a solution than it has been for several years, and there is evidence of greater sanity in its

consideration … Just why a well filled pulpless tooth should have been considered an undoubted menace, it is difficult to understand, in the face of the **clinical fact that countless numbers of such teeth have been retained in the mouths** of patients for many years …

There is **no such thing as a dead tooth** unless it has been extracted … A tooth from which the pulp has been removed may not present any menace to the patient … there are records of many thousands of cases in pulps have been removed and root fillings made which, from all evidence available, do not show any sign of infection after many years.

1928 is the year that the definition of "dead" was rewritten by the editor of the American Dental Association. And so began the idea that a root-canalled tooth is not dead. Retaining a dead tooth in the mouth is *not* evidence of its safety, and most doctors will agree that if the blood supply to any tissue is removed, then that tissue is considered dead. This is a recurring argument, as will be shown later. Even the Australian Society of Endodontology, in 2022, claim that a root-canalled tooth is not a dead tooth (https://www.ase.org.au/resources/). There is not one reference for "all the evidence available".

The brainwashing continues:

March 1930: *JADA* Vol 17, No. 3

… *no other kind of evidence can ever take the place of clinical facts well authenticated* … when this question of the status of the pulpless tooth is finally settled, it will be done in the clinic and the office rather than with the **test tube and the microscope** … **let us study clinical records more and resort to theorising less.**

October 1930: *JADA* Vol 17, No 10, "Shall we abandon our birth right?" by Editor C. N. Johnson

> … at one time dentistry begged to be taken under the wing of medicine and was curtly refused … asserting that 'the art of dentistry has … advanced to an infinitely greater perfection under the present plan than it could possibly as an appendage to another calling … Dentistry has never been well taught in a medical college having a dental department … Dentistry has not built its birth right for nothing … shall all of this be swept away for a **few fanatical hands**? We shall gain little … by the attempt at this late date to attach ourselves to the band wagon of medicine and trail behind like the little dog that has been clipped for the occasion … **Our birthright** means too much to us to go begging to any profession for affiliation … If we had been a failure and our policies had been a mistake, there might have been some logic in begging another profession to mother us … Dentistry has developed specialities in its own field that are outstanding in their service, and it is absurd to try at this advanced stage of its growth to submerge the entire fabric in the body politic of another calling. It cannot be done.

When I was studying dentistry in the 1970s, this argument was presented to the students over and over and over again. By the end of the course, we "knew" that we knew more than any doctor. We had been warned over and over that unless we kept our good clinical records, there was a danger that the legal profession would settle our disputes rather than the clinical experience of us dentists. We *knew* that doctors could not understand what dentistry did. We knew that we were the smartest arses on the planet. *We just knew!*

June 1936: *JADA* 23, No. 6, "Laboratory findings or clinical experience", by Editor C. N. Johnson

> ... *if we cannot trust clinical evidence, we cannot trust anything*. Let us pin our chief faith to the experience that comes to us through actual contact with the daily manifestations that we encounter ***in the mouth***.

November 1937: *JADA* Vol 24, No. 11

> ... we confess that we are a bit weary of the effort that it sometime requires to justify dentistry to the public ... if the teeth are intended to serve any useful purpose in the economy of nature, the efforts to preserve them on the part of the members of our profession are eminently justified and essentially praiseworthy ... ***the pathetic wrecks left by the loss of natural teeth*** have challenged the dental profession to remedy this appalling disaster to humanity ... Let us hold our heads a bit higher, and not mope around in an implied attitude that we are "only a dentist" ... the limit of our possibilities has not been reached, and it never will be reached through the agency of subserviency. We must claim our **legitimate prerogative and prestige** ...

Hitler used similar arguments at the Nuremberg rallies of the same period. The Second World War began in September 1939.

March 1939: *JADA* Vol 26, No. 3

> In 'Educating the Public Dentally,' Editor Anthony bemoans the 'ultra-ethical restrictions that have prevented the profession from publicising the benefits which dentistry can render to humanity.' 'This attitude ... has encouraged and frequently compelled certain classes of the public to obtain their *information on dental health subjects from questionable sources*.'

The only source that should be trusted wears a white coat and is mercury poisoned. I do wonder what these other questionable sources were, considering the Internet and Google didn't exist. These trade organizations are claiming a lofty position that all of mankind should listen to. They create the illusion that they are the only source of information to be trusted.

May 1940: *JADA*

The lead editorial "Why Not Save the Pulp Involved Tooth?" refers to dentistry of twenty years prior having become

> "… hysterically employed in the removal of all teeth in which the pulp was in any way involved, asserting that this fatalistic attitude was **almost wholly without confirmed scientific reason**." "Hunter's diatribe … struck a psychologically hopeful chord" to physicians who could not otherwise address many "more or less intractable conditions."

The editorial offers that with the passing of time and "development of much contradictory evidence," dentistry sought "*a sane and safe position*" which led to the saving of teeth.

> "… the pulp involved tooth can be *restored to usefulness* … without menace to the health of the patient." The article repeatedly emphasizes the *conclusive testimony of clinical experience which argues for saving teeth.*"

> "**… almost wholly without confirmed scientific reason**" means that Price, Rosenow, Mayo, Billings, and many other researchers were clearly lying about their scientific results. Many thousands of rabbits ended badly in the research. By injecting the rabbits with bacteria and their toxins from dental foci, they were able to replicate the disease states of the person from whom the focus was removed. Generally, the patient improved or fully recovered while the poor rabbits

died of the same disease or diseases like that which the donors originally suffered from. When you read the original research, you see that the experiments were not only well controlled but also repeated so often, with the same result, that the conclusion of focal infection became a well understood and treatable concept in medicine. It was not a theory.

As well as redefining the word "dead", dentistry goes on to redefine "infection".

Grossman in stated in 1946, "… the recovery of bacteria from pulpless teeth does not per se indicate that infection is present. **Only when the presence of micro-organisms produces a reaction – inflammation, at least – can infection be said to exist**."

The dictionary definition of "infection" is "The invasion and multiplication of micro-organisms such as bacteria, viruses, and parasites that are not normally present within the body."[27] Infection is not defined by the reaction that it causes. So much for dental textbooks.

Remarkably, in 1951 the American Dental Association was vociferous in their support and understanding of the importance of focal infection. I have no idea why or how this came about, but the understanding published in *JADA* (quoted later) was short-lived.

Other fads discussed at the time were hypnotism, cataphoresis, copper amalgam, analgesia for cavity preparation, the administration of gas for the filling of teeth (resulting in "an unfortunate crop of dead pulps" and dead people), and the use of Emetine for treating pyorrhoea— gum disease. Regarding this last item, Johnson notes, "we can only blush for the extent that this remedy was forced on a helpless public. The fact that it was all done only with the best intentions goes only a short way to ameliorating the embarrassment with which we recall the period of this practice. It is well that a merciful public forgets and forgives …"

I guess it was only those who were not poisoned or killed who could forget and forgive. I hardly consider blushing to be an appropriate response for dentistry's stupidity.

Emetine is a bitter, poisonous white alkaloid obtained from ipecacuanha; the hydrochloride is used to treat amoebic infections. It is lucky that the public are so forgiving or gullible. Emetine is highly toxic, and one study indicates that 50 to 70 per cent of individuals exposed to this substance have very bad side effects. They include heart conditions, nausea, vomiting, diarrhoea, headache, skeletal muscle weakness, stiffness, pain and muscle weakness at the site of injection, and eczematous, urticarial, or purpuric lesions. Prolonged administration may produce systemic toxic reactions, some of which may be serious or even fatal; adverse effects primarily involve the heart and cardiovascular system, the neuromuscular system, the CNS, and the GI tract.[28] It is worth noting that at the time, it, too, was regarded as a state-of-the-art treatment. It remained in use in America till 1990.

The Fabrication of Status

The pedestal which dentistry sits on was created by carefully scripted words, a great deal of arrogance, and some creative vested interests. It was literally created by mercury-poisoned madmen. These are the same mad hatters who claim the mercury from amalgam is safe. These are the same professors who teach dental students to use amalgam while at the same time exposing them to levels of mercury far above the tolerable dose levels of the Occupational Safety and Health Authority (OSHA). These are the same mad people who claim that fluoride in the drinking water stops decay, even though the decay rates in non-fluoridated countries have dropped below those of fluoridated countries. It is more important to be seen to be preventing decay in baby teeth than it is to actually be doing something, such as providing healthy nutritional advice. Reduction of IQs across the whole population is not of any concern to these psychopaths, and it is even welcomed by the politicians, who do not realize that they too are affected. How long has it been since you've seen an intelligent politician? These are the same people who claim total safety of titanium implants even though the dissolution of titanium by fluoride in the drinking water is well published and is a possible cause of the implants getting loose and falling out. These are the same people who are now advocating the injection of botulism toxin for aesthetics. They are the same people who are being given permission to inject medical vaccines.

The professors have no concern for the welfare of their students or the patients. They have little to no regard for science or its findings. Even when I was at university, they spoke of the "noble art" of dentistry. High ethical standards are always espoused. It is always reinforced that we are not under the tutelage of medicine. As dentists, we are better than doctors. Sadly, the ignorance of the medical profession in regard to dental matters is now well established. Medical people generally have *zero* professional knowledge of what dentistry does.

This position of superiority was continued into 1998 by the then dean of dentistry at Sydney University, Emeritus Professor Iven Klineberg, in his welcome message to new students:

"Dentistry is a **noble profession, closely linked with medicine but independent from it** ... is designed to prepare graduates to commence **clinical practice** following graduation and registration ... responsibility on each student and graduate for the delivery of **appropriate clinical treatment ...** Patients will have trust in the **technical and clinical skills** of the clinician as well as their **ethical and moral** standards. The responsibility that rests with each undergraduate and graduate dentist in each of these areas, **requires special understanding, caring and sensitivity.**"

What a shame that dentistry is independent from medicine. Clearly implied is that we have no medical responsibility to our patients. We can poison them relentlessly, but we are independent from medicine! We can cause cancer and MS, but we are independent from medicine. So long as we do "appropriate clinical treatment", our hands will remain clean and noble without regard for the catastrophes we cause. This dean, like all the others, also promoted the poisoning of the public with mercury and fluoride.

He continues to say that the current course will "… reflect much more the biological basis of dentistry and a move from a technology-based discipline that was previously the backbone of dental practice." Now that sounds like a move in the right direction if it weren't for the statement that follows: "The emphasis on preventive care in practice and the fluoridation of water supplies has led to the **virtual elimination of dental caries**. Management of caries in such mouths when it does occur, is a relatively simple procedure …"

Suggesting that decay has been virtually eliminated shows how removed a dean can be from the reality of daily practice. Suggesting that the decline in tooth decay has anything to do with fluoride is completely unscientific and unsupported. Only six countries still fluoridate their water supplies. The others have either stopped or never started. In the whole of the first-world countries, the decay rate has dropped, and the non-fluoridated countries have actually outstripped the fluoridated countries in reduction of tooth decay. Fluoride is not a part of a health equation. It is a part of a financial and biological equation, though. It makes you sick and dumb. So do mercury and the toxins from dead teeth.

Even the NSW State Health Department agrees that water fluoridation does not reduce decay. "Some of these largely unfluoridated countries have reported steep declines in dental caries that parallel declines seen in largely fluoridated countries (Marthaler 2004)."

Another study conducted by NSW Health also demonstrated that fluoride is not a factor causing or preventing decay in rural aboriginal communities.[29] The main factors are socioeconomic and education status.

The damage extends into the medical world as medicine continues to ignore the cause of many of the degenerative diseases it tries to treat. That the medical world has been subjugated to the whims of molar mechanics is beyond comprehension. That the medical profession has relinquished a part of the body to the beliefs of mad hatters is a crime against humanity and medicine itself. We have clear and definite proof of focal infection from dead teeth, yet the medical world never considers dental conditions as causative. Of course, this fits the money-making concerns of big pharma, which makes a fortune treating the created degenerative diseases. In other words, the denial of focal infection has created a litany of treatment models based in fantasy. There is no official known cure for MS, yet I personally have seen several cases of MS disappear relatively quickly after the removal of dead root-canalled teeth. (See chapter 10 for a detailed discussion.) Our doctors send patients away to die miserable deaths because it is "unethical", according to the great and untouchable dental associations, to remove the dead tooth which is causing the disease. As soon as a procedure is pronounced unethical, everyone runs a mile. Our doctors and dentists want to believe the fantasy so strongly that they are willing to ignore the science.

A Rose by Any Other Name

When a procedure is called a "treatment" or "therapy", there will always be an army of dentists willing to jump in. Most dentists do believe that they are looking after the well-being of their patients. If it were just a procedure, it would be looked upon with more objectivity.

Dentists are terrified of their PTOs and dental boards. To step out of line takes a certain amount of madness and a great deal of knowledge. Support by the club in litigious situations is what keeps the majority of dentists toeing the line. When I took out dead teeth, I knew that the dental board were just waiting for a complaint from a patient. They never got one. There is not one endodontist that I know of who would support such procedures. As a side note to dentists: Your dental association needs you more than you need them. There is absolutely no reason to pay a fortune to belong to a corrupt club. You will lose nothing by not belonging. As Groucho Marx once stated, "I sent the club a wire stating, please accept my resignation. I don't want to belong to any club that will accept me as a member."

Many dentists will claim the safety of root canals because they personally have several teeth that are root-canalled in their own mouths. If there were anything wrong, they would know about it— right? (As if this anecdotal observation was a scientific validation of their ignorance.) And we wonder why dentists have the highest suicide rate of all professional groups! I believe another reason for their denial of the possibility of focal infection comes closer to home. Not many dentists will want to take responsibility for the cancer they have caused in their spouse, child, or friends. They cannot accept responsibility for causing leukaemia in their sons or infertility and breast cancer in their wives and daughters. Do you still wonder why I call them mad hatters? These people are seriously crazy, and you want to put your well-being in their hands! Do you really want to trust the "well controlled studies" that these people cherish so dearly but are unable to demonstrate? If you are a dentist reading this, then why not write to your association asking for references to these well-controlled studies? If you're not a dentist, you could do the same. Find out for yourself! "Would you be kind enough to provide me with references to the well-controlled studies which have demonstrated that focal infection theory is wrong." That is all you need to write. If you do get a response, then please send it to me.

To prove cause and effect when only one patient gets "better" after the dead tooth is removed is, of course, unlikely. When this happens several times, though, we'd think that some may start to sit up and take an interest. When this process is repeated literally thousands of times, all that the dental world can do is run for cover. Sadly, it is the rest of the population that suffers. If you are struggling with a degenerative disease that is eventually going to kill or incapacitate you, then what have you got to lose by having a tooth or two removed. You might even consider that removal of a tooth is far preferable to developing cancer or arthritis a few years down the track. Prevention is lots cheaper.

General Knowledge vs. Science

Has anything changed since the time of these great men? So much research and knowledge has flown under the bridges of academia that surely by now the specialist endodontists are able to back up their position. They even have well-thumbed textbooks which support the concepts of their "treatments". A brochure called *Relax—There Is No Need To Lose Your Tooth … Endodontics (Root Canal Therapy) Can Save It For You* was distributed by the Australian Society of Endodontology, in 1996.

Letter to the Australian Society of Endodontology

I wrote to the Australian Society of Endodontology in 1997, asking for references to the wild claims made in the brochure mentioned above, which I, as a GP dentist, was expected to give to patients to convince them of the efficacy and safety of RCPs. The emphasis in my letter below was added by me for the publication of this book.

> 12 April 1997
>
> Dear Dr …
>
> I am writing with a request for information which I hope you, as president of the Australian Society of Endodontology (Inc.), will be able to supply. I am a practicing general dentist in Sydney and have a great interest in the area of Endodontics. My queries are in relation to the patient education pamphlet; "Relax-there

is no need to lose your tooth … ENDODONTICS (Root Canal Therapy) can save it for you."

In paragraph 2 it is written "Once the tooth is fully formed **the main source of nutrition for the tooth comes from the tissues surrounding the root**."

Could you please supply the references for this statement? Would you also be kind enough to explain to me exactly how the tooth is nourished from its surrounding tissues? Is this via the blood supply, the lymph or by osmosis?

In the third paragraph it is written;

"Therefore, a tooth can **function** normally without its pulp and can be kept indefinitely. After endodontic treatment the tooth is **pulpless, but it is NOT a dead tooth**."

Again, I would appreciate references to support this statement. By suggesting that the tooth is not dead, one can only assume that it is alive. For this to be so it must have some vascular supply. If I am not mistaken the very procedure of Root Canal Therapy is to remove the blood supply.

The statement (7th Paragraph) "During endodontic treatment, the infected or damaged pulp is **removed** from the inside (i.e. root canal) of your tooth."

Is it necessary to remove all infected dead pulp tissue from the tooth? If not please supply references which describe the fate and effect of remaining infected tissue.

If so please supply the references which demonstrate that all necrotic and infected tissue can be removed from the tooth.

The 8th Paragraph states: "The root canals are then **cleaned, sterilised** and shaped to a form that can be **completely sealed**." Firstly, I again request references to support this statement. Next would you be kind enough to explain to me;

- the procedure and medication recommended by the society which does **sterilise** a tooth.
- how is sterility of the tooth determined? Is it necessary to take a swab of the tooth for culturing? If so should this be aerobic or anaerobic.
- if anaerobic testing is required could you please inform me of the correct procedures.
- **please supply references** which demonstrate the **complete sealing** of a root canal.

Paragraph 11 talks of the sedative dressings and temporary fillings which are used to settle the tooth "and **destroy** any remaining bacteria". References supporting this statement would be appreciated. Would you also list for me the medicaments which are currently recommended to achieve this outcome?

I appreciate that you may not be the author of this pamphlet and that this is indeed quite a large request. I believe though, that if I am to pass this pamphlet on to my patients, I would like to be in a position to be able to verify each of these statements by published, peer reviewed scientific papers.

If you are unable to furnish the answers to this request, I would appreciate it if you could point me to the author of this paper. I thank you in advance for your response.

Yours sincerely Robert Gammal

Response from the Australian Society of Endodontology

The response I received included some statements which should have been quite embarrassing for such an austere organization. They stated that the pamphlet was written by a committee of endodontists and that the material was based on the *general knowledge* of the committee members. They also stated that ~~no~~ references were used in the creation of the pamphlet. I was also advised to consult any textbook of endodontics to confirm the statements made in their pamphlet.

The Australian gods of endodontics were unable to provide *one* reference to support the blatant and ignorant lies in their brochure—*not one reference* for modern-day dentistry. Only a reliance on textbooks and general knowledge of specialists in the field are needed to make GP dentists toe the line. The "general knowledge" of endodontists is not a scientific position. It's an insult!

The statement "… Once the tooth is fully formed **the main source of nutrition for the tooth comes from the tissues surrounding the root**" flies in the face of the position of the American Dental Association, who stated in 2005, "Inside each tooth is the pulp which provides nutrients and nerves to the tooth …"[30] Thus a pulpless tooth, by their definition, is lacking a nutrient and nerve supply. The tooth does not receive nutrition from the surrounding tissue.

After personally speaking with a number of endodontists to discuss these issues, I can only conclude that this "general knowledge" is one of stupidity, arrogance, and ignorance. This general knowledge underlies a criminal disregard for any published science that contradicts the status quo, as well as the welfare of their patients. Their statement that "no controversial issues are raised in the brochure" is almost funny considering that the whole brochure is based on endless statements that have no scientific validity. Textbooks are not refereed published science. They are also usually not well referenced. They are written to maintain the status quo. Of course, they support each other. This is consistent with the approach of relying on "clinical observation" in preference to published science. The "noble" art of endodontics is not based in science.

In 2022 the Australian Society of Endodontology still maintain the lie on their website. (See https://www.ase.org.au/resources. Click on the "Relax-Endodontics" brochure.) They are a law unto themselves. "The main function of the dental pulp is to regulate the growth and development of the tooth during childhood. Once the tooth is fully formed nutrition for the tooth comes from the tissue surrounding the root. Therefore the tooth can function without its pulp and, in the majority of cases, can be kept indefinitely. After root canal treatment the tooth is pulpless but is not a dead tooth."

The greatest endodontists in the land are telling blatant lies. The function of the dental pulp continues throughout your life. It is responsible for maintaining a continuous fluid flow from the inside of the tooth to the outside, which is the main thing preventing decay in a tooth. It is involved in autonomic regulation of the nervous system. Nerves that are amputated in the root canal procedure may affect the Trigeminal Nucleus in the brain. There is *no* such thing as the tissue surrounding the root providing nutrition to the tooth. It only comes from the blood vessels that enter and leave through the apex of the root. When these blood vessels no longer exist, either because of infection in the tooth or because of their removal in the root canal procedure, the tooth is dead, whether or not it is connected to the rest of the body. Their dedication to mechanics and ignorance is how they justify the idea that a dead, infected, and gangrenous tooth can function normally for the rest of your life. They do not comment that this holy "treatment" may be precisely what shortens your life.

These days there are many 'holistic' dentists. They jumped on the bandwagon of non-amalgam dentistry as they realized that people were looking for more science-based dentistry. They also realized that the holistic label delivered a greater income. They claim to be able to do something called a holistic root canal and always use the words "therapy or treatment". There is *no such thing*. They claim to select their root canal patients on an individual, case-by-case basis. I've not met one who looks at three generations of familial medical histories as Dr Price did! The criteria by which they make their decisions are not written or displayed for anyone to see. Perhaps it may just be the amount of money that they can extract from you instead of extracting the tooth. When they make comments like "We are not sure if complete sterilization of the tooth is necessary", they are simply parroting the American and British Dental Associations' claims that it is unimportant. They are ignoring the science. Their dedication to ignorance maintains their membership in the club and their continued income. This is why I have never referred to myself as holistic. It really is time for science to guide our treatments, rather than the PTOs who have consistently denied the science.

Price–Buckley Debate

On October 12, 1925, a famous debate was held between Dr Price and Dr Buckley before the Odontographic Society of Chicago. Over fifteen hundred dentists attended this meeting! It is a remarkable testament to a great scientist's humanity. Dr Buckley was a past president of the American Dental Association. Sadly, I do not have a copy of the transcript and have not seen one outlining Dr Buckley's side of the debate except for the small bits written below. Both he and Johnson (editor of the *JADA*) used the debate as a means of discrediting Price's research. By the way, this is the same Buckley who introduced a mixture of formaldehyde, cresol, and glycerine as a material with which to "mummify" the pulps of baby teeth. It was called Buckley's Foromocresol, which is still used worldwide to this day by specialist endodontists. Formaldehyde is a *known human carcinogen* associated with nasal sinus cancer, nasopharyngeal cancer, and leukaemia, particularly myeloid leukaemia.[31] I have personally seen a number of children whose leukaemia disappeared soon after the removal of teeth that had been "treated" with Buckley's Formocresol. Clearly

Buckley was very concerned with keeping dead teeth in the head rather than maintaining the health of his patients.

As long as we rely on "clinical judgement" instead of published science, we will not see the patients who die from our treatments.

I have included this section to give a bit of a historical perspective and to demonstrate the ferocity with which Price's findings were denigrated, which continues to this day. Principally, it is to show Dr Price's research findings in his own words. They resonate throughout this book.

Below is a small sample of Dr Buckley's remarks:

... if it becomes necessary for me to speak plainly and to the point in presenting my side of the question, I want the audience to know in advance that there is nothing personal intended.

... the radical stand many men are taking today with reference to the ruthless extraction or so-called surgical removal of pulpless teeth ...

... to assume the responsibility for the radical extraction of pulpless teeth ... he travels too rapidly or does not stay in one place long enough for those of us who are a little sluggish to get our perspective or bearings.

(It's a shame he was intellectually unable to keep up with the information!)

Buckley continued:

... he gives us absolutely no hope of saving a pulpless tooth under any condition. My God, men! Whither are we drifting? There is such a thing as carrying science, so called, far beyond the realm of ridiculous, and plainly toward the limits of criminality.

> … does he report only such as would seem to justify his preconceived ideas? And … does this not prove that as a scientific investigator his is either incompetent or unreliable or both? Certainly, it must be suspected that he lacks the tireless and irresistible courage of complete sincerity and sanity.

> God giving me the strength, I will spend the remainder of my life, if need be, correcting this damnable and criminal practice for which you sir, Dr. Price, whether you realize it or not, are in large measure responsible.[3]

It is worth remembering that ten years earlier it was Dr Frank Billings who was reporting on the work of Dr Rosenow, which showed precisely the results obtained by Dr Price. Billings was similarly denigrated for this by the medical establishment.

Dr. Price, in the opening of his presentation, stated,

> In accepting Dr. Buckley's challenge to meet him in debate on the question- Resolved, that practically all infected pulpless teeth should be removed, I have been controlled by a sense of responsibility to humanity, for I believe with all my heart that humanity needs rescuing, not from a wilful aggressor but from an incorrect interpretation, which has furnished wrong fundamentals for diagnosis, prognosis and treatment.

> I shall probably surprise my opponent and perhaps shock some of my audience when I confess that I hope he will win this debate by furnishing what I have not been able to find: namely, a means for sterilizing and for maintaining sterility of the infected pulpless tooth.

I have searched diligently for the same for more than thirty years.

Dr. Price, concluded with the following:

If, now, we summarize these various presented data, we find that:

- People are not living nearly to the entire span of life, which they have a right to expect.
- Death is occurring even in our most civilized communities largely from the degenerative diseases, chief of which is heart disease.
- Even the mortality statistics of our various communities will at this time give an indication of the level and thought of dental practice with regard to the management of infected pulpless teeth.
- It is practically, if not entirely, a physical impossibility to sterilize infected cementum by treating through the dentin. It is like trying to sterilize infection in the label on the bottle by putting disinfectants in the bottle.
- Root fillings do not continue to fill root canals. The amount of space that ultimately develops is approximately the amount of solvent that was used with the root-filling material, assuming that mechanical filling of every area was possible.
- Individuals are not comparable in their defence against degenerative diseases. Some are susceptible and must have an entirely different preventive program.
- The degenerative diseases are largely symptoms of degenerative processes in the blood stream, an important contributing cause for which is long-continued, usually unsuspected, chronic infection.

The extremely inadequate time and space for this statement prevents the inclusion of similar important evidence, demonstrating that:

- The roentgen rays cannot reveal all the required information, and under old standards will often be misleading.
- The complement fixation method for dental infections can be related to systemic sensitization.
- Chronic dental infections reduce the normal bactericidins of the blood.
- Leukocyte activity is depressed by chronic dental infections.
- Chronic dental infections can produce antigens, to which the sensitized patient may respond with an allergy of severe and very obscure type.
- Dental infections can be demonstrated to have had specific localizing ability for many of the organs and tissues of the body. I have already reported on most of these in my papers and books.

We cannot, therefore, continue in the light of these new truths to give any quarter to the infected pulpless tooth until we can both accomplish its disinfection and insure its continued sterility. Until then, it must be eliminated. By the elimination of dental focal infections, we will eliminate one of the important contributing factors to the shortening of life and loss of health, for it is chiefly the destructive influences of these infection products that have to do with the destroying of the defensive mechanisms of the blood stream and the producing of abnormal levels, chiefly of calcium, which thereby predispose to sensitization reactions, cancer, tuberculosis, diabetes and the anemias, on the one hand, and to the rheumatic group of degenerative diseases on the other, two groups which together constitute the great majority of deaths in the various communities.

A new truth is a new sense, for with it, we can see things that we could not see before and things that cannot be seen by those who do not have that new truth.

In closing, I want you to see with me a little incident that happened in a town in Illinois, a year ago last Christmas. Prior to that time, there had been appearing, in a window, a little hand that seemed to wave to each passing train as if in distress. At night a flickering match took its place, and it was waved frantically as a signal for help.

This got on the nerves and hearts of the trainmen as they passed by; and as they exchanged reports, they decided that there must be someone there in distress. Accordingly, a committee was appointed to go and investigate; and it was found that a little bedridden child lay crippled where she could not see out of the window but where she could reach her hand in front of the window.

On Christmas morning, two trans-continental express trains stopped on the main line in front of this little home, and from them committees of trainmen proceeded to the little home to carry comforts and money to help this afflicted little sister of humanity.

I do not know what she was suffering from, but I do believe that there are many such sufferers who have been important, if not a controlling, contributing factor in dental infection. I am going to ask that every time you place a root-filling in an infected tooth, you shall see that waving hand in the window.

3

Why Do I Need a Root Canal?

· ·

There is nothing more frightening
than active ignorance.

—Goethe

This chapter aims to give you some basic understanding of some of the more common questions I have been asked as a dentist.[32] This includes things like "Why do teeth decay?" "What is an abscess?" "How is a root canal performed?" "Why would you need a root canal?" "What are the options?" and "Do I need fluoride on my teeth?" I hope you will find the answers here. It is a bit like Dentistry 101, for beginners, with minimal jargon.

When my colleagues and I speak about fluoride, the dental world also calls us anti-vaccinationists, and of course when we speak against vaccination, we are also called anti-fluoridationists. Both positions are supposedly so well understood scientifically that to oppose either is the height of stupidity and ignorance and a complete lack of science. This name-calling helps their arguments, which do not have the scientific support that is implied by their prestigious university appointments. It seems that Dr Buckley had a long-standing influence. The words "conspiracy theorists" are used often, and in this new age, it is called "false news".

Fluoride Poison or Protector

This is a very brief introduction. To do this subject justice, we would need several books. I bring it in here only as a means of showing the false thinking in terms of the real causes of decay in the next section. There is much more information on my website, www.realdentalinfo.com.

In the early 1940s there was a secret US military project called the Manhattan Project. This top-secret project used masses of fluoridated water to make what we now know as the atomic bomb. Farms downstream were poisoned. From apple trees to cows to humans, all suffered.

The vested interest was in the war effort, and the medical world was appalled at the idea of allowing people to drink poisoned water. As the continued fluoridation of the downstream water became worse during the development of the bomb, there was a thought from the polluters that people could be told that this fluoride is good for teeth and prevents decay. There was *nothing* scientific or medical in this decision. This decision was purely a political (and military) cover-up. "If the people believe that we are helping their teeth they will accept anything" is how the thinking went. It's all about how the bugs produce acids which dissolve the teeth, and thus, when we add fluoride into the developing teeth, they become stronger and more resistant to acid attack. Parents then won't have to spend their life savings on their kids' teeth. The old advertisement which showed blue dye entering a piece of chalk was all that was needed to convince all parents that this poison was good for their children's teeth—and their own, for that matter. Sadly, a piece of chalk is *not* a tooth, and blue dye is not a schedule 6 poison, as is fluoride. What was known about fluoridation even then was that it produces apathy! You no longer care! As a population you are thus more manageable by less force and more propaganda. Does a reduction in IQ result in more submission?

Apart from anything else, the simple fact is that fluoride, either in the water or applied topically to teeth, makes *no* difference to the decay rate. Studies also exist which demonstrate a reduction of decay rates when the fluoridation programmes have been stopped.[33,34,35,36,37] Epidemiological studies of decay rates around the world show that non-fluoridated countries have decay rates as low as, if not lower than, those of the fluoridated countries(WHO). There are only *six countries* in the world that still add toxic fluoride to their citizens' drinking water. These are Australia, New Zealand, the United Kingdom, South Ireland, the United States, and Hong Kong. The rest have either tried it and then banned it, or never introduced it in the first place.

In the 1940s, there was occasionally more honesty in the medical and dental worlds. In 1943 the *Journal of the American Medical Association* (September 18) published the following warning: "**Fluorides are general protoplasmic poisons**, probably because of their capacity to modify the metabolism of cells by changing the permeability of the cell membrane and by inhibiting certain enzyme systems."

In **1944** the American Dental Association published the following dire warning:

"Drinking water containing as little as **1.2 ppm fluoride will cause developmental disturbances**. We cannot run the risk of producing such serious systemic disturbances. **The potentialities for harm outweigh those for good**."[38]

In 1945, Hiroshima and Nagasaki vanished.

Tooth Decay and Some Preventive Tips

Decay in teeth is also called caries. Dentistry has always taught that decay is caused by bacteria that produce very strong acids which "dissolve" the enamel of our teeth. This implies that the sole cause of decay is external to the tooth. That is why all the emphasis is on oral hygiene and fluoride. I am certainly *not* opposed to good oral hygiene and advocated this to all my patients. Good brushing and flossing are critical, but that is not the whole story. Having clean teeth and mouth will not just help to prevent decay but will also keep your gums and the supporting tissues of your teeth in good health. This is basic. There are many ways to clean those porcelain pillars, but the real point is that they must be kept clean if you wish to stay healthy. This means physically removing the sticky mucous layer called "plaque", which supports the growth of normal oral bacteria in such a way that leads to the production of acids, which dissolve the tooth structure. This needs to be done regularly at a minimum of twice per day and ideally after each meal. There is no getting around this, so get a little toothbrush and start your religious practice today.

Fluoride, on the other hand, is not acceptable. No matter what the story, remember that fluoride is a protoplasmic poison for everyone. In any form and in any propaganda, fluoride remains a poison just like mercury.

There are a few basics that are worth remembering. Firstly, do *not* use fluoridated toothpastes. They only serve to poison you and do nothing to prevent decay. Use a child-sized toothbrush. Anything larger does not fit in the small spaces in your mouth. Dental tape is easier to use than floss, as its thickness stops the shredding effect. If it keeps shredding, then go see a dentist to find out what the sharp bit on your tooth is. Normal teeth do not have sharp bits. Sharp bits are not cleanable and will harbour decay. You do not need expensive mouthwashes; nor do you need whitening toothpastes. (Bleaching agents that are applied to the enamel are very reactive and will also draw large amounts of mercury out of any amalgam fillings you may have.) Do not use fluoridated mouthwashes. Avoid all forms of fluoride, including fluoridated drinking water. Get a reverse osmosis filtering system, at least for your drinking and cooking water, which will remove the fluoride.

You *never* need fluoridated toothpaste.

The dean I suffered under during my undergraduate years was also the man responsible for fluoridating Tamworth and half of NSW.

This criminal denied anything which did not support his fluoridation programme. But who's going to argue with the dean! At the same time this dean was teaching me the values of fluoride, other important and ignored research was being published in the dental journals. Just as we never heard about Price, Rosenow, or Billings at university, so too we did not hear of Dr Ralph Steinman. Decay in teeth is a little more complicated than what the fluoridation mentality would have us believe.

The Real Cause of Decay

In the late 1960s and 70s, Dr Ralph Steinman published research demonstrating that decay in teeth is related to the health of the whole body. Much of his research was published in dental journals and then promptly ignored as the fluoridation circus started to swing into full force. Fluoride does not make a difference except to weaken the body.

Steinman's work showed that a healthy body produces a flow of tissue fluid from the inside of a tooth right out through the dentine and enamel. By injecting blue dyes under the abdominal skin of rabbits, he could demonstrate that same dye coming through the enamel of the teeth in less than a day. With this healthy fluid flow, there was no decay, even when people did not brush their teeth. There was certainly gum disease when brushing didn't happen, but virtually no decay.

As the health of the body is compromised, however, this fluid pressure reduces, and there is a corresponding increase in the amount of decay. Systemic health affects the rate of decay in teeth and is also affected by decay in teeth. It's a two-way street.[39,40,41,42,43,44,45,46,47,48,49,50]

The abstracts of his research are also available on my website, www.realdentalinfo.com

The autonomic nervous system is that part of our nervous system which regulates all the unconscious functions of the body, such as heart rate and digestion. When we are in dangerous situations, the Sympathetic side of this system kicks in, and we have the traditional fight-or-flight response. Blood supply is increased to the legs and arms and is reduced to the gut. The heart and respiratory rates increase, and the pupils in the eyes dilate. It's a bit like flattening the accelerator in your car. When the danger is gone (e.g., you've just left the dentist's office) and you no longer need to stay in this state of stress, the other side of the autonomic system kicks in to gear. This is the Parasympathetic nervous system, which slows your heart and breathing, allows the blood vessels in your arms and legs to reduce in size, and lets the pupils come back into normal light adjustment. You can now rest. Homeostasis is the name of this resting state where everything is balanced.

It became clear to Steinman and other researchers that the blood flow and tissue-fluid flow in a tooth is under the direct control of this autonomic nervous system and that when we are stressed the blood and tissue fluid pressure is reduced in the tooth and decay starts.

"Circulation of blood in the human tooth is affected by evoked changes in autonomic nerve activity, involving activation of both vasodilator and vasoconstrictor nerves to vessels serving the tooth."[51]

Parasympathetic stimulation (that which causes calming) encourages increased fluid flow throughout the tooth. Sympathetic stimulation (as found during stress periods and the fight/flight response) dramatically reduces the fluid flow through the tooth.

The current position of the Australian Society of Endodontology, that the only use for the pulp is in the formation of the tooth, is at best ignorant. The function of the pulp extends throughout life. When the pulp is removed, there is no longer any tissue fluid in the tooth, and this tooth has a much greater chance of decaying.

I saw many patients who came for their regular six-monthly check-up and never had anything for me to do. Sometimes these patients would come a year later and suddenly have lots of decay in their teeth. Almost without fail, there had been a change in their lives or their health. Family separations and deaths of close people can elicit so much stress that we see it in the increased decay rate. This is so common, in fact, that we can see the physical changes in the mouth and know that something major has happened.

Steinman found that the fluid pressure, and hence the decay rate, was dependent principally on *diet* and *stress*.[52] Sugar and white flour were amongst the worst in negatively influencing the body. Both reduce the flow of fluid through the teeth.

This is precisely what Dr Price found and published in 1939. He found that within one generation of introducing sugar and refined flour in the diet of a population, the decay rate in the next generation went from almost non-existent to what we in the wealthy Western countries consider normal.

As Dr Steinman says, "… The logical approach then to caries control is a way of life which includes a sound nutritional program and freedom from stress. For many individuals this would represent a changed way of life. But there is much evidence that the answer to caries lies in nothing less."[53]

There are many studies which discuss the flow of fluids within teeth and their clinical significance.[54,55,56,57,58] This information is not in mainstream dental teaching even though it was published some fifty years ago in dental journals. If we were to accept this, then sugars and refined flour would be off the table and the fluoridation approach would be the laughingstock of the world, as it should be.

If you think the research is old and thus irrelevant, think again. This early research is fully supported by the Australian Dental Association in 2007.

> The outward flow of the dentinal fluid is important in the pulp's defence against the entry of harmful substances because it affects the rate at which toxic substances from the mouth diffuse into the dentinal tubules.[59]

> … the tissue fluid volume in the pulp remains constant. The relatively high pulp tissue pressure results in *an outward flow of fluid in the dentinal tubules,* which helps to dilute toxins and wash out bacteria.[60]

Although not quite as sophisticated as Steinman's research, the point is that the current research is saying the same thing. Definitely clean your teeth. But also consider getting rid of sugars and flours from your diet. If the decay process is underway with a systemic condition, then it only makes sense to keep our bodies as healthy as we can. We could therefore question the sanity of putting fluoride into the drinking water, when it is clear that dental decay is a systemic condition rather than a topical one. There are many studies which have shown that the rate of dental decay is closely related to diet, education, and financial well-being. Reduction in decay rates has *nothing* to do with fluoride. In fact, fluoride, being the toxic poison that it is, causes an increase in decay rates and a host of other systemic disasters. Generally, this information is not given to dental students. Although published by the dental association, it is buried deep, and the significance is thus drained out and sanitized.

An anecdotal comment: I worked in both fluoridated and non-fluoridated areas of Australia. The most decay that I saw in children's teeth was in areas that were fluoridated. The next best were the non-fluoridated areas where the children were drinking city water. The best teeth with the least decay and the healthiest children were those that were drinking mainly rainwater from tanks.

Anatomy of a Tooth

To understand why root therapy may not be such a good idea, it's important understand the anatomy of a tooth and how it relates to the rest of the body. They're *not* just big chunks of inert calcified material, as dentistry would have us believe in their single-dimensional ways of thinking. Teeth are a complex and integral living part of the body.

The Enamel

Enamel is the part of the tooth that we all know as the "crown", with which we eat, bite, and smile. This is the part that many people these days want to make brighter and whiter. It is the toughest part of the tooth and, in fact, the hardest and densest tissue in the whole body. It is the part that is usually visible in the mouth.

Under the enamel in the crown of the tooth, and making up the bulk of the root, is another calcified material called dentine.

Down the centre of the root is a narrow, long space known as the root canal. In the crown part of the tooth, the canal is called the pulp chamber, which is merely a bad description of the pulp in the top of the tooth. The canal opens at the end of the root, called the apex, deep inside the jawbone. Passing through this opening are the nerve fibres and blood vessels, which bring sensation and nutrients to the tooth and take away the toxins. These contents of the canal are collectively called the "dental pulp"—or, in lay terms, the "nerve" of the tooth.

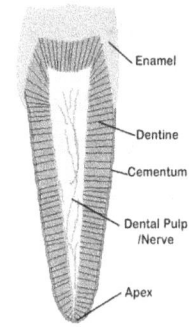

Around the outside of the root is another, slightly softer, calcified tissue called cementum. It's very thin, and its main function is to attach the tooth to the periodontal ligament—the membrane that surrounds the root. This ligament attaches the tooth to the bone and forms a fibrous seal to prevent infection tracking down the outside of the root. It, too, is rich in nerve fibres and blood vessels.

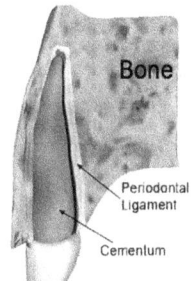

This ligament is the tissue which is most affected by infection and inflammation in the mouth and is also the *critical tissue* that is missing around implants. It is also the tissue that should be carefully removed with every extraction so that proper bone healing can occur.

The tooth is surrounded by bone—which also has a rich blood and nerve supply and vast lymphatic drainage.

~~~~~~~~~~~~~~~~~~~~~

Around the bone, which surrounds the tooth, is the rest of you!

~~~~~~~~~~~~~~~~~~~~~

The Australian Dental Association (2007) have stated, "If you have infection in the pulp you will have infection spreading from the tooth to the bone and then to the rest of your body."[61]

In other words, the bacteria which infect the pulp of a tooth can and will spread from the tooth to the surrounding tissue and the rest of the body—*all* of the rest of the body—from the brain to the toenails.

In the 1920s, Dr Weston Price demonstrated that once the decay had penetrated the enamel, oral bacteria could be found in both the dental pulp and the rest of the bloodstream. Although denied by all the dental PTOs, the above quote is a perfect description of focal infection. Much more about this sore point is later in the book.

Dentine

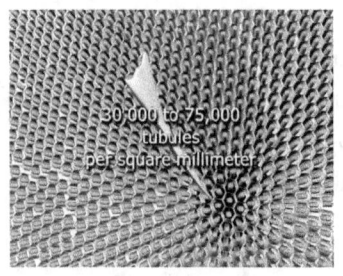

The dentine deserves closer inspection. It makes up the bulk of a tooth. It is *not* a calcified mass. It's made of millions of tubes which run from the surface of the root canal to the enamel and the outer surface of the root. There are 30,000 to 75,000 tubules per square millimetre of dentine.[62,63]

The root canal, running down the centre of the tooth, is lined with a membrane that is only one cell thick. These cells cover the pulp and send an extension of themselves up the middle of the dentine tubules. The extensions are surrounded by tissue fluid and communicate with the sensory nerves in the pulp. When dentine is stimulated with cold air or water, it is these cellular extensions that tell the body that you are feeling pain.

Thus, the bulk mass of any tooth is really a whole bunch of tubes packed tightly together; it's far from solid.

Minute as these tubules are, if you were to place the tubules of a single-rooted tooth (like your front tooth) end to end, you would have about three miles of tubing.[64] (That's about 4.6 kilometres.) One root = 3 miles of tubing. Molars may have up to three roots each.

All the dentine tubules in the root communicate directly with the surrounding tissue—from the cementum to the periodontal ligament and then the bone. In other words, they communicate directly with the whole body, as do the accessory canals.

Each of these tubules is wide enough to contain eight bacteria in cross section. Billions of bacteria can and do live happily in such an environment when a tooth becomes infected. These bacteria will penetrate to the full depth of the dentinal tubules—right out to the edge of the tooth![65,66]

Accessory Canals

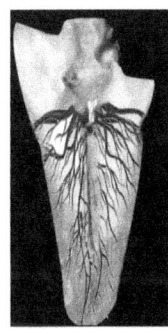

The Accessory Canals are branches of the main canal and will come off it at all sorts of angles and continue through to the cementum on the outside of the tooth. They are branches off the main canal and contain extensions of the dental pulp. The root canal system is *not* a simple tube, as presented in endodontic textbooks. In reality it is more like the taproot of a tree, with branches that reach out to the surface of the root in all three dimensions, all around and down the length of the root, communicating freely with the rest of the body. Towards the apex of the root, the canal often splits into many branches in a way that is like a river which forms many estuaries as it approaches the ocean.

When looking at pictures of teeth and root canal systems, we must remember that we are looking at a two-dimensional representation of a three dimensional object. The same, of course, applies to X-rays. Diagrammatic explanations of RCPs never show these accessory canals, as they present a bit of a problem for the poor specialists and professors. They cannot be eliminated, cleaned, sterilized, or filled. They are so tiny that you couldn't get an instrument down there even if you could see where they were with a microscope. The tissue which remains in them will die and become gangrenous. They are another great seat of infection. Billions of bacteria can fit in any one of these accessory canals and be fed forever by the gangrenous breakdown products of the dead tissue. None of the root canal medicaments will penetrate these accessory canals.

What Is an Abscess?

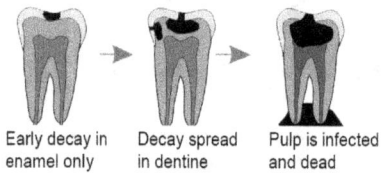

Early decay in enamel only   Decay spread in dentine   Pulp is infected and dead

When the decay in the tooth has penetrated both the enamel and dentine and caused the pulp of the tooth to die, the breakdown products and the infection will leach out of the tooth all the way down the root, but mainly through the opening at the end of the root—the apex. These breakdown products will affect the bone and cause it to break down at the end of the root, thus creating a hole in the bone. The process is called "liquifaction necrosis" of the bone.

If the immune system is strong, it will develop a fibrous capsule to try to quarantine these breakdown products from the rest of the body, and then this hole is very visible on an X-ray. It looks like a dark area surrounded by a white line within the rest of the bone (a condition also called "X-ray Positive".) As you will see later, the abscess may or may not show on an X-ray. It is an area of infected dead bone which has dissolved.

If there is a build-up of pressure in this area, you will experience pain. As you bite down on the tooth or the dentist taps it, this will increase the pressure and thus the pain. Occasionally the abscess will erode the bone around the outside of the tooth with drainage into the gum and thus a swelling in the gum. (This used to be called a "gum boil".) If this happens, you may have pus oozing from the swelling, but usually less

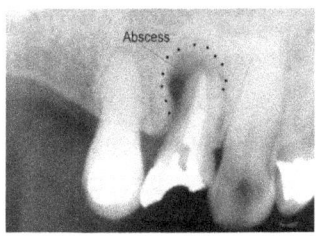

pain, as there is now somewhere for the pressure to be relieved. The term "Apical Periodontitis" is the modern term for what most people and dentists would call an abscess. It is completely inaccurate. There is no inflammation in the periodontal ligament which has been destroyed in this apical part of the tooth by the infective organisms from the root canal. These big words are only used to confuse the patient and to make the dentist seem knowledgeable.

The severe toothache that you may experience from an abscess on the tooth can be relieved by doing what most dentists would consider the beginnings of a root canal procedure. All that is needed is to drill a hole in the top of the tooth, down to the top of the root canal, thus relieving the pressure in the tooth and the bone. Usually you will not even need an anaesthetic for this, as the tooth is already dead.

Often the dentist will then want to put in a medicament and a temporary filling to fill up the hole in the top of the tooth. This is to try to sterilise the tooth and prevent it from getting infected. This is weird thinking, in my opinion. The tooth is already infected and leaving it open will not create a worse infection. Leaving the tooth open is what is needed to relieve the pressure, and thus the pain, till you can have it removed properly. This is against all of the current teaching but is the only way to drain the tooth to relieve the pain. At worst you will have some of the infected pus going into your mouth and gut. This is far better than having it go into your bloodstream and the rest of your body. I can see the endodontists rolling their eyes in disbelief. The teaching is that if the tooth is too infected, it is that much harder to sterilize. This is a perfect example of "mad hatter thinking", as it is impossible to sterilize a tooth anyway, as you will find out. There isn't much logic used in dental thinking, especially by specialists.

Why Would You Need a Root Canal?

There are many reasons you might hear your dentist say that your tooth will need a root canal procedure (which, again, is not a therapy or treatment), which of course assumes that you would believe and agree with this strange being in a white coat. The most common reasons are as follows:

- accidental damage—sport and car injuries
- damage to the tooth caused by amalgam and other filling techniques
- pain—no matter what the cause, even if it is caused by the previous dental treatment
- believe it or not, even to get that perfect smile
- a decayed or dead tooth with or without an abscess (the most common reason)

A Note on Pain

In the bad old days, the only filling material that we had for rear teeth was mercury amalgam. All dentists loved it because it stayed relatively soft for about an hour after it was implanted into the tooth. Patients were told not to eat for that first hour, so as not to break it, for this reason. An advantage of this soft state was that when patients paid their bills for being poisoned in this way, most would unconsciously grind or clench their teeth in shock at the cost. This had the effect of grinding in the bite so that any high spots were ground down.

The more modern white composite fillings are completely set within about twenty seconds, and the only way to fix the bite is for the dentist to grind the filling so that it fits the opposing teeth when they close together. Many dentists leave the bite slightly high—just enough to pound the tooth every time the mouth closes. It may be only $\frac{1}{10}$ of a millimetre too high. This will cause pain on chewing, pain on exposure to heat and cold, and pain in the tooth the rest of the time. If the bite is left high enough, it will cause you to change the way you bite, so that the tooth is not being bashed as much. This has a knock-on effect of changing the alignment of the vertebrae in your neck, and you may end up with headaches, pains and tingling down your arms, and lower back pain. When dentists are confronted with this, they will often assume that the tooth has died and recommend a root canal procedure instead of rechecking the bite. This was a common problem for patients who came to see me with such a diagnosis. All that was needed was to grind the filling, very gently, so that it no longer was being hit by the opposing tooth. When this is done, there is an instant relief for the patient. Within twenty-four hours, the tooth usually stops hurting. If the new filling is the first thing you feel when you close your teeth together, then you can guarantee that the bite needs adjusting.

Brutality is a part of dentistry for some of its practitioners. Instead of picking up a high-speed drill and wiping the filling away very gently, so as not to cause more pain, many will use a slow-speed drill that feels like a jackhammer going off in your brain. These dentists are to be avoided at all costs. They have gone past the point of insanity and aren't coming back.

There is another form of mad hatter that you should be aware of. Occasionally you may come across a dentist who is very well respected, usually in a very wealthy part of town, and who insists that every tooth to be treated will eventually need a root canal so it is better to have it done first. You can identify them by the Botox smiles plastered across their faces and the expensive bits of gold that drip from them. The endodontist buddy gets rich, and the smooth-talking dentist also gets rich on the crowns that need to be made. I've had the misfortune to meet a few of these criminals, who are always well-spoken and well connected. I can only advise everyone to keep well away from them. They usually have friends who sit on the dental boards. Their diagnostic criteria are only how much money they can extract from you.

The Root Canal Procedure Explained

The procedure called "root canal therapy" attempts to remove all dead infected tissue from the inside of a diseased tooth and then attempts to clean, sterilize and fill the canal which runs down the centre of the tooth. The dental profession calls this "saving" a tooth because the tooth will remain in your mouth, and you can still eat and smile with it. (A more visual explanation of this is a part of the film *ROOTED*, which I made in 2006.www.youtube.com/watch?v=I4QVgnN2jD0).

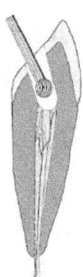

To gain access to the root canal, a large hole is drilled into the tooth from the top of the crown. On a molar or premolar this is done through the biting surface of the tooth, and on a front tooth access is usually gained from the back (palatal or lingual) surface of the tooth. This hole goes all the way into the top area of the pulp, called the "pulp chamber". This chamber in the crown section of the tooth is usually drilled out with large, round slow-speed burs until the top of the root canals can be seen.

The canals are then scraped out, using special files of increasing diameter to remove dead tissue and infected dentine from the inside of the canal. During this process, some of the debris and infected tissue and bacteria will be forced through the end of the root and into the surrounding bone. This happens even if the endodontist is a god-professor or has his or her offices in Macquarie Street in Sydney or Harley Street in London. It is simply a fact of life that this infected debris will be forced through the end of the root. Thus, every time the dentist scrapes the inside of the root, you will get bacteria floating around your body (called a "bacteraemia"), which may not be too good if you have a heart condition or an artificial hip, as it is well reported that such a bacteremia may localise in these tissues.[67,68] This is a well-accepted fact, and yet there is still a denial of focal infection! Further scraping is done to widen and shape the canal for the final filling.

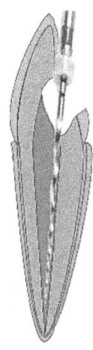

The length of the canal is judged by taking an X-ray of the tooth with a metal file down the inside of the canal. The difference in length between the X-ray view and the actual distance that the file has been pushed into the tooth is then calculated to *estimate* the correct root length and allow the dentist to try to get within one millimetre from the end of the root (on the inside of the root). We are taught that this is the ideal place for the root filling to finish, although no logical reason has ever been given for this. Instead of being a delicate skill gathered over years of practice, it is at best a good guess, as dentistry has still not found a way to measure the length of a root canal with precision. Most of the time, the good guess falls far short of the true root length. I have extracted teeth that have root fillings extending ten to fifteen millimetres from the end of the root. Many were done by endodontists. This "guessed length" forms the basis of the rest of the scraping and creates the "working length" of the canal. It is believed that using the files that do this scraping will remove all of the dead infected tissue. Thus, great efforts are made to work the whole length of the canal completely.

The official endodontic position is that the main goals of this procedure "… are to eliminate microorganisms from the root canal system, to remove pulp tissue that may support microbial growth, and to avoid forcing debris beyond the apical foramen which may sustain inflammation."[69,70]

This mechanical cleaning effort is enhanced by squirting, with a syringe, some reasonably potent medicaments into the tooth. They supposedly wash the main canal of all the debris and start the sterilization process. This is done initially by squirting hydrogen peroxide and sodium hypochlorite into the tooth. (Sodium hypochlorite is exactly the same bleach used for cleaning dirty nappies). Research from 2003 showed that over 94 per cent of endodontists used these materials to wash the canal. The rest used ordinary household bleach, which is about a dollar cheaper per litre![71] When these two liquids are mixed together, a fairly violent chemical reaction occurs which releases oxygen and hydrogen as bubbles, which supposedly will force debris from the canal and out through the hole that was drilled in the tooth.

Sometimes these bubbles and debris go the wrong way and are forced into the bone instead. This will cause the death of a great deal of the surrounding bone, and you may lose much more than just the tooth that has been worked on. This practice of mixing hydrogen peroxide and sodium hypochlorite in the tooth is over one hundred years old. It is conceptualized from a mechanical rather than a biological point of view. It is still done today even though it has never worked as a means of cleaning or sterilizing a tooth, but so long as we are seen to be doing the right thing, we may also be seen to be really good practitioners.

Next, a concoction of antimicrobial medications is placed in the tooth and the tooth is sealed with a temporary filling in the hope that it will become sterile by the time you return for your next appointment. These medicaments are usually changed every week till the tooth is deemed ready to be filled. The most common medicaments used for this are camphor, phenol, menthol, and formaldehyde. These materials are known carcinogens and have been used for over one hundred years. Antibiotics, calcium hydroxide, chlorhexidine, and cortisone are more recently included. They also don't work. This process is repeated until the tooth stops hurting or the dentist runs out of patience.

The recent advent of ozone therapy in dentistry has been praised as the magic bullet of sterilization. Ozone kills bacteria very efficiently. Sadly, it does not kill the bacteria that it cannot reach. It also does nothing about the gangrenous breakdown product of the dead tissue. Sadly also, for the promoters of this approach, the ozone only goes about 0.3 mm into the dentine tubules, which leaves between 2–3 mm untouched. I once had the opportunity to ask the professor who helped to create one of these dental ozone machines how far the ozone penetrated the dentine tubules. He was none too polite when I asked about the other 2–3 mm of untouched dentine. This god-professor, who was an endodontist himself, was interested only in selling his machine. He did not give a damn about the lack of sterility of the tooth, the patient who had to suffer his lies, or the dentists who would spend thousands of dollars on useless equipment. Dentists came from all over the country to hear his lies. The respect that he showed me was to turn his back and walk away. More recently, the use of lasers has become another state-of-the-art means of sterilizing teeth. Do they sterilise teeth? No, but more of that in the next chapter.

When the tooth is considered sterile, it is ready to fill. Believe it or not, the measure of sterility is that the tooth stops hurting and stops smelling. No aerobic or anaerobic samples are ever taken, and thus no laboratory standards are used to test this sterility.

Not one of the god-endodontists has a way of measuring the sterility of the tooth. In fact, there is no measure of sterility at all. It is impossible to sterilize the canal, so there is not really any standard by which we can judge whether the tooth is ready to be filled. Because they had to admit failure regarding their ability to sterilize teeth, they created a new term. They now claim to be able to take the teeth to a state of "physiologic balance". There is no such thing as physiologic balance!

When the tooth is ready to be filled is a guess based on a lack of pain and 'no stinky smell'. The decision to fill the canal and finish the treatment is based only on the dentist's appraisal of how much he or she can get away with. Spending too much time on such a tooth erodes the profit margin. It is neither a scientific nor a logical decision. It is, as the gods require, a "clinical" decision guided by past clinical observation. I know this because, in my stupid days, I used to do precisely this. The supposed general knowledge of endodontists is what separates these specialists from GP dentists. But this special knowledge does not make them any better at any of the procedures in their treatments. No matter how fantastic the endodontist is, your tooth will remain infected!

The filling process uses slow-setting cements which are spun down the canals using a twisty spiral wire (like an Archimedean spiral) and then Gutta Percha (GP) points (which are long, thin, rubber-based, nail-shaped points) that are inserted into the canal and the root-filling cement. They're packed in tightly to try to completely seal the canal. The GP points act as bricks, and the cements are like the mortar around these bricks. This is supposed to stop bacteria from getting into the tooth and reinfecting it. A temporary filling is then placed in the crown of the tooth until the final restoration can be completed.

All that remains is for you to be separated from your hard-earned dollars (or other currency or preferred method of payment).

All materials used in the root canal procedure are toxic. Some will affect the nervous system. Some will affect a developing foetus. Some will cause cancer. There is not one which is biocompatible. All these materials will escape from the tooth and spread around the whole of your body. They can cause all sorts of diseases in any part of your body. Appendix 1 has a list of the most commonly used materials.

Many textbooks have been written about root canals. Thousands of papers have been published. Dental students are forced to waste years learning (badly) how to "save" teeth. The industries that support this procedure are worth billions. The microscopes that can look all the way down a canal make no difference to the fact that the teeth cannot be sterilized or sealed. These huge microscopes are seriously impressive to the patients, because most people are conditioned and brainwashed to think that dentistry is only a mechanical project (just like the dentists who perform these miracles). Thus, if the dentist has the latest and greatest equipment, it surely shows that this dentist keeps up with the latest techniques and, by a silent understanding, the latest knowledge! They are worthless in terms of making the procedure work, yet they cost thousands of dollars. Dentists are willing to spend this sort of money on a machine that is ultimately useless but attracts a willing clientele. Mad hatters are all over the dental world. The whole procedure is a disaster based on mechanics and lies that everyone wants to believe! Perhaps if we all believe hard enough, it will come true?

Two of my best friends are dentists; one works from his refurbished garage using old second-hand equipment. It is his knowledge, skill, and expertise that not only maintain our friendship but also serve as the reason he is one of my preferred dentists. He has patients flying in from all over the country. He makes people well. The other has more modern gear, but everything else is equal. She is a great dentist with more courage than most men could ever muster up. It's not about the equipment. It is about the knowledge and compassion of the dentists, as well as their skills.

4

A Mythical Procedure

● ●

The great enemy of truth is very often not the
lie—deliberate, contrived and dishonest,
but the myth, persistent, persuasive, and unrealistic.
Belief in myths allows the comfort of opinion
without the discomfort of thought.

—John F. Kennedy

~~~~~~~~~~~~~~~

The greatest myth about root canal therapy or treatment is the name.
It is neither a treatment nor is it therapeutic.

There are a few others:

- The root canal procedure is evidence-based and supported by science.
- The root canal procedure saves the tooth.
- The root canal procedure is safe and effective.
- Dead teeth cannot affect your health.

According to the Australian Dental Association in 2007,

The goal of endodontic treatment is to preserve the tooth as a functional unit within a functioning dentition.

… In order to give good advice the dentist will need to exercise clinical judgment that is based on **rational treatment principles**. It is the skill and care with which these judgments are made that distinguish the ***really good dentist from the merely good dentist***.[72 from 73]

~~~~~~~~~~~~~~~~~

I wonder whether there are any really good dental associations or whether they are all just merely good. Perhaps even that is being generous.

Don't we all want to be *Really Good?* Considering that all we need is our own clinical judgement of what "really good" means, then of course each one of us is *Really Good?* The stage was set back in the 1920s. The "rational treatment principles" suggested here must surely be based on published scientific evidence; otherwise, they would not be rational. The possibility of achieving every stage of the procedure must be validated by clear scientific parameters and published research (e.g., Is the tooth sterile or is it not sterile? It's that simple.)

These "Rational treatment principles" have no scientific validation! They are merely a recipe for insanity. Every dentist that I have ever spoken to who does root canals, including myself (for thirteen years), believes that these treatment principles not only exist but also are achievable. Insisting on the principle of clinical observation means that we restrict our vision to the procedures we have done. We are taught to look only at the tooth and the bone around it. Then we are taught to misdiagnose what we are looking at. We are actively instructed to not look at the big picture of the whole person. The world of endodontics is completely myopic. As Victor Frankl said in *Man's Search for Meaning*, "An abnormal reaction to an abnormal situation is normal behavior."

Root canals are the interface of "clinical judgement" and science. It is the interface between the "general knowledge" of the endodontists and the specialized knowledge of great healers in the world of cancer treatments. This is the interface of mad hatters and madness. It's also the interface between health and disease.

This is *not* the interface between a really good dentist and a merely good dentist, as there is not one endodontist or professor who is able to achieve the goals of a "really good root canal procedure."

Like fake news, there is also fake science. A great example is the "Root Canal Safety Fact Sheet" from the American Association of Endodontists.[74] This article is compiled with twenty-two references. Only three of them were published after 2000. The rest go back to 1951, and this particular [75] one is inaccurate. Three refer to the *Textbook of Endodontics*, which is very far from a scientific or truthful document, as shown earlier. Four of the references actually contradict what is said in this fact sheet. All twenty-two references are put forward as a list. They are not referring to any statement in their fact sheet. In other words, this document is not referenced, even though they would like you to think it is. This is nothing but propaganda. Show us all the well-controlled studies that disprove Dr Price's work. They do *not* exist.

It is now a trend at most universities to allow students to use only references that are less than ten years old, as it is presumed that everything that comes before will automatically be taken into consideration. This presumes a thing called honesty, which is sadly lacking in the world of dentistry. I once had an official complaint sent to the Dental Board of NSW about the information on my website. I was informed that it brought down the whole of the fine standing of dentistry, worldwide. The complaint was from a specialist dentist in the UK who promoted both amalgam fillings and root canals without any references. I invited the dental board to read through and critique all that was on my website. I even offered to discuss with them any facts they might find untrue. As it turned out, the only criticism on everything I had written was that many of the references were over ten years old. If you are going to level that complaint against me, you had better level it against the American Association of Endodontists (AAE) as well.

The Australian Society of Endodontology relies on the "general knowledge" of their members for the information that they print in their misinformation brochure. You will see that they are not in any way concerned about verifying their deceitful statements with references. The "general knowledge" of a group of dental specialists is not good enough to support a so-called treatment that is a major cause of cancer and so many other diseases; nor is it good enough to support one that is supposedly based on "rational treatment principles." The general knowledge of endodontists comes from the *mercury-poisoned deans and professors*. It is the blind leading the blind. The general knowledge of specialists is worthless if not supported by published scientific research. As Joseph Campbell stated,

"Myths are public dreams, dreams are private myths."

Clearly Defined Steps: Rational Treatment Principles

The steps involved in root canal procedures are clearly defined. They have not changed in well over one hundred years.

It is essential to

- clean and shape the canal to within one millimetre from the end of the root on the inner side of the end of the root;
- remove *all* dead gangrenous tissue from the whole of the tooth;
- sterilize the tooth—no bacteria, fungi, or yeasts can be allowed to survive, so as not to act as a focus of infection;
- fill and seal the canal completely to within one millimetre of the end of the root (on the inside of the root), completely sealing the tooth so that bugs cannot get in or out of the tooth;

- use only biocompatible materials; and
- restore the crown of the tooth in such a way that prevents bacteria from the mouth getting into the top of the tooth.

The belief that any of the objectives can be achieved is one of the greatest fantasies in dentistry and medicine. There is *no* science to support this belief. I mean it. There is no published scientific research that demonstrates that any of these goals are achievable, yet millions of root canal procedures (RCPs) are done every year around the world in the hope of maintaining the tooth "functionally". There are an endless number of papers published that say that the goals are not achievable. Quite simply,

- it is not possible to remove all dead tissue from the tooth;
- it is not possible to sterilize the tooth.
- all materials used, including the root filling materials, are toxic; and
- it is not possible to seal the canal.

The Australian Dental Association have even published that the goals are unachievable:

> All root canals in the affected tooth must be treated. (1996)

> ... all instrumentation techniques left **35 per cent or more** of the canals dentine surface untouched, with very little difference found between the four instrument types. These findings highlight **the limited ability of endodontic instruments to clean the root canal** ... (2007, my emphasis)

> ... predictable eradication of bacteria from the root canal still remains an **elusive goal** ... (2007, my emphasis)

> **... since no current restorative dental material is able to provide a total** and permanent seal, it is

always possible that micro leakage will occur and bacteria may enter the tooth. (2007 my emphasis)

Dentistry consistently talks about the need to seal the tooth so that bacteria cannot enter it. They never talk about bacteria escaping from the tooth and entering the body! The real outcome of this procedure is a "'Toxin Factory" which leaches poisons into your body all the time. The inability to achieve the goals of RCP were demonstrated by Dr Weston Price in the 1920s. This is not new information.

Just recently (near the end of 2018) a great documentary called *Root Cause* was released. It is well made and talks about the taboo subjects of cancer and heart attacks in relation to dead teeth. Interviews include one of America's leading cardiologists, Dr Thomas Levy, who made it clear that infection from root canals cause heart disease. I agreed with everything presented, and my only regret is that the documentary was not referenced. The dental associations completely freaked out, and here are some of their reactions as reported in the *Guardian* on 4 Feb 2019:

> Dentists, endodontists and dental researchers are warning Netflix, Apple, Amazon and Vimeo to remove a documentary that spreads fear and misinformation about the safety of root canals and extracting wisdom teeth.

> … the American Dental Association (ADA), American Association of Endodontists (AAE) and American Association of Dental Research (AADR) warned the media companies in a private letter sent late last month that continuing to host the film could harm the viewing public by spreading long-disproven claims.

> The premise the film is based on dates back to research conducted in the 1920s which was later disproved *because the original conditions for the experiments were poorly controlled and performed in non-sterile*

environments. Perhaps most importantly, other researchers have not been able to duplicate the results from the original experiment. Why portray information demonstrated to be incorrect as fact?

This line of propaganda has been sold repeatedly, and no evidence is ever proffered to support their claims. The claim that dentists are concerned for the poor people who will die from having a tooth out is beyond ludicrous. Dentists are taking teeth out every day, and people generally continue to live healthy, productive lives. No one has died from losing a tooth. (Many have died from keeping them.)

It is common practice for the PTOs to threaten and manipulate the media. Political and media censorship is also not new. It didn't take long for Netflix to bow to the pressure of the American Dental Association and take *Root Cause* off. It is no longer available. I am hoping that enough people have downloaded it to be able to keep sharing this vital information. One can only guess at the machinations behind this decision, which clearly was not based on published science.

Dr. Price was the leading dental researcher at the turn of the twentieth century. He demonstrated thousands of times the creation of diseases from non-vital teeth. He demonstrated how every belief about the root canal procedure held by the dental community at the time was based on a complete lack of scientific understanding. They were myths based on the writings of just a few influential dentists. The current dental communities have now set these beliefs as concrete truths, and still there is *no* published research to support them. When Dr Price finally published his research in 1923 and tried bringing the new information to the dental world, he was ostracized.

The techniques, most of the materials, and some of the instruments that were used in the early 1900s are identical to those used today. The aims have not changed in this time, and the diagnostic teaching has sadly also not changed. The medicaments used to "sterilize" teeth then are still being used today: camphor, phenol, formaldehyde, and menthol.

There is not one bit of Dr Price's research that has been shown to be wrong. Every one of his findings has been validated many times over in the last one hundred years. Even some of the recent deans and professors have come to the same conclusions as he did. Their papers are published. It is current. There is no disagreement.

The work of people like Dr. Patrick Störtebeker, Associate Professor of Neural Surgery at Karolinska University in Sweden [76,77,78,79] and the work of Dr. Eugene Ratner [80,81] in the United States verify many of Price's findings. Cancer specialists like Dr Joseph Issels and Professor Daunderer in Germany support the findings of Dr Price. The work of Lida Mattman verifies the findings of pleomorphic change, which Dr Price was able to demonstrate in the early 1900s. [82,83,84] Of course, the work of Rosenow in particular supports Price's findings.

If all that you need to know is that none of the goals of this procedure are achievable, then I am telling you this right here. I have now just saved you the task of reading through the next chapter. These are big statements, so the next chapter contains the references to support them. One of the greatest myths about root canal procedures is that the procedure is based in well-proven science.

5

Science or Clinical Observation

The fact that millions of people
share the same vices does not make these vices virtues,
the fact that they share so many errors
does not make the errors to be truths,
and the fact that millions of people share the same form
of mental pathology does not make these people sane.

—Erich Fromm, in *The Sane Society 1955*

Belief

We dentists undergo years of "training" so that we "know" that what we are taught is correct and true. Our beliefs are based in all the stuff that we sweated over to pass the exams. There is no room to judge or question this holy information. Most would not even consider this as an option. We treat our beliefs as though they have a scientific foundation, and we are taught to scoff at any arguments against these beliefs. We repeat the mantra daily to ourselves and our patients.

The previous chapter contains many sweeping statements. Unlike the dental associations and other PTOs who regularly give sweeping statements without support, this chapter aims to give the scientific support for those sweeping and unbelievable statements. For some dentists this may produce a cognitive dissonance. If so, there are plenty of references to check what I am writing, and I encourage everyone to do just that. I apologize for the use of jargon in this chapter, but I will be using many quotes which include foreign words. I will try to explain them as we go along or in the glossary at the end of the book. The repetition you will find in this chapter is to reinforce the concepts. As Nietzsche once said,

"There are two different types of people in the world, those who want to know, and those who want to believe."

X-Rays

X-rays are used in endodontics to demonstrate everything from infection to success of the treatment. They are used to measure the length of the root canal and to prove to the patient and other colleagues how good the dentist is in his or her clinically observed outcomes. They are also a part of the dentist's legal records. If you will forgive the pun, the little that dentists learn about X-rays is very black and white. Many radiologists don't have a clue what they are looking at on a dental X-ray. Usually they can see that teeth are present or not. I had the pleasure of meeting one radiologist in Sydney who not only could see what I was talking about but also understood the significance of it. To him the subtleties were clear. Dentists are not taught to look at the subtle changes let alone interpret them correctly.

X-Rays Problem 1: Interpretation

Success of the root canal procedure is determined only by lack of pain and the way the tooth and bone appear on the X-ray. Dentistry teaches that if the bone at the end of the root looks normal and there is no visible big black area, then there is no infection in the tooth. This is considered a good outcome. The conclusion that there is no infection present is, of course, ridiculous, as X-rays do not show bacteria or any other bugs. (This is covered more completely below.) The conclusion drawn is based merely on how the bone looks on the X-ray.

We are taught that when the big, dark abscess disappears from the X-ray a few months after the RCP, this is a great outcome and the healing is good. We are taught that this means there is no more infection in the tooth. On the X-ray, the bone around the tooth looks normal. The periodontal ligament also seems to be normal on the X-ray. The tooth stops hurting, and there is no pressure sensitivity. This interpretation has many flaws that are not discussed in the profession.

This "good outcome" is precisely what Drs Price, Rosenow, Issels, and many others see as a serious failure of the procedure. Dr Price found the following:

- If the X-ray shows a well-defined dark abscess (radiolucent area), then the person has a high resistance (good immune system) and is trying to quarantine the infection from the rest of the body (X-ray Positive).
- If the X-ray shows a dark abscess but the margins are *not* well defined, it is difficult to judge where the abscess starts and stops. This means the person's resistance is becoming weaker (perhaps because of a compromised immune system) and different disease patterns begin to emerge (X-ray Positive).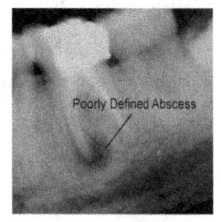
- If the X-ray shows, instead of bone loss, a condensation of the bone (condensing osteitis) around the end of the root, then this is a sign of poor to no resistance to the toxins coming from the tooth (a collapsed immune system) and is accompanied by far worse diseases, such as cancer and MS (X-ray Negative).

I have seen this in many of my patients, and seeing condensing osteitis became a loud alarm bell for a patient with serious health issues. These days, the idea of condensing osteitis is shunned, since dental implants are often associated with this weakened immune response. Instead, the dental world calls this reaction "osseointegration" to make it sound as if the implant and bone are now one integrated unit—a rose by any other name!

Dr Issels published similar information in 1999, from the perspective of a highly respected German Oncologist with one of the highest treatment success rates in Germany at the time.

> If the body's local resistance is intact, the inflammation is enclosed by a capsule of connective tissue known as the dental granuloma. This membranous cyst prevents its toxic contents from spreading into the organism. Radiographs of these teeth show granuloma cysts as more or less marked transparencies at the apex of the root. This type of tooth is called **X-ray positive.**

> If the body's local resistance is weakened to such an extent that the inflammatory process cannot be encapsulated by the granuloma cyst, the toxins will be able to advance unhindered into the marrow spaces, the tonsils, and into the body. In this case, it is proof that the organism has become largely incapable of reaction. Radiographs of these teeth as a rule show no transparencies and are therefore called **X-ray negative.**

> In my cancer patients, I have found that such non-encapsulated foci - that is those who show X-ray negative - were particularly common, as one would expect from people whose body resistance has been lowered.[85]

As stated in his research, Dr Price was able to associate many disease states with the X-ray view of the reaction of the bone around the end of a root and with the individual's perceived susceptibility.

All root-canalled teeth are infected. The bone around all of these teeth is infected. No matter how good it looks on the X-ray, it is still infected. There are even many holistic dentists who claim a successful root canal procedure if the bone looks like it is healing on the X-ray!

Why are dental students deprived of this knowledge? If dental X-rays were interpreted correctly, it would be possible to pick up medical conditions long before they became clinical disasters. It would also then be possible to relate the teeth as causative of these health changes. This gives the dentist a critical role in medical diagnosis. These vital clues on the X-ray may prevent diseases and even save lives. Yes, a dead tooth can be fatal, and it may take a long and painful time to kill!

It is a desperate shame and a crime that cardiologists, oncologists and most other medical "ologists" are unable to read or interpret dental X-rays. It is *critical* knowledge for everyone in the health care profession.

Bone Changes Dr Price	**Rarefying Osteitis** **– Decalcification** **(Dark** 'abscess' visible on X-ray)	**Condensing Osteitis around rarefying Osteitis** (Abscess area surrounded by dense bone)	**Condensing Osteitis**
Susceptibility Group	**Absent Susceptibility** (High resistance)	**Acquired Susceptibility** (Resistance is being challenged)	**Inherited Susceptibility** (Very low resistance)
Heart			*
Arthritis			*
Caries		*	*
Rheumatism		*	*
Kidneys		*	*
Stroke		*	*
Nervous Breakdown		*	*
Degenerative Arthritis		*	
Neuritis		*	
Skin Conditions.		*	

Rhinitis		*	
Asthma		*	
Periodontal	*	*	
Hay Fever	*	*	
Diabetes	*	*	
The bracketed comments are my explanatory additions.			

Dr Joseph Issels stated the following:

> My clinical experience has produced evidence of a causal connection between foci and tumour development ... From this it is clear that the advisable treatment for devitalised teeth is extraction.
>
> A survey conducted at my clinic found that, on admission, ninety-eight percent of the adult cancer patients had between two and ten dead teeth, each one a dangerous toxin producing "factory." Very often we are confronted with X-ray negative dead teeth, root remnants, and residual ostitis which had not been diagnosed and therefore had not been removed.
>
> If total treatment is to be performed, it is necessary to remove not only any devitalised teeth but also any hidden dental foci remaining in the jaw.
>
> The dentist should always remember that he has a vital role to prevent the development of chronic illness and, most important of all, to decisively reduce the hazard of cancer.[86]

X-Rays Problem 2: The Shadow and the Angle

X-rays are at best a two-dimensional representation of a three-dimensional body. Consequently, they may not give an accurate picture of what is happening in the bone or the tooth. The problem is that in the mouth we can take an X-ray from only one angle (i.e., from the outside to the inside). We cannot get a picture from back to front. This is now changing with three-dimensional cone beam X-rays, but the resolution is still far from acceptable for real diagnosis.

Whatever may be in the shadow of the root will not be seen. There may be nothing, or there may be a great big abscess.

An eminent and respected endodontist, Dr I. Bender, in 1997, made the following statements:

- X-rays "may not detect the presence of inflammatory lesions or neoplasms causing bone destruction."
- "Often radiographs give negative results even when cortical bone is involved"
- "Changes in angulation of the X-ray beam produced an increase, a decrease, or an elimination of radiolucent areas"[87]

If the bone loss is above the root, you may see a dark area on the X-ray.

If the bone loss is behind and in the shadow of the root, the X-ray will look normal. The bone loss which is present will be missed.

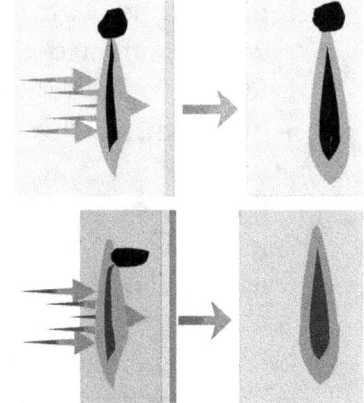

It is also common for a canal to split into multiple canals. These are nearly impossible to see and always impossible to treat. If a root has more than one canal, or if the canal divides halfway down the root, it is often missed as a result of the shadow effect on the X-ray.

X-Rays Problem 3: Root Length Measurements

X-rays of teeth in the mouth can be shot from only one angle, as mentioned above. Measurements of teeth are made from images in this view only.

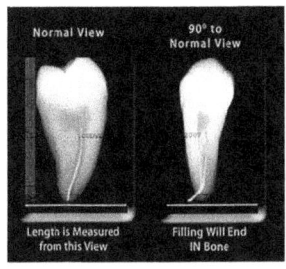

"When a canal is filled flush with the radiographic apex, it is in reality likely to be overfilled, since the apical foramen is seldom located at the radiographic apex."[88] This little bit of knowledge has been known since 1958, and yet to this day, the X-ray is relied on to measure the tooth! To this day also, the inaccuracy of this technique remains consistent.

Often the canal finishes short of the end of the root, but this would only be seen if the tooth were rotated 90 degrees. Thus, for the root filling to appear to be at the end of the root in the normal view, it will in end in the bone.

X-rays are an especially poor method for measuring the length of a root canal. Considering that the canal should be treated to within one millimetre of the end of the canal, and that the canal itself may sometimes finish two millimetres short of the end of the root, and that the angle of the X-ray may lengthen or shorten the appearance of the tooth, how is it possible to achieve the above objective?

One patient was seriously compromised with recuring sinusitis and an ever-increasing variety of allergies. The root filling looked, on the x-ray, as though a good job had been done. The bone at the end of the roots appeared normal. I usually separated the roots to do such an extraction, as doing so is far gentler and produces better healing. After the roots came out, I thought to X-ray it again so that we could get a different view at 90 degrees to the original one. This clearly showed huge voids in the root filling and areas that were not filled at all. It also clearly showed that the root filling in one of the roots went down only about two thirds the length of the root! Her health returned to normal within a month.

Relying on X-rays to show the success of the root canal treatments is like Lord Nelson at the Battle of Copenhagen in 1801, where he ignored orders to cease action by putting the telescope to his blind eye and claiming he couldn't see the signal.[89]

One experiment that Dr Price conducted was to see how good the dentists of his time were. (There was no such thing as an endodontic specialty at the time.) He took a series of extracted single-rooted teeth and mounted them with their roots embedded in a plaster block. These teeth were then sent to dentists to do root canal procedures on. Their being mounted in a block of plaster instead of the jaw meant that the dentists were able to take X-rays of these teeth from any angle. The teeth in blocks were then returned to Dr Price, who knocked off the plaster and examined the root fillings that had been performed. He found that 17 per cent were overfilled.

At least 17 per cent of all root canals are still overfilled, including those done by endodontic specialists. Price published his findings in 1923. More recent research has found that the current rate of overfilling for endodontists is also 17 per cent.[90,91]

Of these overfilled teeth, 100 per cent are accompanied by death of the surrounding bone—called "liquefaction necrosis" in dentistry. The bone dies and becomes liquefied. It appears on the X-ray like an abscess. This dead tissue and the decomposition toxins will spread to the rest of the body.

These days, even the endodontic textbooks display images of overfilled root canals and claim that these are great outcomes. Some of these great volumes are priced upward of US$250. For that sort of money, any dentist will accept what is written. Easily visible on the X-ray is the root-filling cement protuding through the end of the root canal and also through the accessory canals. Clearly the teaching of endodontics has no regard for published science!

I once asked an endodontist whether he was concerned that the root filling he had placed in an upper molar extended well over 1 cm into the maxillary sinus. His response was that it should not present a problem. He based this belief upon his "clinical observation" and, clearly, his "general" knowledge. He was offended when I pointed out that all overfilled canals are accompanied by death of the surrounding bone.

Although a specialist, he was not aware of the literature published in his own endodontic journals. The patient received a refund the next day. The argument that "these things happen" is just an excuse for sloppy work and an impossible dream.

X-Rays Problem 4: Infection

Dental schools teach that if an X-ray shows bone loss around the end of the root, then there *is* an infection in the tooth, and that if the bone looks normal, then there is *no* infection. The word "infection" means the invasion of a body tissue by disease-causing organisms, such as bacteria, viruses, and fungal and yeast forms. To comment on the sterility or not of a tissue by X-ray appearance is nonsense. As mentioned earlier, the abscess, or lack thereof, is the body's reaction to the invading microorganisms. By the time decay has penetrated the enamel, bacteria can be found in the pulp and, thus, the rest of the body.[92] The tooth is infected at this stage. This does not mean that the tooth will die, as there is still a very active blood supply and an immune response that usually can handle it for a little while.

If X-rays could show infection, we wouldn't need petri dishes and microscopes. X-rays do not show infection, and as demonstrated earlier, their misdiagnosis cannot interpret whether there is an infection present or not.

A study from 2017 looked at 349 extracted root-canalled teeth and their surrounding bone. All samples were reported on by a USA Board-Certified pathologist. All displayed infection and a chronic to acute reaction around the end of the root into the bone. They also revealed starlike microorganisms in colonies called actinomyces bacteria. Over 50 per cent of implants removed and studied in this way also showed an infection of actinomyces. (These are gram-positive anaerobes.) These organisms are found in nature and in the mouth and are responsible for the breakdown of dead tissue, whether it be in the compost bin or the root canal or around the implant. From 2017:

As the dead tooth degrades, it gives off various chemicals such as putresciene, cadaverine, thioethers, and what we call endotoxins ...

Actinomyces species reside on mucosal surfaces and gain access to deeper tissues via trauma, surgical procedures, or foreign bodies, which disrupt the mucosal barrier.[93]

Dr Price pointed this out in 1920:

Roentgenograms do not reveal infection and may or may not reveal its effects.

The extent of the absorption does not express the extent of the infection, except in part as the individual's reaction to the infection is understood.

An area of absorption of the supporting tissue at the apex of a tooth or laterally, may not be disclosed because of any of the following conditions;

1. being hidden by a part of that tooth, such as another root.
2. a heavy mass of bone such as the malar bone.
3. a layer of condensing osteitis obscuring the area of rarefying osteitis."

Research from 2001 supports Dr Price's position.

An asymptomatic tooth that appears normal on a periapical radiograph usually indicates that endodontic treatment has been successful.

It has been shown, however, that even if a periapical area seems to have been resolved on a radiograph, microorganisms may persist indefinitely.

Dentists are **unable to test the sterility of a tooth's apex**. Therefore, an asymptomatic endodontically treated tooth may be harbouring a chronic infection, which may be the cause of implant failure.[94]

The tooth cannot be sterilized no matter how hard you dream. Even when it looks great on that X-ray, it will be infected. There is no way around this except to deny it.

Dentistry teaches that when there is a condensation of bone about the end of the root, this is a great outcome for their treatments. The reality is that teeth showing a "Condensing Osteitis" are demonstrating that the body's immune system is incapable of quarantining the infection locally.[95] These are often the teeth which cause the greatest systemic effects, such as cancer and MS. "The author is confident that this body of experimental factual information is ample evidence corroborating Dr Voll's assertion electronically over 33 years ago, that 'endo-teeth' are energetic liabilities working against human health and should be removed."[96]

The tools that dentistry has, with which to make these clinical diagnostic assumptions, are limited to the way the X-ray looks and whether the tooth hurts when you tap it. Tools such as those used for electrodermal and infrared screening are not permitted in Australia. These tools are awesome and give information that the standard head-in-the-sand approach of dentistry doesn't come near. Dr Voll's pioneering and ground-breaking work in the area of electro-acupuncture has never been acknowledged by the drug company medical world of the West. More of Voll's work will be discussed in the chapter on Neural Therapy.

> X-rays do not and cannot demonstratethe
> presence or absence of infection

Dredging the Canals: Mechanical Cleansing

"All root canals in the affected tooth must be treated," according to the Australian Dental Association and most other dental associations.[97] It was true in 1900 and in 1996 and is still true now. In other words, all dead tissue must be removed from the tooth. This is a well-known and well-stated dictum of endodontics. If not completely removed, the dead tissue will be nourishment for any bugs that remain in the tooth and will also be a source of gangrenous breakdown products, which will spread to the rest of the body. This is extremely dangerous, as it could kill you. If a big toe is gangrenous, it is removed fairly quickly before the dangerous toxins can spread too far.

Most dentists would agree that this goal needs to be achieved. This is a two-stage approach involving mechanical filing of the canal and then using a variety of chemicals to try to kill the bugs.

To try to achieve this mechanical cleansing, dentistry has come up with the most amazing array of miniature files and reamers. Some are hand operated, and some are drill operated. Some are made from stainless steel, and some from nickel titanium. All varieties come in increasing diameter sizes so that the canals can be carefully scraped out and widened and shaped to a nice funnel shape. The presumption is that we can convert an irregularly shaped ovoid canal—which may have a variety of bends, connections, and divisions in it—into a perfect round cylinder. This should get rid of *all* dead tissue from the canal, as well as a large amount of infected dentine. It looks impressive as a two-dimensional diagram. I am talking here about the main root canals only—not the splits and branches, and not the dentine tubules.

Research, however, clearly showed that when teeth were cleaned and filed with every known technique, **"Large amounts of decomposing tissue were left in the canal."**[98] This is in the main canal. The accessory canals and dentine tubules are always left untouched, and as they constitute the largest part of the tooth, it is fair to say that very little of the pulp tissue is ever removed from the dead tooth. The rest breaks down into a gangrenous infected mess. No blood supply means that the cells of the immune system don't have a chance of getting rid of this dead tissue. There is still no way of removing all the dead tissue from the main canal, let alone the accessory canals.

The Australian Dental Association acknowledged this in 2007.[99] "… all instrumentation techniques left **35 per cent or more** of the canals dentine surface untouched, … These findings highlight **the limited ability of endodontic instruments to clean the root canal** …"

In other words, the ADA is now clearly stating that the aforementioned goal is impossible to achieve. No matter which technique was used, from 35 per cent to 50 per cent of the inside of the main canal was left untouched. A large amount of dead tissue always remains in the main canal itself. Many studies have been performed which demonstrate that it is impossible to remove all dead tissue from the main canal, let alone the accessory canals or the dentine tubules.[100,101,102] Yes, I am repeating this intentionally because the endodontic approach completely ignores the research, yet endodontists carry on regardless.

Another issue that should concern dentists and patients alike is that the actual process of scraping the inside of the canal and using the "cleaning" materials that are placed in these teeth substantially weakens the dentine.[103,104,105,106,107,108]

Hence the ease with which these teeth can break after completion of the RCP. Fractured roots after such a procedure are common.

The actual root canal is only a tiny part of the volume of the tooth. The dentine and its contents constitute the greatest bulk and thus the greatest amount of dead tissue in the tooth. It is physically impossible to remove any dead tissue from the dentine tubules and accessory canals. No matter what the dentist claims, most of the dead tissue is left in the tooth. There are *no* methods of fully cleaning even the main root canal.

The toxic breakdown products leach out of the tooth all the time. Some come out of the main canal, but a larger amount leaches from the dentine tubules and accessory canals directly into the periodontal ligament and the bone along the whole length of the root, and then throughout the body.[10]

Another major problem with all forms of mechanical preparation is that debris can be, and usually is, forced through the end of the root—this debris comprises bacteria and their toxins, as well as the gangrenous breakdown materials and the dead dentine shavings produced in this process. These bacteria can localize in other parts of the body and produce disease in other tissues.[10,109] "**... endodontic treatment can be the cause of anaerobic bacteremia and fungemia.**"[110] This is, of course, not too big a problem for anyone with a good immune system that can take care of this bacterial overload. If, on the other hand, you have a faulty mitral valve in your heart, an implant in your hip, or a stent in your aorta, this procedure could be life threatening. Bacterial infection in such situations is well reported, as you will see in the next chapter.

It is physically impossible to remove
all dead, gangrenous tissue from the tooth.
All root canal procedures cause a flood of
anaerobic bacteria and toxins throughout the body.
A root canal which does not cause a bacteremia does not exist.

Dr Issels puts it this way:

Even the most perfect preservation will only reach the most vertical intermediary trunk of the root canal system. In no way will it reach the lateral branches or the numerous dental canaliculi, which likewise takes its exit from the root canal. Even after the most precise preparation of the root canal, there will always remain protein in the adjoining areas. This protein is usually infected and denatured by filling materials, whereby toxic decomposition products will be formed ... the dental canaliculi exhibit an exuberant bacterial flora. The decomposition toxins produced by these microbes can, with a dental root filling, no longer empty into the oral cavity. They can only be derived via the cross connection and the unsealed branches of the root canal finally reaching the pulper spaces of the jaw and thereby the flowing systems of the organism. Because of the devitalising and preservation procedures, the tooth has become a toxin factory by which the organism (the person) will be continually damaged. [This is an English translation from the original German]

Some Mechanical Stuff-Ups

As mentioned earlier, there are a whole range of reamers and files that are used to try to scrape out and shape the inside of the canal. Some of these instruments are handheld and some sit on the end of the drill and rotate into the canal. Most canals have weird shapes and difficult bends, let alone the labyrinth of micro-branches towards the end of the root—a bit like the estuaries of a river as it meets the ocean.

Tunnel to Nowhere

A common problem when using rotary files is that sometimes they don't bend the way they should. They just keep going straight ahead. Sometimes the dentist will realize the mistake when an X-ray shows the file coming out the side of the tooth. Instead of following the bend of the canal, it just drills another tunnel in an almost straight line through the root. This is no drama for our fearless specialist, who will have it fixed up with a bit of Portland Cement. No, I am not joking. The area of the perforation is surgically exposed deep in the bone, and the hole is bogged up with Portland cement. Side effects are discussed later. It will probably add to the cost of the "treatment", as you will need to see an oral surgeon to get this bad job patched. Oh, how exciting to be the ping-pong ball between the god-specialists! The more gods that are involved, the greater their ability to disperse the blame for their failures and your wealth. Portland Cement is carcinogenic, according to its manufacturer.

Blame the Tools

Endodontic files are supposed to be disposable, but as they cost about 0.5% of the fee charged to you, they are usually sterilised and reused.

Heating them in an autoclave weakens the metal. Thus, it is relatively easy for one of these files to get stuck and then break inside the canal. This will happen if done by hand or with an engine-driven file. This is so common that the profession accepts it as a sort of side effect—just a bit of collateral damage. "Not what anyone wants, but it happens." It is so common, in fact, that you will find many YouTube videos about how to fix this issue. One of them that I watched claims that the rate of breakage is up to 10 per cent. Considering the years of training that the specialist undertakes, I believe that a 10 per cent failure rate blamed on the tools is pathetic.

These broken bits of the file are usually impossible to remove and thus 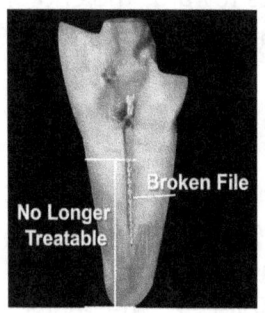 remain stuck in the canal. This very effectively prevents any further "treatment" beyond this broken instrument. You cannot ream and file it, you cannot get any medicaments beyond it, and neither can you fill the canal beyond it. You cannot work beyond the broken instrument. If nothing can happen beyond this broken bit of metal, then the tooth will be left with an empty canal, which in any textbook of endodontics is unacceptable. It is a major problem for any dentist, as it means that the job embarked upon now cannot be done. Perhaps the file was damaged by being overused. Perhaps the dentist was a bit too rough. Perhaps it would have just happened, as these things do! Regardless, the fact remains that the tooth is now stuffed, according to any of the principles espoused by the root canal specialists. It should be removed.

On the other hand, the endodontists take a different view. From their clinical observation point of view,

> "Broken, separated, or disarticulated instruments can occur during the day-to-day practice of endodontics … broken instruments are not the direct cause of endodontic therapy failure … Breaking files

is not malpractice; however, failing to inform a patient that a separation has occurred is. Here's how to best manage this situation: Calmly inform the patient that, during treatment, a sterile piece of the instrument separated from the file and …"[111]

Once in the tooth, the broken bit of file is no longer *sterile*. The bloody thing *broke*. It did not just separate or "disarticulate", whatever that is supposed to mean. *it is stuck in the tooth*, and it is *infected* by the bugs in the tooth!

It seems that the general knowledge of endodontists does not have a problem calling it part of the treatment! Most endodontists and dentists will carry on regardless and pretend to clean, sterilize, and fill down to the broken file. They will then claim that the procedure is completed and charge you for this service. They will charge you whether they have stuffed it up or not. Clearly the aims of the root canal procedure are impossible to achieve beyond the broken instrument.

Why bother at all with this procedure when the endodontic specialist is willing to leave canals "untreated" and pretend that this is okay? The next time you call a plumber to unclog some pipes, make sure that you pay for the service whether the pipes are unblocked or not. There are very few tradespeople who can get away with blaming their tools for a lousy job. Why should the highly paid specialists be allowed to get away with it?

I can only advise that you keep your money in your pocket and instead register a formal complaint against the person who stuffed it up, whether he or she is a specialist or not. Clearly by now you have the message that the tooth should have been pulled out in the first place, but at least keep them a bit more honest. It is like paying for your car service after the clutch has been removed. The only finding that an examination board can conclude is that the job was not done correctly. Thus, why should you pay for it? Dentists continue to charge a fortune for stuffing up your teeth. Even an endodontist will pretend that it is okay and send you the bill anyway. Do *not* pay. Instead sue for poor workmanship.

Breaking an instrument in a tooth is a lousy job. Just because it happens so often that it has become normal does not stop it being a lousy job. Just because one of the gods did it does not stop it being a lousy job. Make the endodontist pay the oral surgeon to take your tooth out. This is the best of both worlds, as far as I am concerned!

What about the Bugs?

One of the basic principles of a successful root canal procedure is that the tooth is to be made sterile. All bacteria that inhabit the tooth must be eradicated. Even Grossman's textbook states this as an essential goal—a sort of deforestation with agent orange! A veritable genocide of all bacteria is to occur before filling and preserving the tooth. The whole of the profession has been forced to take a big step sideways on this issue. They have been forced at last to admit that sterility of a tooth is an impossible dream. Some holistic dentists even go so far as to question whether sterility of the tooth is necessary at all. They claim that the jury is out on this issue, which allows them to pretend that they can do the job properly. Very few of these holistic dentists have read any of the science. They prefer to sit on the fence, rake in the income, and still remain part of that "old boys' club".

In 1920, Dr Price wrote, "The entire problem of whether or not infected pulpless teeth should be extracted or may be treated should perhaps be settled right on this fundamental premise; for if this cannot be done there is no basis for argument."

In 1996, the Australian Dental Association agreed with Dr Price: "… the role played by micro-organisms has been demonstrated and cannot be emphasized enough. Elimination or destruction of all organisms within the entire tooth is essential for long term success."[112]

In 2007, the Australian Dental Association continues to agree.[113] "The classic studies by …[114,115,116,117,118,119,120,121] have clearly established that most pulp and periapical diseases are a result of the presence of bacteria within the tooth, and particularly within the root canal system. Therefore, the main principles of endodontic treatment should be aimed at eliminating all bacteria from the tooth, and then attempting to maintain the tooth in this disinfected state by preventing any further ingress of bacteria during and after treatment."

Clearly the *success* of an RCP is very dependent on *sterilizing* the tooth and keeping it that way. This basic knowledge has been known for 120 years.

When faced with an impossible goal, the next best thing to do is change the language. Instead of sterilization, the endodontic world speaks of *disinfection*. A disinfected tooth is not necessarily a sterile tooth. The difference between the two is like the difference between a vaccine that is injected into the baby at birth and the immunization that you hope to create with this vaccine. Thus, we hear about immunization programmes instead of vaccination programmes. It's subtle but very effective in propagandizing the wished-for outcome.

The bacteria in the dentine can migrate to the full depth of the dentine tubules.[122,123,124] These tubules, in the crown part of the tooth, end where the dentine finishes and the enamel starts. In the root of the tooth, the tubules end at the surface of the root. So too do the accessory canals, which end in the periodontal ligament. In effect, they finish where the rest of the body starts. There is easy communication through the periodontal ligament to the rest of the body.

How Many Bugs Is a Lot?

Imagine a distance of three miles (nearly five kilometres). (Note that at sea level the horizon is about eight kilometres away) It may be the distance to your favourite restaurant or your lover. If you live in the country, it may be the distance to a far-off hill you can see. Try to imagine walking this whole distance. This is the distance that all the dentine tubules from a front tooth with only one root, lined up end to end, would span. Now imagine that there is a continuous line of bacteria all along this distance, with no spaces in between. Now imagine eight of these lines of bacteria. Make sure that you can see them as you stroll along this three-mile path of infection. Well, that is the number of bacteria that fit in the dentine tubules.[125] Lower molars usually have two roots, and upper molars usually three roots. Without doing the maths, I am sure we can all agree that this constitutes billions of bacteria. Remember that there are between thirty-five thousand and seventy-five thousand dentine tubules per square millimetre of dentine.[126,127] The bacteria inhabiting the tooth will penetrate to the full depth of these dentinal tubules.

In the *Journal of the Australian Dental Association,* March 2007, we find the following text.[128] (And this is agreed upon by other research.[129,130]) "It has been estimated that as much as 50% of the canal wall may remain uninstrumented during preparation. The remaining necrotic tissue remnants may provide a source of nutrition for any surviving bacteria. In addition, bacteria are likely to remain in dentinal tubules after instrumentation."

Most dentists will argue that by filling the canal appropriately, these bugs will not be able to escape and then will die, just as in mummies in the deserts of Egypt. This was the nonsense that I was taught and that is still taught today. This concept also does not have any evidence base to back it up. "The long standing popular notion of entombment and perishing of intraradicular microbes following treatment lacks scientific validity."[131,132]

"Intraradicular microbes" is just another way of saying "bugs that are living happily in the dentine tubules in your tooth". This completely blows the myth that is being taught at most universities and which is considered a form of religious truth by most of the dental profession.

The belief is that if it is buried in the tooth, it will no longer be a problem. The bugs in the tooth do *not* die when "entombed" in the tooth. These bugs are mainly anaerobic bacteria that live happily in a dead tooth that has been sealed up. They will leave the tooth via the main canal, the accessory canals, and the dentine and go for a stroll around your body. If they find a nice new home, they will colonize it, just as the British did for so many years. They are also very good at adapting to changing conditions in which they live. As mentioned previously, the concept of pleomorphic change is well established. This translates as disease in your body. It's a bit like former prime minister Howard's desire to bury the world's radiation waste in the Simpson Desert! It also does not just go away.

Multicultural Colonies

According to the Australian Dental Association, "Bacteria are everywhere, but the environment selects. An anaerobic milieu, inter-actions between microbial factors and the availability of nutrition are principal factors that define the composition of the microbial flora."[10, 133]

In other words, it is the environment which determines the bacterial flora within the tooth.[134,135,136,137]

In the oral cavity there are an estimated 100 billion bacteria comprising more than five hundred different kinds of microorganisms.[138] All of these are searching for a place where they will be happy to live, eat, and multiply.

It is a shame we humans cannot learn to live with each other in the same way that bacteria create happy multicultural communities within a tooth. As you can see, the official position states that there is a wide variety of bacteria, and lots of them, invading a tooth. These are almost all anaerobic organisms. They do *not* rely on oxygen to live.[10,139,140,141,142,143,144,145,146]

One particularly nasty inhabitant of many dead teeth is a little bug called *E. faecalis*. This little bug has many remarkable and distinct features which make it an exceptional survivor. It can

- live and persist in the nutrient-poor environment of endodontically treated teeth;

- survive in the presence of several medications: sodium hypochlorite, clindamycin, and calcium hydroxide, the latter being a much-loved root-filling cement of holistic dentists;
- form biofilms in medicated canals;
- invade and metabolize fluids within the dentinal tubules and adhere to collagen in the presence of human serum;
- endure prolonged periods of starvation and utilize tissue fluids (human serum) that flow from the periodontal ligament and bathe alveolar bone to recover;
- establish monoclonal-infections in medicated roots;
- acquire gene-encoding antibiotic resistance combined with natural resistance to various antimicrobial agents;
- survive in extreme environments with low pH, high salinity, and high temperatures;
- acquire plasmid-encoded resistant genes from other bacteria, which results in intra-species propagation of antibiotic resistance (which is a major issue with this bacterial species); and
- have a prevalence of 12 to 70 per cent of microbial flora in dead teeth.

E. faecalis is a normal intestinal organism and may inhabit the oral cavity and gingival sulcus. In its intestinal environment, it is considered a commensal organism that contributes to carbohydrate, amino acid, and vitamin metabolism. However, a subset of this species appears to be pathogenic because it has acquired a number of genes which confer infectivity and virulence, plus resistance to multiple antibiotics.[147]

These organisms are intrinsically resistant to many antimicrobial agents, including cephalosporins, clindamycin, penicillinase-resistant penicillins, vancomycin, and aminoglycosides.

In addition to these intrinsic resistances, they have also acquired genetic resistance to many classes of antimicrobials, including tetracycline, doxycycline, erythromycin, chloramphenicol, ciprofloxacin, and vancomycin.

E. Faecalis is one nasty little bug that can survive just about anything, and that includes everything dentistry can throw at it. Dentistry does not have any compound that will eradicate it. It can support the survival of other organisms. It easily becomes antibiotic resistant and passes this resistance on to other bacteria. How many yet unidentified organisms, which may do the same thing, exist in a dead tooth?[148, 149] There are lots to choose from.

Research published in 2006 concludes that "the endodontic bacterial biodiversity is greater than previously described by culture methods ..."[150]

Weston Price was saying precisely this in 1923!

Beyond the scope of the dental profession's research, there is a wealth of further research demonstrating that under certain conditions, bacteria and other microorganisms are able to change form. As mentioned earlier, Dr Price demonstrated in 1920 that if oxygen is removed gradually from aerobic bacteria, they will become anaerobic. This is called pleomorphic change. The concept of pleomorphism is ignored in the dental literature, although current medical research demonstrates this reality. A quick search in Medline will reveal hundreds of references related to pleomorphic changes in bacteria.[151,152,153,154,155,156,157,158] What this means is that even though a huge range of bacteria have been found in dead teeth, the conditions in the teeth are ripe for any of these organisms to change form, depending on the environment. The environment inside a tooth is not static; it is changing all the time at a chemical level and in terms of the amount of oxygen in various parts of the tooth. Microorganisms do have the ability to adapt to the environment and to chemicals that are used to try to kill them.

Current research shows that bacteria and other non-virus microorganisms can cause cancer. Much of this literature stresses the likely involvement of highly pleomorphic bacteria as causing cancer.[159] Considering this finding, it would be wise for dental researchers to acknowledge that the organisms which remain in the teeth can cause cancer.

A friend of mine who owned a pathology lab examined a wide variety of extracted root-treated teeth that I had sent her. Each tooth demonstrated a range of microbial forms which could only fall into the category of "cell-wall-deficient forms." These findings have been linked with various stages and forms of cancer.[160] This information is rarely mentioned in dental literature, with very few dentists or professors being aware of it. In fact, current dental philosophy strenuously denies the link to cancer.

Cell-wall-deficient forms have also been described, through the use of dark-field microscopy, as being associated with dead teeth. They have been found in both the teeth and the blood of the same patients. They pose serious threats to health.

> The dangers of these organisms become obvious when you consider that the enzymes produced by the CWD form that maintains their lack of a cell wall, also would break down the cell walls of the red and white blood cells. Even more alarming is the understanding that these organisms not only parasitize our immune cells but can enter into our nervous system and travel to the brain. These Chips have been verified by Dr Lida Mattman in the cerebral fluid of patients with MS and in a high percentage of cases oral spirochetes were seen in massive amounts in the brain.

> ... while these organisms are observable in the bloodstream, the surgical extraction of root canalled teeth and the cleansing of osteonecrotic sites nearly always heal with a recurring osteonecrotic lesion. Again, this would make absolute sense when one realizes that the infection of CWD forms produce enzymes that use and break down cells that are newly forming the bony matrix. Antibiotics that work by disrupting the cell wall of bacteria are not only ineffective but contribute to the formation of the offending CWD forms.[161]

This information is not taught to dental students or dentists!

Death to Bacteria—Maybe!

For a root canal procedure to be successful, the tooth must be sterile. No bacteria should survive. This has always been one of the basic principles of root canal procedures. Dr Price found it impossible to sterilize a tooth without causing serious harm to the patient. The only way that he could sterilise a tooth was to boil it for half an hour. Many of the antibacterial materials used in Dr Price's time are still in use today. Dr Price even tried pouring fuming formaldehyde down the root canals of extracted teeth and was still able to culture anaerobic organisms from the depths of the dentine tubules.

In his own words,

a) Infected teeth can be completely sterilised in the mouth only with great difficulty, or by the use of medicaments whose irritability readily injures the vitality of the supporting structures of the teeth.

d) Many of the usual methods used for the sterilisation of infected teeth do serious injury to the supporting structures about the teeth.

We have, for example, allowed fuming concentrated solution of formaldehyde to trickle through the pulp canal of a tooth which had the infected cementum protected with a rubber dam above and below, until 10 c.c. had passed through, and the cementum was still infected; ... the neutralized tooth was planted beneath the skin of a rabbit under surgical conditions, and an abscess developed containing pure cultures of streptococci.[162]

The bacteria inside a tooth can grow on anything, including formaldehyde! Formaldehyde is one of the most carcinogenic compounds known. It is routinely placed inside teeth. Some materials do not contain formaldehyde to start with, but it may be one of the breakdown products of the root-filling cement. Bacteria are able to grow on formaldehyde-soaked dressings that are placed inside teeth. What justification does dentistry have for their continued use of this chemical when it has been clearly shown to be useless in killing the bacteria found in dead teeth? Dr Price demonstrated this nearly one hundred years ago, yet the procedure is carried on to this day.

> In more than 95% of cases in which we have placed a medicament in a canal on a dressing, … we have in forty eight hours, been able to grow cultures from the dressing that was placed in the tooth, regardless of the medicament that was placed on the dressing.

The dental literature from 1981 agrees with Dr Price's research.

> In the case of an acutely infected tooth there is no natural process of drainage and there is no mechanism by which the antibiotics which have been administered can reach the bacteria inside the tooth

> It is now known that complete sterilization of an infected root canal is very difficult to achieve and complete removal of all pulp tissue remnants frequently is not possible.

> The micro-organisms are isolated and protected inside the canal from the phagocytic activity of the defensive elements of the body and the presence of necrotic tissue fragments can serve as a source of nutrients that will continue in maintaining their viability.[163]

Even the Australian Dental Association now concedes that this is correct.[55] There is not one or any combination of medicaments which can kill the bacteria in the tooth.

Many medicaments have been used in an attempt to achieve the above aims but no single preparation has been found to be predictable or effective.

Current medicaments used in association with instrumentation and irrigation are **unlikely to predictably achieve a bacteria-free root canal system**.[12]

Following are some snippets from the Journal of the Australian Dental Association special endodontic supplement of 2007. According to this organization, there is nothing that will achieve sterility of a tooth.

- "… teeth with pulps are much more resistant to bacterial invasion into the dentinal tubules than are teeth with root canal fillings.[164] … In teeth with pulps, the dentinal tubules are occupied by dentinal fluid and odontoblastic processes, which may behave collectively as a positively charged hydrogel.[165,166] The hydrogel is capable of arresting a great number of the bacteria that enter the pulp."
- "The outward flow of the dentinal fluid is important in the pulp's defense against the entry of harmful substances because it affects the rate at which toxic substances from the mouth diffuse into the dentinal tubules."[167,168]
- "Thus, in view of its limited action on faecalis and Candida, calcium hydroxide cannot be considered as a panacea for all cases of infected root canals."
- "Ledermix and Septomicine: Neither of these can be considered as suitable for use against the commonly reported endodontic bacteria because of their inappropriate spectra of activity."
- "The antibacterial action of phenolic materials may not persist for prolonged periods of time. Hence some bacteria may survive and have the opportunity to multiply and persist in the root canal system. **CMCP can diffuse beyond the apical foramen …**" (my emphasis)

- "The authors cautioned against using Cresophene due to its known **cytotoxic and possible carcinogenic, mutagenic and teratogenic** properties." (my emphasis)
- "CMCP is the most toxic and irritating phenolic antiseptic agent followed by Cresatin, Formocresol, and Camphorated Phenol (CP)"
- "It is estimated that bacteria grown in a biofilm have a 1000-1500 times greater resistance to antibiotics than planktonically-grown bacteria."
- "E. faecalis has been shown to form biofilms in the root canals of human teeth, with or without intracanal medicaments,"
- "**Only a few cells need to survive** treatment so that **when the canal is closed, the anaerobic milieu will be restored, and the bacteria can re-multiply.**" (my emphasis)
- "… bacteria cannot be completely eliminated after thorough instrumentation and irrigation regardless of the technique."
- "Microbes grow as biofilms in the root canal system and may be located in areas that are inaccessible to instrumentation such as dentine tubules or accessory canals."
- "**Thus, on the basis of currently available information there is insufficient scientific support for the idea that it is possible to eliminate infection by apical enlargement of the canal space.**" (my emphasis)

Effectively they are saying that there is *no* mechanical or chemical means of sterilizing a tooth. They are agreeing that *the most important principle of a good root canal procedure is impossible to achieve.* They are agreeing with Dr Price from 1923! They are disagreeing with themselves!

Antibiotic Resistance

Dentistry has used a variety of antibiotics to try to kill the bacteria in a tooth. Not only do they not work, but they are presented to the bacteria in such low dosages that the bacteria are very easily able to form resistance against them. It appears that the bacteria are quite able to form resistance to *all* the materials used in endodontics, and this will of course present as a serious risk as they multiply. Thus, the use of suboptimal antibacterial substances, including antibiotics in ever-increasing numbers of people, may put these patients in grave danger if a systemic infection is caused by these bacteria. The root canal procedure is thus a cause of antibiotic-resistant bacteria in the human body.

This is again confirmed by the ADA:[10]

> … sub-optimal biocide concentrations may result in the emergence of non-susceptible organisms which could also be resistant to antibiotics.

> Bacterial resistance to tetracycline usually results in cross resistance to other tetracyclines … Enterococcus, Staphlococcus and Lactobacillus species contributed to the majority of strains that were resistant and they also had the highest degree of multiple antibiotic resistance.

> Sub-lethal concentrations of antibiotics (tetracycline and chloramphenicol) can act as inducers of multi-drug resistance. It is possible that during root canal therapy, only sub-lethal doses may be in contact with the infecting organisms, particularly in the narrow and more inaccessible parts of the canals.

To make matters worse, it is now well accepted that bacteria have the ability to share genes. This enables them to share and spread the ability to become resistant to antibiotics.[169]

Sterility Impossible

In 1996, the British Dental Association stated, "It is well known that total sterility of the root canal system is impossible and that the aim is thorough cleansing and obturation."[170]

"Obturation" refers to filling and sealing the canal, which is also an impossible goal. I have no idea what "thorough cleansing" means.

In 2007 the Australian Dental Association conceded that it is impossible to sterilize a tooth:

> Current medicaments used in association with instrumentation and irrigation are unlikely to predictably achieve a bacteria-free root canal system.
>
> **... predictable eradication of bacteria from the root canal *still remains an elusive goal* ...** (my emphasis)

In response to the question "Which endodontic irrigants are most effective?" the British Dental Association published a whole paper which explored the various irrigants used in RCPs to sterilize the tooth.[171] It has a simple conclusion: "There is currently insufficient reliable evidence showing the superiority of one irrigant over another."

As Richard P. Feynman said, "**I would rather have questions that can't be answered than answers that can't be questioned.**"

A more recent review of endodontic procedures from 2017 compares just about all methods of trying to sterilize a tooth and still comes up with the fact that they cannot achieve this goal.[172]

Bacteria remaining in a tooth multiply rapidly and escape from the tooth and enter the rest of the body. Sadly, endodontists do not advise their patients of this.

The Latest and the Greatest

Cleaning Techniques—Ozone and Laser

In the last ten years, there has been an increased use of ozone and laser to attempt to sterilise the canal. These are certainly innovative, and they actually do kill bacteria and other microorganisms when the bacteria and microorganisms are suitably exposed. Another paper from 2006 looked at the use of laser to sterilise a tooth, and even that was an abysmal failure. "Neither the laser nor the rotary instrumentation was able to eliminate endodontic infection."[173]

I truly admire the dentists who have invested many thousands of dollars to purchase the necessary equipment in an attempt to treat their patients with the most up-to-date methods to try to achieve success. Sadly, the research shows that ozone will penetrate the dentine tubules only to a depth of three hundred microns, or a third of a millimetre. Laser is better, but it can go only about 0.5 millimetres into the dentine.[174] There are a couple of articles that claim a bacterial reduction to a depth of a whole one millimetre into the dentine, which is further than any other method I have come across.[175,176,]

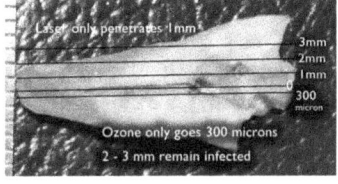

No one dares to talk about the other two to three millimetres of dentine that is left untouched and therefore contaminated.

Much of the research has also suggested that laser is about equal to sodium hypochlorite in reducing the bacterial load. In other words, it is no better than the old tried, tested, and failed methods of attempting sterilization of the canal system with nappy bleach. In fact, they go on to say that "there is insufficient evidence to suggest that any specific laser is superior to the traditional endodontic treatment."[177]

Irrigation with old-fashioned sodium hypochlorite shows similar results to using laser treatment.[178,179,180] I might say that this is great confirmation for how to treat soiled nappies. Keeping your baby healthy with sodium hypochlorite for the nappy wash certainly can work. I don't recommend using a laser on your baby or on a tooth. Another study showed that chlorhexidine was significantly more effective at killing bacteria than laser.[181] Similar studies have shown a great reduction in the bacterial count in narrow sections of dentine, but still they demonstrate that the bacteria were not 100 per cent eliminated. Thus, the canals were not sterile.[182,183,184,185,186,187,188,189,190]

It is also worth mentioning that there have been several adverse effects from the use of laser in dentistry, such as histopathological changes and infection transmission due to laser smoke. During dental procedures, necrosis of the pulp, periodontal ligament, and odontoblasts, cemental lysis, bone resorption, hypo/hyperpigmentation, burns, itching, and scarring might occur. In addition, laser can weaken the dentine by inducing surface cracks.[191]

Realistically, no matter how holistic the dentist is, the use of ozone or laser is neither useful nor effective. There is *no* known way of sterilizing a tooth aside from autoclaving or boiling it for thirty minutes. Neither method has a high patient acceptance.

That Last Millimetre

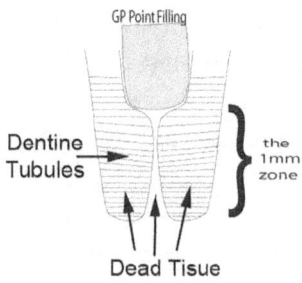

I would like to quickly comment on that last little millimetre of root that should be left untouched. The only reason that I have ever found for preserving this last one millimetre of root tip is that this will supposedly prevent the root filling from being pushed through the end of the root; it is *purely a mechanical consideration*.

Considering that the dentine in this area is also infected, it makes no sense to leave this part of the root untouched & 'untreated'. If the dental gods are screaming that the entire tooth is to be sterilized, then why leave this most critical part of the root untouched. It makes no sense; the pulp in this area is left alone (i.e., dead tissue in this area is left alone). Bacteria in this area are left alone. Medicaments are not supposed to be placed in this area, and the root filling should not extend into this area. I know that it is only one millimetre, but surely in this case size does not matter. This one millimetre, like the rest of the tooth anatomy, is a serious issue for the dental profession.

Endodontists have never been able to work out what to do about it. It is incredible the volumes that have been written about what should be done to this little one millimetre of root. Most, if not all, of the suggestions are contradictory. In other words, you could literally do anything to this little one millimetre of root and find a reference somewhere in the endodontic literature that both supports and contradicts the approach.

Physiological Balance

A common way that dentistry sidesteps an unsolvable problem is to either rename it or reconstruct it. We have just seen the British Dental Association call for a "thorough cleansing" of the root canal instead of completely sterilizing it. This issue is so huge that the endodontists can no longer keep living in denial; nor can they accept failure.

They have therefore created a new name for a new concept. Instead of cleaning, disinfecting, or sterilizing the canal, they now claim to be able to achieve a state of "physiological balance" in the dead infected tooth.

This concept is problematic for a number of reasons:

- No one has ever defined how to assess this mythical state.
- No one has demonstrated how this mythical state can be achieved or maintained after completion of the procedure.
- No one has stated what happens to the bacteria and other organisms that are happily living and multiplying in this "anaerobic milieu" a year or two after this mythical state has been achieved.

"Physiological Balance" is a fantasy created by an incompetent profession to disguise its total inability to achieve the single and most basic requirement of a root canal procedure. It is nothing but smoke and mirrors by the top professors and specialists. It is a disgusting attempt to conceal their ineptitude and maintain their income.

The Final Root Filling

Dentists are taught that the correct placement of that final filling is also critical for the long-term success of the procedure. The filling must completely seal the canal. The idea is to lock in (entomb) the toxins and bacteria. This should prevent them from either entering or escaping from the tooth via the hole at the end of the root canal. There have been great advances in the techniques and materials used to try to achieve this. Volumes have been written about how important this part of the procedure is. To demonstrate how good the root filling is, the only method a dentist has relies on the appearance of the finished job on an X-ray.

All root fillings leave large voids of unfilled space in the main canal of the tooth.[192] These are not usually visible on an X-ray. Often the X-ray does not show the root filling extending out of the end of the root. As mentioned earlier, at least 17 per cent of all root fillings are overextended into the surrounding bone.

Most endodontists don't seem to have an issue with this—possibly because most are guilty of doing it. They blatantly disregard their own journals to keep doing the same bad work. They pretend that this will not cause a problem to the patient. Well, the dental literature does *not* agree with this general knowledge of these endodontists![193,194,195,196,197,198,199,200,201,202]

Even the dental journals have reported on the effects of overfilling the canal.

- The maxillary sinus can be affected from an over filled root canal.[203]
- Bacteria are forced into the surrounding tissue and thus the rest of the body.[204]
- Nerve damage and numbness of the Mental nerve (the nerve that supplies sensation to the lower lip and the gum on the outside of the lower front teeth) can occur.[205,206,207]

- Nerve damage of the inferior alveolar nerve (the nerve that supplies sensation to the lower teeth and branches off to create the Mental Nerve) can occur.[208]
- Infection of the maxillary sinus with Aspergillus mycetoma can occur.[209,210]
- Disabling pain may present after overfilling into the inferior dental canal. (This canal runs along the lower jaw to allow the Inferior Alveolar Nerve and blood vessels to be distributed to the teeth, periodontal ligament, lower lips, and gums.)[211]
- Root- filling cements overextended into the bone are transported great distances through the bone and thus throughout the body.[212]
- An injury of the inferior alveolar nerve is not uncommon.[213,214]
- Overfilling with calcium hydroxide elicits calcium hydroxide resorption and the ingrowth of periapical connective tissue into the root canal [215]
- Overfilling of the root canal is one of the *most common errors* encountered in dental practice.[216]

Whether overfilled or not, the fact remains that none of the filling techniques work, and this fact is simply ignored. There is not one technique which completely fills the canal or seals it. The research from the endodontic journals shows that all root fillings leak to varying degrees.[217,218,219,220,221,222,223,224,225,226,227,228,229,230]

The Australian Dental Association even agreed as recently as 1998 that it is impossible to completely seal a root canal.[231]

If the canal leaks, then it can and does leak in both directions. Bacteria can find their way into a dead tooth, and the bacteria and their toxins will leak out into the bone and the rest of the body. Accessory canals, dentine tubules, and secondary canals are ignored in the filling process, as though they don't exist. This means the bulk of the tooth is left unfilled and infected, as well as having necrotic dead tissue left inside it![232,233,234,235] This is otherwise known as a *toxin factory*.

As good as the X-ray looks, it does not provide any indication of the sealing ability of the root filling. In fact, according to Professor Abbott and the ADA, all of the literature of the last forty years *cannot* be used to assess the filling and sealing ability of any of the techniques or the materials used. "… since no current restorative dental material is able to provide a total and permanent seal, it is always possible that micro leakage will occur, and bacteria may enter the tooth … Once bacteria have entered the tooth, there are thousands of potential direct pathways to the pulp chamber or root canal via the dentinal tubules which are wide enough for bacteria to migrate through."[18]

There is more chance of recurrent infection associated with root-filled rather than non-root-filled teeth.[236] This doesn't say much for the success rate of this insanity. All root fillings leak. There is not one material or technique capable of completely sealing the main root canal, let alone the accessory canals or dentine tubules.[237,238,239]

Clearly, we cannot remove all dead tissue; nor can we file the whole of the inside of a canal or sterilize the tooth. Nor can we completely fill or seal the canal. The ADA is stating that the dental literature of the past forty odd years is completely *unreliable!* What an admission! This, from our leading organizations and teachers, is acknowledgement that what they are teaching dental students to do is impossible to achieve.

In 2007 the International Endodontic Journal published the following: "The manner of execution of treatment procedure(s) is so diverse even within prescribed protocols that it is difficult to define it any more precisely and it is accepted that this treatment intervention is not by its nature standardizable."[240]

The Measure of Success

The success of the root canal procedure is based on the following criteria:

- It looks well filled on an X-ray.

- Abscess in the bone disappears.
- There is no pain.

The lack of pain as a sign of success has been disputed for 120 years. Dr Price stated, "Local comfort ... may constitute both what is probably one of the greatest paradoxes and one of the costliest diagnostic mistakes through injury to health, that exists in dental and medical practice ... the absence of this local reaction and the consequent destruction by the infection products, permits them to pass through the body to irritate and break down that patient's most susceptible tissue."

Paradoxically, it is precisely these painless teeth that look good on an X-ray that are the most dangerous, being strongly associated with cancers and other degenerative diseases. It is only the dental profession which refuses to accept this basic concept.

We know that all materials, microorganisms, and their toxins are transported directly from the tooth back to the brain via the blood and by transport along the nerve fibres.[241,242,243,244] Many other research articles have shown that whatever you put in a tooth can be transported to the rest of the body, and horrifyingly quickly.[245,246,247,248]

A root canal procedure which does not plant a focus does not exist.

Titanium Implants Do Have a Use

The creation of our bionic selves is well underway. Titanium can be implanted anywhere there is bone in our bodies. There is much more detail about these things a bit later, but for now it is worth remembering that on an evidence-based measure, these dental implants do not do well. Some of these implants are inserted into the bone next to a tooth with a root canal.

In 2001, a paper was published in the *Journal of the American Dental Association* which demonstrated the disaster that root canals are. The researchers looked at implant failures caused by infection in the bone around them. These implants were inserted in bone adjacent to root-canalled teeth. The paper is titled "Implant Failures Associated with Asymptomatic Endodontically Treated Teeth." In each case, the root canal looked perfect on the X-ray. Each patient demonstrated signs of infection after initial implant placement. The common factor in each failing implant was its placement next to a root-canalled tooth with no clinical or X-ray evidence of pathology, and no pain symptoms.

> Usually an x-ray that does not disclose a big abscess is regarded as a sign that the treatment was successful, but this research clearly demonstrates the bacterial contamination even when the x-ray looks good and that the microorganisms may persist indefinitely.
>
> The inability to consistently identify endodontically treated teeth that have potential microbial contamination has resulted in new dilemma surrounding implant cases.[249]

The dead tooth is always harbouring a chronic infection which spreads from it to the bone around the implant, causing its failure.[250,251,252]

The research is clearly telling us that it is better to extract a root-canalled tooth before placing an implant in the area, as it is impossible to determine the extent of infection in a dead tooth no matter how good the X-ray looks. They clearly state that these good looking X-rays of dead teeth are shielding the main cause of infection around foreign bodies called titanium implants. The problem, though, is not limited to titanium implants in the mouth. No matter how good the tooth looks on an X-ray, it will still be infected.

For the bone surrounding the implant to become infected from this source, the bacteria have to have "escaped" from the dead tooth and penetrated the bone. If they are in the bone, then they will be carried everywhere else in the body. If these bugs decide that your heart is a good home, then you might just have a heart attack. They might decide to inhabit your brain instead and create neurological cancers or MS. They might localize in your ears and cause deafness. All bacteria and the toxins they produce can and do travel out of the tooth to the rest of your body. It is not just the implant that might fail in this case. In any language, this is a focal infection arising from the source, which is a root-canalled tooth that looks good on an X-ray! Focal infection does exist!

The bacteria can and do travel to other weakened areas in the body and can infect this tissue. Thus, implants in the hips and knees can be and are infected by oral bacteria. "Such infections carry an enormous and crippling morbidity."[253]

Those of you contemplating implants had best discuss this research with your dentist. Remember that an answer like "In all my years of doing this, I have never seen it happen" is *not* a scientific answer. Nor does it even rate as anecdotal. It just means that the dentist hasn't seen it (maybe). The next question I would ask is "Did you ever look?" If you really are contemplating getting an implant, I would strongly advise you to read the entire website at www.melisa.org and the section on implants later in this book. (See also www.realdentalinfo.com.)

I have finally found a use for titanium implants. They demonstrate what has been known for so long—that root canal procedures do not work. The whole concept is flawed from beginning to end.

Down the Rabbit Hole

Dr Weston Price published his findings in 1923. They have not been shown to be wrong. They have not been discredited or vilified by later research. Everything that Dr Price discovered has, in fact, been supported by current research and even by the Australian Dental Association as late as 2007!

All the procedures that must be fulfilled in stages are totally unachievable. The dental associations have stated this. The professors have stated this. Voluminous research has demonstrated this. The specialist endodontists have admitted they have no references to support any of their claimed "general knowledge."

Yet every dental school in the world teaches students that root canal treatment is essential to maintain health. Every procedure is painstakingly taught and examined. Millions of dentists around the world are pretending. The teaching includes the *fact* that specialist endodontists sit on the left side of God. The right side is reserved for the oral surgeons.

The world of medicine and dentistry is full of contradictory research, concepts, and even evidence. If people's lives and finances were not affected, we could all enjoy the stupidity of these contradictions by well-spoken and almost well-published experts. As stated by Mason Cooley "Ultimately, blind faith is the only kind."

To Summarize

- It is impossible to clean the dead tissue out of a tooth.
- It is impossible to sterilize the tooth.
- It is impossible to see infection on an X-ray.
- It is impossible to measure the true length of the root canal.
- It is impossible to fill or seal the tooth.
- It is impossible to entomb the bacteria within the tooth.
- It is impossible to achieve any of the goals of root canal procedures.
- It is impossible to demonstrate that this is a therapeutic treatment.

I saw many patients who did not want their dead teeth removed and preferred to have a referral to an endodontist to have this job done properly. This was their choice, which I always respected. Usually they said things like "But send me to a really good one please, Rob." I always replied that a really good endodontist is the one who no longer does root canal procedures. Dr George Meinig is the only one I have heard of who falls into this category.

Clearly the current research is in total agreement with the research of Dr Weston Price, Dr Edward Rosenow, Dr Cecil Mayo, Dr Frank Billings, and so many others. The dental institutions are misleading the public and their own members by claiming otherwise.

6

Do Dead Teeth Affect Your Health?

● ●

I am the only guinea pig I have.

—Buckminster Fuller

This chapter should be read by dentists and doctors as well as everyone else. Many diseases can be prevented with an intelligent approach to dentistry.[254]

Many treatment approaches used throughout the history of medicine and dentistry were later shown to be disasters. Syphilis used to be "treated" by placing people in baths of mercury. What was once called Tertiary Syphilis, or "end-stage syphilis" was later shown to be *severe and lethal mercury poisoning!* Treatment for teething pain was a teething powder that contained mercury and caused Pink's Disease (Acrodynia). It caused the infants to turn *pink!* Many thousands of infants died, and many more who lived suffered a variety of horrible symptoms for the rest of their lives. The effects of this were far more dramatic for the ensuing three generations. "Staggeringly, we found that 1 in 25 grandchildren of pink disease survivors aged 6-12 had been diagnosed with an autism spectrum disorder. This compares to the current Australian prevalence rate for that age group of 1 in 160" (in 2011).[255]

That is over six times the incidence compared to the rest of the population! What is done to one generation may affect many in the following generations. That flu shot which contains mercury is injected into pregnant women to prevent a minor illness that may have repercussions over the next few generations. The flu shot has been shown to be completely ineffective at preventing the flu.

A vaccine is now advocated for the treatment for cervical cancer, which is killing and harming more women than are affected by the cancer itself. Current cancer treatments pour toxic immune-destroying chemicals into the body.

Polio, which is caused by a neurological toxin in pesticides, is "treated" by vaccinating against the virus while at the same time putting monkey viruses into the body from the vaccine. These viruses, called SV40, are known to cause human cancers. The SV40 problem was known at the initial time of manufacturing the vaccine in the 1950s. Monkey tissue is still being used today to manufacture polio vaccine. It is still contaminated with SV40.

To this day, the advised treatment for a hole in your tooth is to plug it with metals that contain mercury and release that mercury into your body.

A treatment for morning sickness was Thalidomide. How many thousands of deformed babies were needed before it was taken off the market? There was no compensation.

Dentists can learn from a vast bibliography and an array of published material on how all the various diseases affect the mouth and teeth. It is well known that diabetic patients will need to be very vigilant regarding their oral hygiene, as they are more susceptible than others to gum disease. If, as a child, you had a systemic disease like chicken pox, you may have striations across your teeth. If you had certain antibiotics as a child, you might have discolouration of the teeth. If you were fluoride poisoned as a child, this will appear as white to brown discolouration called "fluorosis".

Dentists are taught that their Noble Art cannot cause any disease. The denial is from the teachers and the PTOs. Considering that the dental journals themselves have published that this is not the case, the continued denial by the dental establishment can be seen only as blatantly criminal. This denial must surely be seen as a crime against humanity.

Just one short list published in the *International Endodontic Journal*, titled "Root canal treatment and general health: a review of the literature," is testimony to this:

> "There has been an increase in the number of case reports published in the <u>medical literature citing dental infection</u> as an associated factor in several systemic illnesses including;
>
> - uveitis [Sela & Sharav 1979] (inflammation of the middle layer of tissue in the eye)
> - intracranial abscess [Holin et al. 1967, Henig et al. 1978, Ingham et al. 1978, Churton & Green 1980, Aldous et al. 1987, Marks et al. 1988, Saal et al. 1988] (brain abscess)
> - childhood hemiplegia [Hamlyn 1978], cerebral infarction [Syrjanen et al. 1989], acteriospermia and subfertility [Bieniek & Riedel 1993] (brain damage or spinal cord injury that leads to paralysis on one side of the body)
> - necrotizing fasciitis [Gallia & Johnson 1981, Steel 1987, Stoykewych et al. 1978] (a bacterial infection that results in the death of parts of the body's soft tissue. It is a severe disease of sudden onset that spreads rapidly.)
> - mediastinitis [Hendler & Quinn 1978, Zachariades et al. 1988, Musgrove & Malden 1989] (inflammation or infection of the mediastinum)
> - fatal endocarditis [Kralovic et al. 1995] (infection of the lining of the heart)
> - toxic shock syndrome [Egbert et al. 1987, Navazesh et al. 1994] (acute septicaemia typically caused by bacterial infection)
> Septicaemia [Lee 1984] (Bacterial Blood Poisoning) [256]

I'm sure that many dentists do consider themselves part of a "noble and ethical profession" and as long as they continue to do what the establishment teaches, they will maintain this status quo. They really are trying to do the best they can for their patients. I don't give the teachers and politicians of dentistry the same grace.

A New Language

Keeping up with current trends in dentistry requires some understanding of the rhetoric used to support the status quo. When certain ideas and trends are no longer fashionable, they are simply dropped. However, when it becomes impossible to maintain the denial of a problem, there is a different way of dealing with it. Dropping the idea is not good enough, because people like me will keep reminding the world. Instead it must first be accepted as "known all along": "Of course, we have known for *years* that we cannot sterilise a tooth!" "Everybody knows." It is then necessary to normalise this new and old knowledge. A statement from the website of the American Dental Association in 2005 reads, "… microbes do remain in the dentinal tubules of endodontically treated teeth *but pose no health hazard.*"

If it is unachievable, it's simply no longer a problem. Again, everybody knows! The same lie has been used for over one hundred years.

A common ploy that dentistry uses to dissociate itself from the reality of undeniable disasters is the addition to the English language of new words—big words that sound scientific, such as Monty Python's "Biggus Dicus". Ideally there are no comparable words that a dictionary can even associate with the new ones. There is *no* definition for these words aside from what dentistry *implies*. These are the red flags of dentistry which let everyone know that there is a major problem. In other words, it is the language used to hide the impossible dream.

- "Peri-implantitis"—the infection in the gum and bone that surrounds implants that no one has yet been able to deal with.

Almost *all* implants are affected, whether titanium or zirconia. This is one of the main causes of implant failures.

- "Pulpless"—the state of a tooth that has had the pulp removed, leaving the tooth only a little bit dead. This is the same as "non-vital".
- "Physiologic balance"—a nonsense term used to try to hide the fact that sterilisation of a tooth is impossible. There is no such thing as physiological balance.
- "Oseointegration"—the supposed reaction of the bone to accept an implant and heal without any other stuff-ups. The bone and implant become 'one'. This is otherwise known as condensing osteitis.
- "Unintentional Replantation"—This describes the unintentional extraction of a tooth (e.g., when an old bridge is being removed and one of the teeth comes with the bridge instead of staying in the jaw), followed by a root canal procedure done out of the mouth and then the reimplantation of the dead tooth back into the jawbone. The reason such a tooth comes out is that the bone which was supporting it has already been destroyed by periodontal disease! All I can say is "YUKKK!"!
- "Coronectomy"—the removal of the crown of the tooth while leaving the dead infected root in the jawbone. Instead of removing the whole tooth, just the crown away in this procedure, leaving the roots to rot in the bone.

These procedures are not based on *any* evidence. Nor do they rest on *any* scientific research. There is no scientific basis supporting the achievable success of such procedures. The only basis for them is clinical observation! They cannot be labelled "Safe" or "Effective". Dentists who truly value the well-being of their patients must surely question the wisdom of continuing to attempt to get a different result by repeating the same old adage.

Mechanisms of Disease

There are several ways that dead, root-canalled teeth can affect the health of your body and mind.

- Toxic Chemicals implanted into your tooth
- Allergies arising from the contents of the tooth
- Focal Infection
- Neural Interference

Each of these mechanisms needs exploring, as it is only with this deeper understanding that we get to make sense of the variety and sometimes bizarre nature of the symptoms and diseases presenting themselves. Following is only a brief overview, but I hope it will fill the cavernous gaps left by our current dental teachers. Neural interference is dealt with in a later chapter.

Toxic Insertions—The Ffirst Way

All of the medicaments used to fill a root canal have been approved by the TGA and the FDA. This supposedly allows them to be used as "safe and effective". This allows the dental establishments to claim them as "biocompatible". There are many other drugs and medicaments that in the past have also been approved by these government organizations and later withdrawn as a result of their disastrous health effects. For example, Thalidomide, Mercurochrome, Cerivastatin, Valdecoxib, and so many more. Interestingly, the use of mercury as an additive in many products, including vaccines, is still allowed to continue. It is worth searching the lists of drugs that have been removed from the market after having been approved.

Many health authorities who try to cover the devastating effects of a plethora of toxins added to the environment will claim that "Dose makes the poison," implying that only a little bit will be easily tolerated by most of the population. This may be true but is only half of the equation. The other half is that each person's sensitivity will determine the poisonous nature of the substance. Repeated exposure to various toxins will eventually increase your sensitivity to most toxins.

Patients are not told that the materials used in the root canal procedure, may be carcinogenic (cancer causing), teratogenic (causing developmental malformations), embryotoxic (poisonous to foetuses), allergenic (causing allergies) and neurotoxic (poisonous and damaging to the nervous system). Patients are not informed that all these medicaments and materials will pass through and out of the tooth and be transported throughout the body. Informed consent to place these materials into the body should be sought in every case. Patients are not informed of the detrimental health hazards of these substances. The white-coated specialists probably don't know either, because they rely *only* on clinical judgement. Very few have read the Material Safety Data Sheets associated with the materials they are implanting into people's bodies.

The endodontic literature itself states that biocompatible materials must be used in this procedure. Some of these substances are used temporarily to try to sterilize the tooth before it is filled. Others are permanently implanted into the tooth as the root filling material. Of all the materials that I have researched, I have not found one that could be considered biocompatible. Some of these are dangerous to the local tissue in and around the tooth, and some have toxicity which will affect the foetus. Most are environmental toxins and carry warnings that they should not be disposed of in any water like sewerage, as it will kill the fish.

Some of the materials implanted in the tooth are neurotoxic (i.e., toxic to nerve tissue). They are transported along nerves back to the brain. They are as toxic in the brain as they are to the peripheral nerves. These toxins can easily affect nerve transmission. They can cause paraesthesia (numbness) in the affected nerve. In other cases, these toxic materials may sensitize the nerve, causing it to overreact to stimuli, and clinically we see things like Trigeminal Neuralgia. The neurotoxicity of root-filling materials is well published.

All materials used to try to sterilize a tooth will travel throughout the body. Not one of them alone or in combination will achieve the sterility or sealing ability that they are used for. The authors of a 2005 study say that they should "expect clinical outcomes with new materials that are at least as good as those obtained with the old."[257] We could therefore expect all of these new materials and techniques to be as useless as the old. We could also expect them to be as toxic as the old materials.

Joseph Issels states the following in *Cancer: a Second Opinion*: "… the gangrenous contents of an inflamed pulp cavity and its adjoining spaces" have been shown to spread throughout the body. "… the German researcher Spreter von Kreudenstein showed that drugs injected intravenously were, four to five hours later, discernible within the intradental capillary ducts (dentinal tubules), and in a concentration only slightly lower than in the blood."

Also, "If radio-iodine, I-131, is deposited in an evacuated pulp cavity which is then sealed off with a filling, the iodine will appear in the thyroid some twenty hours later, as can be demonstrated by taking a scintograph (see glossary) of the thyroid region. Similarly, dyes can be washed out of a sealed pulp cavity. (Bartelstone (USA) and Djerassi (Bulgaria)."[258]

The two materials that are most commonly and routinely used to attempt to sterilize, clean, disinfect, and wash the canal are hydrogen peroxide and sodium hypochlorite (Milton's Solution). Milton's solution is the bleach that you buy at the supermarket to bleach nappies. When the dentist has had enough of filing the inside of the canal, they will wash it by squirting hydrogen peroxide into the canal, followed by a squirt or two of Milton's Solution. The reaction of these chemicals produces lots of gas that bubbles out of the tooth and carries with it all the debris created by the filing process.

This can go terribly wrong when these chemicals are injected beyond the end of the canal, or they bubble through the wrong orifice. This happens far more often than is reported. In severe cases, they are injected into the maxillary sinus (the sinus above your upper teeth and below your eye), with devastating long-term pain and destruction of the lining of the sinus. Sometimes they are injected through the lower teeth and into the inferior dental canal, which wipes out the nerve that resides there and produces permanent numbness of the lower lip. It may also damage the vein and artery that supply the lower jaw and the teeth, with consequent effects. It may also cause necrosis (death) of the surrounding bone, and it is not uncommon in these cases to lose adjacent teeth and half the jawbone. Needless to say, the patients usually win the court cases that result. There is a financial payout for the patient, which will never fix the permanent damage, but the dentist is not even reprimanded, as the profession regards such disasters as collateral damage.

All other materials that are sealed into the tooth for the sake of creating "physiological balance" (which used to be called "sterility") during the procedure may stay in the tooth for weeks to months. They are placed there in an attempt to disinfect the tooth. This constitutes a chronic, long-term exposure.

Camphor, phenol, menthol, and formaldehyde have been used without any success for over one hundred years! They are all carcinogenic and allergenic. They are all still being used. Did your dentist tell you about this? (See MSDSs in appendix 1.)

The dental associations claim that implanting these materials into your body is ethical. It is considered ethical by them even though they know that these materials will travel to the brain and the uterus. They will have profound effects on the development of a child in utero.

One of the most dangerous materials that can be implanted into your body is formaldehyde. A root-filling product called N2 is almost completely made of paraformaldehyde, which forms formaldehyde when water touches it. The use of this root-filling cement was made popular by a dental mad hatter called Angelo Sargenti, a Swiss dentist who introduced this material in 1954. He died in 1999 after profiting enormously from his carcinogenic paste that was put in people's teeth, as it still is today. The term "Sargenti Technique" has been applied to the use of N2, and, incredibly, a whole endodontic society has been set up to promote the use of this material and technique. The American Endodontic Society is set up to promote the placement of a known carcinogen into your body.

Following is what the manufacturer of N2 says about the formaldehyde in its product—it is a copy of the Material Safety Data Sheet (MSDS). MSDSs are information brochures about the properties of products; these brochures are issued to government organizations and must be publicly available.

Formaldehyde

WARNING:

POISON! DANGER! SUSPECT CANCER HAZARD. MAY CAUSE CANCER. Risk of cancer depends on level and duration of exposure. VAPOR HARMFUL. HARMFUL IF INHALED OR ABSORBED THROUGH SKIN. CAUSES IRRITATION TO SKIN, EYES AND RESPIRATORY TRACT. STRONG SENSITIZER. MAY BE FATAL OR CAUSE BLINDNESS IF SWALLOWED. CANNOT BE MADE NONPOISONOUS. FLAMMABLE LIQUID AND VAPOR.

Tumorigen, mutagen, reproductive effector;

Causes burns. Very toxic by inhalation, ingestion and through skin absorption. Readily absorbed through skin. Probable human carcinogen. Mutagen. May cause damage to kidneys. May cause allergic reactions. May cause sensitisation. May cause heritable genetic damage. Lachrymator at levels from less than 20 ppm upwards. Very destructive of mucous membranes and upper respiratory tract, eyes and skin.

Acute Exposure; Death if inhaled or absorbed; severe eye irritation and burns. Allergic dermatitis, skin burns; bronchitis pulmonary oedema; headache dizziness nausea vomiting, abdominal pain; blindness.

Chronic Exposure: Nasal Cancer, respiratory tract irritation, reproductive disorders, asthma, dermatitis, multiple organ damage. Carcinogen

Toxic fumes of: carbon monoxide, carbon dioxide

Effects may be delayed

Most formulations of formaldehyde also contain Methanol; Repeated or prolonged exposure to methanol could result in visual impairment and central nervous system effects.

KNOWN TO THE STATE OF CALIFORNIA TO CAUSE CANCER."

If a material is sealed into a tooth as a final root filling, this constitutes a chronic long-term exposure. To pretend that it stays sealed into the tooth and cannot get out, affecting the rest of the body, is the thinking of the fools that have been poisoned by mercury. Any other motive is even too horrifying for me to comprehend. "Clinical studies involving chronic topical application of formalin have demonstrated the induction of leukoplakia and lesions resembling carcinoma in situ. The respiratory tract may be the area for the greatest risk of the development of tumors. Animal studies demonstrate that formaldehyde may affect reproduction potential. Formaldehyde should be considered a potential carcinogen in humans. Formaldehyde poses problems to systemic health via ingestion routes, interaction in air with other aldehydes, and in final breakdown products of formalin in the body. If formaldehyde is clearly not necessary, why is it used at all, particularly in light of its deleterious effects?"[259]

This is what the American Association of Endodontists (the opposition specialist group) say about the use of formaldehyde known as the Sargenti Method:

> ... the AAE does recommend *against* the use of paraformaldehyde-containing materials as they have proven to be both unsafe and ineffective.
>
> Paraformaldehyde-containing endodontic filling materials or sealers (frequently known as Sargenti pastes, N-2, N-2 Universal, RC-2B or RC-2B White) should not be used for endodontic treatment because those materials are unsafe. Extensive scientific research has proven unequivocally that paraformaldehyde-containing filling materials and sealers can cause irreversible damage to tissues near the root canal system including the following: destruction of connective tissue and bone; intractable pain; paresthesia and dysthesia of the mandibular and maxillary nerves; and chronic infections of the maxillary sinus. Moreover, scientific evidence has demonstrated that the damage from paraformaldehyde-containing filling materials and sealers is not necessarily confined

to tissues near the root canal. The active ingredients of these filling materials and sealers have been found to travel throughout the body and have been shown to infiltrate the blood, lymph nodes, adrenal glands, kidney, spleen, liver and brain.[260]

What grand hypocrisy. On the one hand, they deny the ability of anything travelling from the tooth throughout the body, and on the other hand they clearly admit that everything travels from the tooth through the body and has been shown "to infiltrate the blood, lymph nodes, adrenal glands, kidney, spleen, liver and brain." Some other materials used to fill the root canals also break down to formaldehyde.

All these materials and breakdown products travel throughout the body.[261,262,263]

Two other materials, AH26 and Endomethasone, are the most commonly used root-filling materials in the world, and one of the breakdown products of these materials is formaldehyde! AH26 comes with some interesting warnings. The following comes from its MSDS:

> Danger to drinking water if even small quantities leak into the ground. Also poisonous for fish and plankton in water bodies. Avoid contact with eyes and skin. Skin Irritant, Eye Irritant, Sensitization by Skin contact.

> After Swallowing: Rinse mouth thoroughly and then drink plenty of water. Call a doctor immediately.

Dentistry considers these materials to be okay to place permanently into your body, knowing the effects on your health, yet always denying the possibility of creating disease. What more could we expect, though, from the same maniacs who espouse the value of implanting mercury into your brain and who set the concepts of ethics in the profession. It is unethical to suggest that a dead tooth may be causing your disease, but it is perfectly ethical to implant poisonous carcinogens into your body.

The reason for implanting these toxic chemicals is an attempt at sterilizing the tooth and filling up and sealing the root canal. That these goals are unachievable with any material is rarely spoken of. In 1923, when Dr Price was warning the dental world of exactly the same information, nobody wanted to listen. They are still not listening.

All materials placed in dead teeth are poisonous.[264,265,266,267,268,269,270,271, 272,273, 274, 275,276,277,278,]

The Sargenti technique is loved by so many dentists because the materials are cheap, the procedure requires minimal work in the actual root canal, and the N2 paste acts as the permanent root filling. It is all done in one session, with a great profit margin! It is the most common root-filling material in the UK and other countries that have national health care schemes. What the government pays for RCPs is so little that none would be done if they used any other technique. Another way of seeing this could be that the British government and the British Dental Association condone the poisoning of its population with this carcinogen. No warnings are demanded, contrary to the case in California under Proposition 65.

This "treatment" is recommended for everyone, from children through to the elderly and frail, in order to save their teeth. It matters not if you have a compromised immune system; nor does it matter if you have atherosclerosis or cancer, or if you're pregnant. The sacred "root canal treatment" is the procedure of choice. Dentists believe that the part of the body they are legally allowed to treat is from the lips to the tonsillar folds at the back of the mouth. This area, then, is the only one that dental treatment could have an impact on—the rest of the body just does not exist.

The rest of the body is the domain of the medical profession, and never the two shall meet. The doctors know their place in this hierarchy, and thus a dead tooth remains only a "pulpless or non-vital tooth", or one which has had a root canal "therapy", which is necessary for chewing and looking good. Recently the role of the dentist has been expanded a little bit. We are now allowed to inject botulin into your wrinkles so that the expensive crown and bridgework that have just been inserted will look their best. I love the idea of ageing disgracefully is acceptable.

A variation of the N2 and Formocresol madness is called "Russian Red Endodontic Therapy." It contains two potentially toxic components, formaldehyde (liquid) and resorcinol (powder). Zinc oxide or barium sulphate may also be added. "… resorcinol resins and glues have also been shown to have toxic side effects."[279] Incredibly, the same study describes the technique used: "A RF resin-soaked piece of asbestos or similar material is sealed into the pulp chamber to replenish the resin on the floor of the chamber …" This technique is becoming available in the United States.

To complete a regular root filling (not the Sargenti Technique), the dentist will spin a runny cement down into the canal and then pack in a series of rubbery points called Gutta Percha points". Gutta Percha is derived from a plant and of itself is fairly harmless. Dentists are taught that these points are inert and non-toxic. The research, though, does not agree. "All GP points tested were toxic at longer observation periods, and the toxicity was attributed to leakage of zinc ions into the fluids."[280]

In their final form, gutta percha points consist of some 20 per cent gutta percha (GP)and up to 80 per cent zinc oxide. A dye and metal salts are added for colour and to make them visible on X-rays.[281]

Gutta Percha is a form of latex. It's just too bad that the dentist does not care whether you have a latex allergy. Such allergies are *not* taken into consideration. Most dentists have no idea that GP will cause an allergic reaction in the latex-sensitive individual.

A 1995 journal article states the following regarding the runny cements that are used: "Zinc oxide-eugenol, Tubli seal, and Endoflas F.S. were severely toxic at 48h and 7 days."[282]

AH26 and Endomethasone are the most common sealing cements.

Another material called Pro Root MTA is used to try to seal the end of the canal after the end of the root has been surgically removed, in a procedure called apicectomy. Admittedly, it is less toxic than mercury amalgam, which was the go-to material for this procedure in the past. Pro Root MTA is also used to seal up holes that are accidentally made in the root by a "merely bad dentist." It is a form of Portland Cement.

This material is placed at the end of the root and in other holes in the root. They are therefore implanted in the jawbone. This material is thus exposed directly to the body fluids and blood and nerve supply in the bone. The MSDS for Pro Root MTA states the following:

> The major components of Pro Root (calcium silicate compounds, and calcium compounds containing aluminium oxide and gypsum) are considered Hazardous.
>
> **This product contains chemicals (trace metals) known to the state of California to cause cancer, birth defects or other reproductive harm.**
>
> **INCOMPATIBILITY**
>
> Wet ProRoot MTA Root Canal Repair Material is alkaline (caustic/basic). It is incompatible with acids, ammonia, ammonia nitrate, ammonium salts, aluminum metal and chlorine.
>
> (Living bone is wet! See later how this reacts with some root filling materials.)
>
> **Effects resulting from skin contact:**
>
> Discomfort or pain cannot be relied upon to alert a person to a hazardous skin exposure ... Exposed persons may not feel discomfort until hours after the

exposure and, in this case, significant injury may have already occurred ... Dry powder contacting wet skin or exposure to moist or wet material may cause more severe skin effects due to caustic nature.

Effects resulting from inhalation:

It also may cause delayed lung injury including silicosis, a disabling and potentially fatal lung disease, and/or other diseases.

Effects resulting from ingestion:

Although small quantities of dust are not known to be harmful, ill effects are possible if larger quantities are consumed. Take care not to eat any of this product.

Carcinogenic potential:

The ingredients used to manufacture ProRoot MTA Root Canal Repair Material are not listed as carcinogens by NTP, OSHA or IARC. It may, however, contain trace amounts of substances listed as carcinogens by these organizations.

Crystalline silica, a potential trace level contaminant, is now classified by IARC as a known human carcinogen (Group I). NTP has characterized respirable silica as "reasonably anticipated to be a carcinogen."

Regarding the Arsenic contamination of Pro Root MTA, studies have shown the concentration of Arsenic in Pro Root MTA is 1.16 ppm (or 1.16 mg/L).[283] This 116 times above what the Centers for Disease Control considers unsafe. Arsenic levels above .01 mg/l are considered unsafe by the CDC.

Arsenic ingestion has been linked to both cancerous and non-cancerous health effects. These include cancer of the bladder, lungs, skin, kidney, nasal passages, liver, and prostate. Arsenic ingestion has also been linked to cardiovascular, pulmonary, immunological, and neurological effects.[284]

Cancerous effects: skin, bladder, lung, kidney, nasal passages, liver and prostate cancer

Non-cancerous effects: cardiovascular, pulmonary, immunological, neurological and endocrine disruption effects.[285]

The US EPA's final arsenic rule was issued in 2001. It revises the Maximum Contaminant Level (MCL) from 50 µg/L to 10 µg/L and sets the maximum contaminant level goal (MCLG) to zero in drinking water.

Well, you can't eat it, breathe it, touch it, or put it anywhere wet, but implanted into your bone, a couple of inches from your brain, is okay! This is what the manufacturer is saying about its own product. Dentistry ignores these warnings and is placing this material into living bone daily. This material is placed into living children daily! Dentistry considers this rubbish as a state-of-the-art filling material for the roots of baby teeth. Dentistry does not consider the arsenic contained in this material to be a problem.[286,287,288,289] Dentistry also does not consider mercury from amalgam to be a problem. Mercury is the third most toxic element known to science. Arsenic is the "first" most toxic. Lead is somewhere in between. There is *no* amount of arsenic that is safe. None.

The manufacturer states that this material causes cancer. Why in the name of sanity does a health care profession want to implant it into living bodies? Why do the TGA and FDA give approval for its use, especially in children? Perhaps it is in line with the edicts of the Society for the Control of Cancer set up in 1923.

I wonder how many patients have been asked whether they want this cancer-producing substance placed into their bodies. How many women get pregnant having had this material put in a tooth, with the risk of birth defects and reproductive harm? How many parents are given this information before the specialist pedodontist puts it into their children's teeth? I'm sure that most cancer patients would want to know this information. I'm sure that everybody, whether they have diagnosed cancers or not, would want to know. Proposition 65 in California requires a notice to be given if people are being subjected to toxic substances: "**This product contains chemicals (trace metals) known to the state of California to cause cancer, birth defects or other reproductive harm.**" How many specialist endodontists and oral surgeons give this information to their patients? How many dentists actually *know* this information? Most accept what they are told by the sales reps and their godlike specialist endodontists and professors. Some keep up to date with what the dental literature offers. Most are oblivious. All are subjected to the comparative types of studies that show the effects of materials against each other instead of against the effects on a healthy person. For example, "It has been shown previously that MTA is less toxic than other root-end-filling materials tested … "The finding that these materials also are toxic to glial cells is of less obvious practical concern."[290]

As I mentioned before, the other root-end-filling material was dental amalgam, which releases mercury 24-7 directly into your brain and the rest of your body. No wonder that it is less toxic than its alternative.

"Less toxic" is a far cry from *non*-toxic. It is an even further cry from "biocompatible." The manufacturer admits that no toxicity studies have been done! These authors are stating that there is no practical concern that this material is toxic to the most prolific cells in your brain. They have no concern that it could cause a type of brain cancer called glioblastoma. They have no concern that dental personnel already have twice the rate of Glioblastomas than the rest of the population.[291] These researchers also found that amalgam is not toxic if it does not have zinc in it! Have they not heard about mercury? Papers like this do nothing but create confusion and misrepresent and downplay the serious issues at hand. They do *not* provide the information that a dentist needs to decide what to implant into your body. These sorts of papers actively, and I believe intentionally, misinform most dental professionals. They do *not* provide the information that patients need to make an informed choice.

As Carl Sagan said, "The absence of evidence is not evidence of absence."

Case studies, although anecdotal, provide some insight that the dental profession denies. Mary was eleven years old when she came to see me with her distraught mother. When she was nine, she had a pulpotomy performed on a lower left molar tooth. This procedure involves scraping out the top of the nerve of the tooth (pulp chamber) on a baby tooth, instead of performing a full root canal procedure. The remains of the nerve (pulp) of the tooth going down the root are bathed in a strong solution of formaldehyde, and a piece of formaldehyde-soaked cotton wool is sealed into the crown of the tooth. (This is the Buckley's Formocresol mentioned earlier, which was created by Dr Buckley, who was also president of the American Dental Association.) The tooth was covered by a stainless-steel metal crown that releases nickel into the body. Nickel alone is highly carcinogenic and immune reactive.

She was always a skinny, robust, and athletic kid, according to her mum. One year later, when she came to see me, she was very overweight, had constant kidney pain, and was emotionally and intellectually vague and quite depressed. She was being treated by an endocrinologist who insisted that the steroid treatment she was on would one day start to work. Mum told me that she had never been like this before the dental "treatment". The most distressing symptom, though, was that from the day of the dental procedure, she began to wet the bed at nights, something that she had not done since she was a baby. It was every night. She was so embarrassed that things like sleepovers at friends' were not even a consideration. She again spent her nights in nappies. Apart from being a known carcinogen, formaldehyde has many other side effects. It can cause physical deformities, can retard growth and development, and is embryotoxic and teratogenic, to name but a few. Mum, Mary, and I decided that the tooth should not be there, whether or not it was the cause of the bed-wetting. They were relieved to have found someone in the dental world who agreed with them. Every other dentist and doctor had told them that it was psychological or systemic but could not have anything to do with the previous dental treatment. It was simply not an option! I would like to mention here, as well as later, that I have never made a promise to anyone to fix up any medical condition. The possibility was always discussed but never promised.

I took the tooth out for her on the day of the first appointment. It was simple, and she was really relaxed about the procedure. (*No pain* is a good thing). Literally from that day on, the bed-wetting stopped and she returned to a healthier lifestyle. The endocrinologist insisted that the steroids were finally working even though she stopped the steroid medication soon after the extraction. One year later, she came in to say hello. There had been no return of the bed-wetting, and she had returned to her normal thin and healthy tree-climbing self.

Another substance called Ferric Sulphate is now being used to replace Buckley's Formocresol in baby teeth, still in the hope of mummifying the remaining pulp tissue. This is the new material of choice for the Pedodontists.

The MSDS for Ferric Sulphate states the following:

> WARNING! HARMFUL IF SWALLOWED OR INHALED. CAUSES IRRITATION TO SKIN, EYES AND RESPIRATORY TRACT. AFFECTS THE LIVER. Low dosages may cause nausea, vomiting, diarrhea, and black stool. Pink urine discoloration is a strong indicator of iron poisoning. Liver damage, coma, and death from iron poisoning has been recorded.

Interestingly, dentists who become specialist pedodontists do so because they love working with children. Most of the time though, the kids that are referred to the pedodontist are the ones that are too difficult (or expensive) for the regular dentist to handle. If you think a specialist is going to affect his or her income by spending the time that should be spent with terrified children, you are sadly mistaken. Almost all the kids seen by the pedodontist are given a general anaesthetic for the work to be carried out. It is not uncommon therefore to try to maximize the profit in this session by doing all the work that the child needs at once. Your child might come home with three or four teeth containing formaldehyde or Ferric Sulphate, a number of mercury-releasing amalgam fillings, and some nickel-releasing stainless-steel crowns over the now dead teeth—all of this in one to one and a half hours or less. Do you really think your child will ever be the same? Parents accept this sort of treatment plan, being already conditioned by the vaccine industry that multiple shots in one session gets it over with quickly for the poor child who hates the needle. The legal profession needs to create a word that describes this type of "institutionalized child abuse".

Calcium Hydroxide is another root-filling cement. It is a very popular and well-researched material. It is regarded by some holistic dentists as the panacea for root filling. It has been shown to migrate easily and far from the root canal, and it causes chronic inflammatory reactions in the tissue around the end of the root (i.e., the periodontal ligament and the bone).[292,293] It also swells in the tooth and can crack the root. By the way, chronic inflammation is related to cardiac disease and the development of cancers.

All materials placed in a root canal either temporarily or permanently are *toxic*.[294,295,296] Some are neurotoxic and harm the nervous system. Some are teratogenic and harm the unborn foetus. Some interfere with neurologic development of the foetus. Some are straight-out causes of cancer.

All these materials will leak out of the root-canalled tooth. All these materials will spread throughout your body. All these materials will affect your health, whether or not you display clinical symptoms. These materials will, in some cases, attach to proteins of your body and end up causing an autoimmune disease. Endodontists don't give a damn, because what they do is supported by their trade organizations. It's great to have a powerful organization that you can point the finger at and get away with doing what is proclaimed by that organization to be correct. No one takes responsibility.

If you are being offered a root canal by your local dentist, it may be a good idea to write down the names of all the materials that are to be used in your tooth, from the irrigant solutions, to the antimicrobials that will be in your tooth for a month or so, to the final root-filling materials that will be there forever. Then take this list and check it against the list in Appendix 1 (also at www.realdentalinfo.com). The information here is from the material safety data sheets that the manufacturer supplies with the products. If you have a product that is not listed, simply go to a search engine and type in "[product name] + msds." Pay close attention to the toxicological and environmental sections. If you have a latex allergy, then remember that the gutta percha point in your tooth could set off a permanent allergic reaction. Once you have read this information, you can decide whether you want to go ahead with the proposed "treatment". You might decide to go back and question your dentist about it. Be aware also that all of these materials are approved by the TGA and FDA, just as they approve of amalgam and vaccines containing mercury.

Remember also that at least 17 per cent of all root fillings will extend far beyond the end of the root. These materials are consequently inserted directly into the bone.

The Allergic Way—The Second Way

In 1951 The American Dental Association published a statement that "The bacteria at the focus may undergo autolysis or dissolution. Some of the products of this dissolution, diffusing into the blood or lymph, may sensitise in an allergic sense, various tissues of the body ... A later diffusion of these products on reaching the sensitized tissue may call forth an allergic reaction."

Dr Joseph Issels states, "Antibodies are formed to fight these substances, (the neurotoxins) eventually leading to the destructive processes in toxified cells. Since the organ-destroying antibodies or defence enzymes are excreted by the kidneys, they can be diagnosed in the urine. These toxins can easily begin the process of autoimmune diseases."

Everybody knows this, so why is it still a question? Anything in the tooth—the toxic, gangrenous breakdown products, the endotoxins produced by the bacteria, and the toxic materials that are implanted into the tooth—can create an allergic reaction. This reaction may be as simple as an annoying rash or as complex as full-blown autoimmune diseases! Very few medical people would consider a dead tooth as a cause of Crohn's or Hashimoto's disease. Causes are rarely looked for. They would not consider a dead tooth as a cause of eczema or persistent rashes.

Latex allergies are common in our industrialized world. Gutta Percha Points are largely latex. They are cemented into the root canal to fill it. They too often extend far beyond the root into the bone. This ancient thinking means exposure for many allergic patients without any consideration by the dentists. They do not consider latex and GP as the same. I have seen several patients where this has been an issue. After removing just the root filling for one of my patients, most of her allergic symptoms disappeared in a couple of weeks. They completely disappeared when the tooth came out. Any of the ingredients in any of the materials can set off an allergic reaction.

No one knows the interactions of all the materials implanted in a dead tooth, so no one can make such a diagnosis. I believe that the only real way of doing this is with electro-dermal screening, which is almost illegal in Australia. Isn't it a little bit interesting why these wonderful diagnostic tools are so heavily suppressed?

Ethics and Bugs

Research published in the *Journal of Endodontics* in 1992 tells us that the most frequently isolated bacteria from dead teeth will cause a very wide range of diseases.[297]

In 2005, however, the American Dental Association was happy to admit that it is impossible to sterilize a tooth and is *not* in the slightest concerned about the anaerobic infections that remain: "Microbes do remain in the dentinal tubules of endodontically treated teeth but pose no health hazard."[298]

E. faecalis is not a health threat, according to this bastion of ethics. Neither are any other organisms that live in a tooth! Neither do they care about the endotoxins produced by the microbes which spread through your body. In fact, the whole idea that bugs in a tooth could affect your health has been whitewashed for as long as root canal procedures have existed.

In 1996, the British Dental Association expressed similar views. Their statements are a little more emphatic. "The British Dental Association is satisfied that there are no grounds for believing that endodontic treatment **could cause general health problems**." "… none of this research has found any link between pulpless or endodontically-treated teeth and any of the **so-called degenerative diseases**." "It is **well known** that total sterility of the root canal system is impossible and that the **aim is thorough cleansing** and **obturation**." (Obturation means filling and sealing) "The healthy patient's immune system will then cope with any **transient bacteraemia**. Those patients at risk due to an existing medical condition can be given **antibiotic** protection." "**Infective endocarditis** arising from a dental procedure is also **not a focal infection** because the bacteraemia occurs at the time of treatment and is not due to the presence of a pulpless or root-filled tooth." "Dentists who are asked to extract a tooth on the grounds of press reports about the focal theory will refuse to do so, on **ethical grounds**. It would also be unethical of a dentist to promote extraction of root-filled teeth as a means of **alleviating illness**."[299]

The mere mention of ethics instils fear into the profession, and everyone runs a mile. How else do you maintain a position of superiority and control. If the PTO considers a treatment unethical, the dentists know that if they oppose this position and treat anyway, they will not have much legal support if there is a complaint.

In another universe, the term "ethical" could mean telling the patient that the dead tooth can cause cancer. "Ethical" could mean telling the patient that none of the aims of RCP are achievable. "Ethical" could mean that the dentist must display a sign, as in the state of California, that says, "Root canal treatments and restorations, including fillings, crowns and bridges, use chemicals known to the state of California to cause cancer."[300] "Ethical" could mean explaining to the patient the repercussions of a tooth loaded with anaerobic bacteria and their toxins, which escape from the tooth all of the time, creating a permanent (not a transient) bacteraemia. Usually the immune system is *not able to cope* with this situation, as the toxins that the anaerobes produce are very effective at destroying the immune system. I know this may seem like a strange concept, but ethics could also mean telling the truth!

"It is <u>well known</u> that total sterility of the root canal system is impossible."

Now that this has become a well-known fact, we no longer have to worry about it. If there is nothing that you can do about something, then just ignore it, as though the aim of sterilization is now a wrong approach! They are rewriting the textbooks! They recommend a "thorough cleansing" instead of sterilization. They should define what a "thorough cleansing" is and then explain how they know that they have achieved it. Is it a "really good" cleansing or a "merely good" one? Why do we even bother with autoclaves when such an austere organization takes such a cavalier attitude to infection control?

"Just do your best and make sure the canal is well sealed." Oops, they forgot to mention that the well-sealed canal is also an illusion.

At least the BDA had the decency to tell the truth about bacteria being forced through the end of the root during root canal procedures. Bacteria and their toxins, and a whole range of debris particles of dead tissue, are forced through the end of the root and into the bone, and thereafter to the rest of the body via the blood and lymph. This occurs *every time the dentist is filing the tooth.*

The Mayo Clinic defines bacterial Endocarditis as "an infection of the endocardium, which is the inner lining of your heart chambers and heart valves. Endocarditis generally occurs when bacteria, fungi or other germs from another part of your body, such as your mouth, spread through your bloodstream and attach to damaged areas in your heart. If it's not treated quickly, endocarditis can damage or destroy your heart valves and can lead to life-threatening complications."[301]

By denying that this is a focal infection, the BDA are disagreeing not only with the Mayo Clinic but with most of the medical world and research published in their own journals. I'm not sure whether their position is very brave or just very stupid. Bacterial endocarditis is only one of the many possible outcomes of bacteria spreading from the dead tooth to the rest of the body. *It is a focal infection.*

The bacterial spread from the tooth does not just happen when they are forced through the end of the root. Bacteria are coming from the dead tooth *all* the time. They and their toxins are constantly coming out of the tooth and floating around in your body. This is a *permanent bacteraemia*, and to pretend it isn't constitutes ignorance at best and possibly criminal intent at worst! There is nothing transient about this infective process. It is a 24-7 exposure just like mercury from amalgam. The immune system will eventually give up on the fight against this permanent bacteraemia.

How long do you want to keep taking antibiotics to cope with the permanent bacterial flood into your bloodstream? The BDA suggests this only for people who are medically compromised, whatever the hell that means. If you have one amalgam filling in your teeth, your kidneys' filtration system will be reduced by about 60 per cent.[302] Is that enough to be medically compromised? If you are drinking fluoridated water, you're medically compromised. The BDA seems to have no concern about wiping out your good gut bacteria for the sake of keeping an infected toxin factory in your mouth. Overprescription of antibiotics is strongly associated with antibiotic resistance in all sorts of bacteria, but this great PTO is not concerned about that either. Mercury in the mouth or at the end of the root will also create antibiotic-resistant bacteria.[303,304,305] The BDA certainly doesn't have a problem with this, not even ethically.

Unfortunately, most dentists reading the PTO propaganda will believe every word. They will even believe that their interpretation of ethics is correct. They will even repeat it word for word to their patients.

At least the folks at the BDA are satisfied in their knowledge that a dead tooth cannot in any way affect one's health. That is certainly reassuring! The gospel will not be questioned. I wonder whether the well-known evangelist of the 1960s, Billy Graham, took instruction from these organizations?

This BDA statement was released at a time when most dentists in Britain, who were working on the National Health Scheme, used the material called "N2" as the final filling for root canals. Clearly the BDA have no problem with this carcinogen being implanted into literally thousands of British citizens every year. It must be ethical to cause widespread cancer.

A paper published in the *European Journal of Oral Science*, also from 1996, regarding bacteria coming from the tooth, states that the "anaerobic microorganisms will be found in the blood, and the source in each case is the dead tooth."[306]

This study used some of the most current and sophisticated diagnostic testing, which proved that the bacteria inside a tooth will travel throughout the body. It also demonstrated that the actual *procedure of root therapy will force bacteria from the tooth into the rest of the body.*

The statement from the BDA is also from 1996. Getting with the times is obviously *not* one of the strengths of this private trade organization!

Focal Infection—The Third Way

The clear statement from the American Dental Association from 1951, is denied in their 2005 position statement: "Root canal fillings are safe. The Focal Theory of Infection does not apply as related to endodontically treated teeth."

One thing to be clear about is that Focal Infection is *not* a theory. Neither is focal infection a conspiracy. It is a fact rather than a theory. The acceptance and understanding of focal infection has been around for well over one hundred years. The work of Rosenow, Billings, and Price, has never been shown to be flawed.

> Following is a partial listing of disease conditions addressed in the literature of Dr E. C. Rosenow, as discussed in a 1953 survey article.[307] (Rosenow, E.C., Streptococci in etiology of diverse diseases, including diseases of nervous system, J. Nerv. And Ment. Dis. 117: 415-428, May 1953.) Thanks to Dr S. H. Shakman for this compilation.

- Arthritis
- Cholecystitis
- Convulsions, post-influenzal
- Cystitis
- Diabetes
- Encephalomyelitis, equine
- Encephalomeningoradiculitis
- Erythema nodosum
- Ether convulsions, post-op.
- Eye diseases (lesions, ocular—iritis uveitis, etc.)
- Gastroenteritis
- Goiter and thyroiditis,
- exophthalmic
- Gynecology cystic ovaries
- Herpes simplex
- Herpes zoster
- Hiccup, epidemic (and post-operative)
- Mental Illness
- Multiple sclerosis

- Mumps (epidemic parotitis)
- Myasthenia gravis
- Myocardial lesions
- Myositis
- Nervous system diseases
- Neuritis
- Neuralgia, intercostal and trigeminal
- Parotitis (mumps)
- Pulmonary diseases
- Respiratory tract infections and diseases
- Rheumatic fever
- Sclerosis
- Sneezing
- Spasmodic neuralgia and torticollis
- Sydenham's Chorea or St. Vitus' dance
- Transverse myelitis
- Ulcerative colitis
- Ulcer, stomach
- Urinary calculus
- Vegatonic neurosis

A small taste of the current literature shows that dead teeth can cause a wide range of diseases:[308]

- immune system diseases [309]
- infection of hip replacements [310]
- abscess of eyes [311]
- cervical cellulites and mediastenitis [312]
- Necrotizing fascititis [313]
- coronary atherosclerosis [314]
- sinusitis [315]
- Multiple Sclerosis [316]
- brain abscess [317,318]
- brain cancer [319]
- central nervous system damage [320, 321, 322,323]
- Trigeminal Neuralgia [324,325,326,327,328,329]

In 1996, a special supplement written by Professor Paul Abbott appeared in the Australian Dental Association news bulletin:

> … one of the major advances in dentistry was the recognition of the role of micro-organisms in the pathogenesis of pulpal and periapical diseases although this discovery did have some detrimental effects on the practise of dentistry when Hunter (1911) popularized the *theory* of focal infection. This theory stated that a focus of infection in the oral cavity could lead to various systemic diseases. Many operators claimed that all infected teeth and apical radiolucencies were harmful and should be removed since these teeth were a 'menace to health and happiness'. Subsequently, the focal infection *theory* became severely criticized with *well-controlled research* leading to the dismissal of this *theory* and a return to a more conservative approach to dentistry.[330]

The *"well-controlled research* leading to the dismissal of this theory" is nothing but smoke and mirrors. Where are these well-controlled studies? No one has ever seen them. I asked twenty years ago where they are but have not yet received a reply from Professor Abbott or anyone else. It is really fantastic that the role of microorganisms in disease was acknowledged until that bad man called Hunter came along and demonstrated that dead teeth were a great source of focal infection. Suddenly the focal infection "theory" started costing the dentists lots of money as the world was plunged into the dark ages of tooth extraction and gummy smiles. Suddenly, focal infection does not apply to root-canalled teeth. "Conservative approach", I think, refers to doing the same as you always have and making sure you give dead teeth a good cleaning. This will ensure that big pharma will continue to profit from the diseases that we dentists are creating in our millions of root canal procedures each year. As George Orwell stated, "In a time of universal deceit, telling the truth is a revolutionary act."

Dr Huggins, in an interview, was asked whether all root-canalled teeth should be removed. He replied, "… only if the patient had a concern for their health."

It is well accepted that any form of oral surgery will produce a bacteraemia and that this may cause infections in susceptible tissues, especially the heart. What is less accepted is that other sources of sepsis exist in the mouth. These include

    a) Periodontal infections,
    b) Cavitations in the bone,
    c) Peri-implantitis around the implants, and
    e) Dead teeth—root-canalled or not!

Just eleven years after writing that the focal infection "theory" had been debunked by well-controlled research, Professor Abbott quotes from a paper written by the then Dean of Dentistry at Queensland University, Prof L Walsh. This paper clearly demonstrates the validity of the focal infection and shows that infection spreading from teeth may cause the following:[331]

- Osteomyelitis of the mandible
- Maxillary sinusitis and orbital abscess
- Wound botulism
- Ludwig's angina (Heart)
- Necrotizing fasciitis
- Cavernous sinus thrombosis (brain)
- Persistent pyrexia of unknown origin (high temperature)
- Septicaemia—*Streptococcus milleri* and *Pseudomonas*
- Septicaemia with disseminated intravascular coagulation
- Pulmonary abscess (lung)
- Pyogenic hepatic abscess (liver)
- Brain abscess
- Brain abscess and acute meningitis
- Paraspinal abscess and paraplegia (spine)
- Bacterial endocarditis (heart)

- Splenic abscess (spleen)
- Mediastinal abscess and pneumonia (chest)

(Professor Walsh's paper was also used as a reference listed at National Naval Medical Centre in Bethesda, Maryland, as part of their reading requirement. I guess they must be taking it seriously?)

Professor Abbott seems to want to have his pie and eat it too. I wonder who he really agrees with. Sadly, this situation in dentistry is all too common and leaves the general practitioner floundering in the quagmire of indecision and conflicting information, from the same revered professor. Perhaps it is a good thing that so many dentists are mercury poisoned and cannot remember what was said eleven years earlier?

In his paper, Professor Walsh clearly states that abscesses on dead teeth can cause both bad health and death. He goes on to list a number of disorders of the immune system which will make patients more susceptible to these dental infections:

> Low neutrophil count, cancer treatment with chemotherapy or radiotherapy, cyclic neutropenia, cytotoxic therapy, benign chronic neutropenia, depressed neutrophil function, Down's syndrome, poorly controlled diabetes mellitus, Crohn's disease,

> Chediak-Higashi syndrome, generalized depression of cell mediated immunity, leukaemias, advanced HIV disease advanced malignancy, bone marrow transplant recipients, organ transplant recipients, treatment of auto-immune diseases with immunosuppressive agents such as cyclosporin A, poor tissue healing, localized radiotherapy (e.g., for head and neck cancer) malnutrition.

These conditions allow for an increased chance of infection spreading from a dead tooth. Clearly these conditions should be taken into account when deciding what to do with the tooth. Clearly these conditions should preclude RCP on any tooth. This information is *not* considered by endodontists, oral surgeons, or any other dentists. It is also not considered by oncologists. Neither is there mention of the cancers that are directly caused by medicaments placed inside the tooth, and the thioethers and methyl mercaptans from the anaerobic bacteria in the tooth.

Quintessence International, one of the most highly respected dental journals in the world, stated in 1997, "The detrimental effect of focal infection on general health has been known for decades. Chronic dental infections may worsen the condition of medically compromised patients."[332]

So where is the "well controlled research"? The above quotes come from people who are well respected leaders of dentistry in Australia. They make the rules for the dentists to follow. They contradict and support each other, to the detriment of any logic being taught to the students.

In October 1996, the *Journal of Periodontology* devoted a whole issue to this subject. It showed that periodontal disease was a major cause of systemic diseases, which include coronary heart disease, diabetes, and low birth weight. Many other published articles are now appearing with this information.

A marker known as C-reactive protein, or CRP, can now identify the systemic low-grade infections causing systemic inflammation. It is always elevated in patients with periodontitis.

Chronic or acute inflammation of the periodontal ligament (the tissue around a tooth joining it to the bone) may lead to heart disease because it might cause this low-level systemic inflammation. Since the chemical by-products of the degradation itself, along with the autoimmune response, may spill over into the bloodstream and lymphatic system, triggering the liver to make other proteins that *inflame the arterial walls and clot blood, atherosclerosis* and ultimately, *heart attack* may result.[333]

Note that the same bugs that are in periodontal disease are also in dead teeth. A root-canalled tooth will always have inflammation in the periodontal ligament at the end of the root, whether this is visible or not on an X-ray. This is true 100 per cent of the time!

> The organisms that spread from a dental focus include bacterial, viral, and fungal organisms that survive in such foci.[334,335,336,337,338,339,340] It will also include the toxins called endotoxins, produced by anaerobic organisms in the foci.[341,342,343,344,345,346]

> "… The ability of oral bacteria and their toxins to spread from a site of focal infection, not only in the mouth, but also to other sites in the body is well documented in the scientific and medical literature … Any oral bacteria which can migrate throughout the whole body and cause a variety of systemic diseases, as numerous studies have shown …"[347] (Prof Boyd Haley)

The following diseases are listed in a paper entitled "Systemic Diseases Caused By Oral Infection", published in 2000: "Cardiovascular disease, coronary heart disease: atherosclerosis and myocardial infarction, stroke, infective endocarditis, bacterial pneumonia, low birth weight & diabetes mellitus, cerebral infarction, acute myocardial infarction, abnormal pregnancy outcome, persistent pyrexia, idiopathic trigeminal neuralgia, toxic shock syndrome, systemic granulocytic cell defects, chronic meningitis."[348] (Published in Microbiology Reviews - This paper is referenced with 158 references)

The bacteria in a tooth can and do travel throughout the body. There is now research which demonstrates the presence of oral bacteria in the uterus and amniotic fluid. These uterine infections can lead to preterm birth in pregnant women.[349,350]

Arthritis is one of the most common conditions associated with dead teeth. A relevant case study appears in the 2002 literature.

> This report describes a remission of rheumatoid arthritis (RA) of 16 years duration, apparently caused by the extraction of endodontically well-treated, healthy looking teeth. The only clue that the teeth were contributing to the disease pathogenesis in this case of RA was that the patient was able to reproducibly induce severe attacks of arthritis after prolonged, heavy pressure on some of his teeth treated with root canal fillings. After extraction, a small pus layer was found to cover the apices of the clinically healthy looking teeth. The rheumatoid factor (RF) became negative and the patient remained symptom free for the next 16 years.[351]

So the perfect-looking root-filled teeth were far from perfect when examined after extraction. They all showed a pus layer, indicating a chronic infection coming from the tooth. The X-ray image showed a normal-looking tooth without an abscess. The perfect-looking root-canalled tooth is so far from safe it should be an embarrassment to the whole of modern dentistry and medicine. When the patient bit down hard, the roots acted like pistons, which forced the toxins from this pus layer to be distributed to the rest of the body. Surely that's not so hard for the professors to understand! Do rheumatologists have any idea about the diseases they are treating?

Arthritis, in its various manifestations, is one of the most common end results of the poisons from dead teeth. Just as headaches and migraines tend to disappear when amalgam is removed and the body detoxifies, so, too, does arthritis often improve after the dead teeth are removed. Did you know that taking Boron and Magnesium will assist arthritic conditions more than most anti-inflammatory drugs? It's not only the elderly and frail that succumb to dental infections. Dr Issels relates some other research about children:

Above all, bacterial dissemination tends to produce microfoci or microthrombi in veins, and they in turn have a tendency to thrombosis or thrombophlebitis, possibly with concomitant embolism.

A Russian scientist Shakow carried out an investigation involving more than "1200 young pupils at a boarding school. Over a period of six years, it was seen that students with devitalized teeth had three times as many illnesses as those with healthy dentition. By removing devitalized teeth in these young patients, up to eighty percent of their illnesses were cured … there is no root treatment which does not inevitably produce foci."

The medical literature is replete with references to focal infection. As of February 2019, Medline, the largest source of published scientific medical studies, lists 2,023 entries for "Focal Infection and 2,222 for 'Focal Infection Dental'. There were 408 publications from 2007 till 2019. They clearly do not exist as far as the dental PTOs are concerned. There is a very complete list on my website.

An Adelaide coroner has warned people not to neglect their dental health after finding that a simple infected tooth led to the death of a man in 2002.[352]

Now and Then

The term torticollis is derived from the Latin words *tortus* for twisted and *column* for neck. It is a condition in which the muscles on one side of the neck are in spasm and you cannot turn your head. It is difficult to live with and can be quite painful. The modern neurological way of treating this is to inject botulism into the effected muscles. This makes them relax. Botox has gained attention in weird places. Now we can treat without ever looking for a cause.

Dr Price had such a patient who suffered greatly for many years. He found a dead tooth in her mouth. He removed the tooth, and the woman improved overnight. He also took a biopsy of the neck muscle. From the extracted tooth and from the muscle tissue in the biopsy, he prepared a filtrate of dissolved materials. This liquid he injected under the abdominal skin of a number of rabbits. Of these rabbits, 100 per cent developed paralysis from the mid-spine down, and all died within six weeks. He repeated these types of experiments with many rabbits and with dead teeth from various people with many different health conditions. In every case, the results were similar. The rabbits rapidly developed the diseases that were evident in the patients from which the teeth were extracted. These experiments were meticulously done and recorded over many years. These were similar to the results obtained by Rosenow, Mayo, and Billings. The creation of the similar disease state is called "elective localization." As mentioned earlier, this elective localization was demonstrated literally thousands of times by these researchers.

Just a small sampling of the recent research demonstrates the accuracy and correctness of Price's findings and shows the relationship of infection from dead teeth and the following conditions:

- Infection of the orbit of the eye caused by oral bacterial infection [353]
- Managing periorbital space abscess, Secondary to dentoalveolar abscess [354]
- Abscess of the orbit arising 48 hours after root canal treatment of a maxillary first molar [355]
- *T. Denticola* … substantiating its importance in oral and linked systemic conditions [356]
- … the detection, identification, and quantification of a defined phylotype of archaea in infected root canals [357]
- Organisms found in common dental plaque are capable of producing abscesses at a variety of sites in the body [358]
- Cystic Fibrosis has also been associated with oral bacteria [359]
- Many oral bacteria have been shown to be able to cause premature and low birth weight children. [360] Oral infections can Induce Premature and Term Stillbirths [361]

- *Fusobacterium nucleatum* is a gram-negative anaerobe ubiquitous to the oral cavity. It is associated with periodontal disease. It is also associated with preterm birth and has been isolated from the amniotic fluid, placenta, and chorioamnionic membranes of women delivering prematurely[362]
- Transmission of an uncultivated *Bergeyella* Strain from the oral avity to Amniotic Fluid in a Case of Preterm birth[363]
- Oral bacteria can migrate into the uterus during pregnancy[364]
- Sperm are also susceptible – "A direct causal relationship between dental primary diseases and asymptomatic bacteriosperms, which probably leads to subfertility, must be concluded. ..."[365]
- Infection of pulpally involved teeth near the maxillary sinus sometimes spreads into the sinus and causes serious complications - persistent pathological antral alterations[366]
- Brain Abscess following Dental Infection after root treatment of teeth #22 & #35[367]
- A case is reported here which implicated an endodontically treated primary molar in the aetiology of a brain abscess in a boy with congenital cyanotic heart disease[368]
- Some brain cancers can be caused by infection in a tooth[369]
- There is now evidence of demyelenation of the Gasserian Ganglion after damage as far away as a tooth pulp.[370,371,372,373]
- Preclampsia associated with infection by oral bacteria[374]
- Brain and liver abscesses caused by oral infection[375,376,377,378,379,380]
- Molecular and immunological evidence of oral Treponema in the human brain and their association with Alzheimer's disease[381]
- Three cases of infection of total hip replacements following root canal therapy in 2 cases and periodontal surgery in 1 case[382]
- The association between periodontal disease and joint destruction in rheumatoid arthritis is supported in the current literature. A strong association was found between wrist and periodontal bone destruction[383]
- There is a relationship between diabetes in pregnant and non-pregnant women and oral infections[384]

- These data suggest that type 2 diabetes is associated with an increased risk of Parkinson's disease.[385]
- In 118 patients with deep-space head and neck infections, it was found that over 70% had the initial site of infection in the mouth.[386]
- At least 10% to 12% of sinusitis is caused by dental infections.[387] There is a linear relationship between the incidence of sinusitis and that of Multiple Sclerosis.
- *S. mutans* as a possible causative agent of cardiovascular disease.[388,389]
- Periodontal disease is associated with the development of early atherosclerotic carotid lesions [390]
- A Positive Association Between Periodontal Disease And Coronary Heart Disease [391]
- Oral bacterial infection promotes coronary artery and aortic atherosclerosis [392,393,394,395,396]
- "This study shows that elimination of advanced periodontitis by full-mouth tooth extraction reduces systemic inflammatory and thrombotic markers of cardiovascular risk."[397]
- Atherosclerosis and coronary heart disease [398,399,400,401,402]
- A wide variety of bacteria, including oral bacteria, was found to colonize aortic aneurysms and may play a role in their development. Several of these microorganisms have not yet been cultivated.[403,404]
- Acute Coronary Syndrome linked to periodontal infections [405,406]
- "... *viable E. faecalis* entombed at the time of root filling could provide a long-term nidus for subsequent infection."[407]
- "Neither single- nor multiple-visit root canal treatment, eliminated E. faecalis completely from dentinal tubules."[408]
- Dental disease contributes to increased risk of stroke [409]
- Toxins found in dead teeth and periodontal pockets could induce liver injury including inflammation and oxidative damage [410]
- Oral infections can cause dermatitis [411]
- Cervical cellulitis and mediastinitis caused by odontogenic infections [412]

- Cervical necrotizing fasciitis of odontogenic origin [413]
- Various immunologic diseases may be associated with Pulpal-Periapical Disease [414]

There are very few areas of the body that are not affected. Of the fifty-four sources provided for the items above, twenty-four of them come straight out of the dental journals themselves. The rest are medical journals. Don't any specialists read their own journals, or is it all in the "too hard" basket? Surely the deans and professors would keep up to date with the literature; otherwise, they could not be teaching properly.

In 2006, the *International Endodontic Journal* published the following: "… long-standing inflammation may have systemic effects and influence general health … long-standing inflammation has been related to the risk of cardiovascular diseases."[162] published that:

"Long-standing inflammation" is what is found at the end of *every* single root-filled tooth. *All* dead teeth, whether root filled or not, have inflammation about the end of the root no matter what the X-ray looks like. *All* dead teeth, whether root filled or not, can give you a heart attack!

I have not yet met a cardiologist who could hear this information. It always produced a cognitive dissonance!

Cardiovascular disease is the number one killer in America and Australia, yet our glorious professors and deans are happy to promote the creation of this situation. Of course, you will never hear them admit to this. The best anyone gets out of them is that the possibility is still being researched and the jury is still out on this and just about any subject that might detract from their incomes.

And it goes ON AND ON AND ON!!! Lifting the lid on this Pandora's box clearly demonstrates the spread of infection from teeth to the rest of the body, *and* the dental profession's arrogant dismissal of published scientific research.

I highly recommend the books from Drs Robert Kulacz and Thomas Levy *"The Roots of Disease," "The Toxic Tooth,"* and Dr Levy's book *"Curing the Incurable."* Dr Levy is an American Cardiologist. His list of certifications and publications is impressive: https://www.peakenergy.com/About-Dr-Levy.php. Dr Robert Kulacz is a well-respected American Oral Surgeon. He stepped across the dental association's line in the sand.

Dr Kulacz is now listed on "Dentalwatch," a site dedicated to demonizing anyone that goes against the system. Several years ago, I and many others were listed on a similar site called "Quackwatch." At one stage I put a link to Quackwatch on the front page of my website. I introduced it with "This site has one of the most comprehensive lists of superb medical and dental practitioners in the world." I was honoured to be in such good company. The same author called Stephen Barrett wrote the articles for Quackwatch and Dentalwatch. I should mention that these sites did not waste time with people whose treatments didn't work. Only those who were becoming known for helping people heal. Dr Kulacz practises the way an oral surgeon should. You can read about what Dr Kulacz says regarding Stephen Barrett at https://coletrex.com/articles/stephen-barrett-and-quackwatch. I must say I am looking forward to Stephen Barrett reviewing this book.

The Australian Dental Association admits that bacteria are *not* entombed inside a root-filled tooth. They escape easily and spread throughout the body! The spread of bacteria, other microorganisms, and their toxins from a dead tooth will happen whether the tooth is root-canalled or not. In 2006, the *International Endodontic Journal* published the following: "… it may be concluded that there is insufficient evidence to support the assumption that residual bacteria are entombed in the canal system in vivo by placement of a root filling."[415]

A Train to the Brain

The Trigeminal Nerve is the 5th cranial nerve emanating from the base of the skull and supplying sensation to the face, head, neck, and teeth.

It also has a variety of motor functions. It has the largest ganglion of all the cranial nerves and a huge area of the body to draw from. "Virtually any irritation of the dental pulp or 'amputation stump' has the potential of transporting alegesic toxins throughout the Trigeminal system whether they be of chemical or bacterial origin."[416,417,418]

"Amputation stump" refers to the bit of nerve that is left after the main canal is supposedly cleaned out (that last one millimetre).

Some of the toxins and bacteria are carried directly back to the brain by what is called "retrograde transport" along nerve fibres.[419,420,421] Back in 1973, it was demonstrated that these toxins can be transported back to the brain along nerve fibres at a rate of about 250 millimetres per day.[422]

Bacteria can also enter the brain via the non-valved venous plexus, as Professor Stortebecker demonstrated so vividly. Dye was injected into the bone of the mandible (lower jaw) and within minutes filled the whole of the venous system inside the skull.[423,424,425]

There is also evidence of transport of bacteria via the macrophages. These are white cells of the immune system, which are able to cross the blood–brain barrier.[426] They carry heavy metals, such as mercury and aluminium, as well as bacteria and toxins across the blood–brain barrier and deposit them in the brain.

Everything that is in the tooth can spread throughout the body, and this includes the brain. Brain tumours are seen as the realm of the brain surgeon and oncologist. These people look at the end result and decide how to remove the tumours or not. They never look at the cause, which is often a dead tooth. They never look at oral X-rays. Dental diagnosis and interpretation of dental X-rays should be a part of every medical student's undergraduate training.

The medical world must begin to take responsibility for the mouth even if dentists don't. As Dr Hal Huggins stated, "Root canals are only dangerous if you have a concern for your health."

A Cat Amongst the Pigeons

Honesty in the dental world is rare, but oh, so refreshing when it happens.

In 1976, the *Journal of Endodontics* published that spread of infection from a tooth may result in cases of "… debilitation or dehydration, diabetes, cancer, blood dyscrasias, malnutrition, vitamin deficiency, leukaemia, multiple myeloma, and diseases of the liver or kidney."[427]

In 1996, the *Journal of Dental Research* published a landmark study by Professor Hubert N. Newman. It was edited by Professor Irwin Mandel, the Associate Dean for Research at the Columbia University School of Dental and Oral Surgery. Thus, it is well authored by highly respectable people. This paper has over two hundred references and concludes with **"Focal Infection should be a major concern in dentistry."** The author states,

> "From the oral foci, microorganisms—bacterial, viral, or other—or their products, may gain entry to the deeper tissues directly, by spreading along fascial planes, through bony cavities, or even along blood or lymph vessels or nerves, or via salivary gland mucous surfaces. Can one die of such simple chronic infection? One may cite the coroner's court, but there is also extensive literature evidence.

> "… earlier workers had considered that different organisms selectively colonized specific loci - the theory of elective localization [Rosenow, 1919, 1921, 1923]. By this hypothesis, bacteria would localize from the source focus to the distant, systemic focus, and Rosenow demonstrated a targeting process in a series of experiments, reviewed by Hughes (1994). This should not surprise us. Micro-organisms cause infections of tissues, organs, or systems, clearly depending on an ability to survive and grow better in those loci - a clear extension of the principles of microbial ecology in general."

> "… perhaps the earliest relevant reference, none other than Hippocrates, whom he quotes as reporting a patient whose arthritis was cured by extraction of an infected tooth [Mayo, 1922]. Further, while we may think it a modern discovery that bacterial products rather than the whole cells are the source of focal infection, the same point was made many years ago [Swift et al., 1928], with further proof through the years [Schwab and Cromartie, 1957; Ebringer et al., 1989]. Lens and Beertsen (1988) showed that injection of an antigen into the gingiva produced (mouse) knee joint inflammation. Focal infection has been cited in arthritis of the knee [Morer, 1975] and infected joint prostheses [Rubin et al., 1976; Schurman et al., 1976; Jacobsen and Murray, 1980; Lindqvist et al., 1989]."[428]

Professor Newman lists many diseases associated with the spread of infection from teeth:

- Intracranial infections and Brain abscesses (often resistant to antibiotics)
- Meningitis
- Hemiplegia
- Metastatic paraspinal abscess
- Paraplegia
- Solitary lung abscesses (rare in the absence of teeth)
- Aspiration pneumonia of oral microbial origin
- Infective endocarditis (which remains the clearest instance of focal infection)
- Myocardial infarction
- Liver infections
- Inflammatory bowel disease
- Risk for low birth weight babies
- Nerves themselves may be affected, including such problems as actinomycosis of the Gasserian ganglion and trigeminal nerve anaesthesia

In his paper entitled "Serious complications of endodontic infections: some cautionary tales."[78] the past dean of dentistry at Queensland

University, Professor Walsh, states, "… diseases in the pulp will invariably extend through the apical foramen into the surrounding bone causing further problems."

How much more damning can we get? He is stating that disease in the tooth *will cause disease in the rest of the body*. His paper agrees with the writings of Dr Price in 1923. It agrees with the research of Rosenow and Billings. Yet he still teaches dental students to keep doing this procedure! A "noble" profession indeed! These "further problems" are exacerbated if the bacteria which escape from the tooth into the rest of the body are also antibiotic resistant.

Clearly the concept of Focal Infection is far from disproven by recent experiments. The literature ranging from 1920 to the present is definitive. Microorganisms and their toxins can escape from a tooth and localize in other tissues and create a new disease state. The ability of the toxins to sensitize a person to many other allergic states has also been confirmed. Whether the tooth has had a root canal procedure performed is irrelevant to the spread of these microorganisms and their toxins.

It's inconceivable that any dental association or dental school would dare suggest that focal infection is not a problem in endodontics. Yet they continue to teach this fallacious belief and procedure to dental students and dentists. Go to your dentist and ask him or her to remove a root-canalled tooth. Most likely you will be referred to a psychiatrist instead of an oral surgeon!

The German physician and cancer specialist, Professor Max Daunderer, was very vocal about the association between dental conditions and general health or lack of it. In an interview in 1998, he stated,

"The dental work we get from dentists is not something biological or medical. I'd say it is a technical thing, and the techniques give the dentists a number of very strong poisons to be implanted in the mouth. If you kill the tooth and then fill its root canal with mercury, formaldehyde, cortisone, streptomycin, arsenic, you are not doing a healthy thing. All this dentistry is just a sin against the biology of the body and a sin against the 'real' medicine."

A sobering comment by one of Germany's leading medical oncology professors.

7

Neural Medicine

• •

It is better to learn
what is probable about important matters,
than to be certain about trivial ones.

—Stevenson

There is another way that dead teeth may affect your health. It's time to dip our toes into the world of energetic fields and the interconnectedness of all life, at every level of interaction. Although the medical and dental worlds in Australia and America completely deny the information which follows, Neural Medicine is taught widely to undergraduate medical students in Germany.

Neural Focal Therapy: Energetic Interference and Medicine

Neural Focal Medicine originated in Germany about sixty-five years ago through a fortunate accident made by two brothers: Drs. Ferdinand and Walter Huneke.

The brothers were trying to help their sister, who suffered from severe migraines. Even with all of the various medications they tried over the years, her condition did not improve. Then one day one of the brothers accidentally injected a drug which contained a local anaesthetic into her vein. This medication was intended as an injection into the muscle, not the vein. Instead of killing her, it completely cured her migraines. This was the first time they witnessed such a profound cure through the use of an anaesthetic drug. It was called Procaine and was the first synthetic anaesthetic that followed the use of Cocaine. (The first local anaesthetic that was ever used was cocaine and it was injected around the eyeball by a very famous ophthalmologist called Sigmund Freud. I wonder if that is where psychiatry actually originated.)

The Hunekes continued to research this phenomenon, and some years later they were treating another patient and again by chance stumbled across what they termed a "Lightning Reaction" or in German the "Blitzkrieg Reaction," later to be called the "Huneke Reaction." This particular patient had for many years suffered from pains in her right shoulder and immobility of the shoulder and arm. No treatment had any effect to reduce the pain or mobility. On this day, she came to the Hunekes because a very old scar on her left leg had become inflamed, red, itchy, and generally uncomfortable. They injected Procaine superficially into the scar to try to reduce the discomfort. To their shock, they experienced the first lightning reaction. As though a light switch had been turned off, the pain in her right shoulder vanished completely, and immediately she regained the complete movement of her shoulder and arm.

Thus began a whole new understanding of the body's regulatory mechanisms.

From their findings, a new modality of medicine has developed, called Neural Medicine.

Anything which interferes with a pattern of health is called a Focus of Neural Interference. By interfering with the body's regulatory systems, the focus of interference will create a disease state in a different part of the body. The paradigm on which this is based needs to be fully understood and accepted and taught in medical and dental schools. If this is the first time you are reading the following quote, I warn you that it is a lot to get your head around. Persevere, because you will gain a new understanding of some of the most critical and subtle parts of what regulates our bodies. I've lost count of the number of times that I have read this, and each time different thoughts, memories, and connections happen. We are electrical entities and subtle energies. The best and most succinct description of what Neural Medicineis, and how it works, comes from Dr Peter Dosch, one of the world's leading experts in this field. He states in his book,

> Life is related not only to material aspects but also to energy. The nervous system is a power grid that links all cells and all organs, over which every item of information and all regulating impulses are transmitted and exchanged. Every single cell in the body is a tiny battery with a charge of 40 to 90 millivolts. Any stimulus (such as heat, cold, chemicals, injuries, etc) causes this potential to collapse. The cell's oxygen metabolism supplies it with the energy for immediately recharging itself to the normal voltage. After excessive stimuli (surgery, injuries, inflammatory reactions) it sometimes no longer succeeds in doing so completely. A cell that has become sick due to a permanent irritation has a lower membrane resting potential and can no longer restore itself to normality by its own endeavours. Accordingly, it can no longer fulfill its functions. Such a diseased region, e. g. a scar that has healed but still possesses some residual irritant capability, can send out irritant salvoes that overwhelm the stimulus-absorbing systems and can act as an interference transmitter. Congenitally weak organs, or organs weakened by a previous illness, have a reduced selectivity, like an old radio receiver

which receives the signals of several stations at the same time. They process the irrational information from the interference transmitter that they receive together with the correct signals and transform it into pathogenic circulatory dysfunctions and regulatory disorders.

An interference field produces a change in the cell environment and hence in the reactive capacity of individual organs and of the organism as a whole.[429]

The most common interference fields are the tonsils, followed closely by teeth and other dental conditions. This can be any dead tooth with or without a root canal, or it may be an impacted tooth or a cavitation deep in the bone. Impacted wisdom teeth can have a profound effect on the rest of the body. "Each individual has inherited or acquired weak points, and these are the first to come under stress when an interference field becomes active in the body. This also explains why the same interference field, for example chronically inflamed tonsils, can give rise to totally different disorders in different individuals; one may suffer from articular rheumatism, another may have glaucoma, a third may present with a slipped disc or asthma, and so on." [Dr Dosch]

These interference fields can either produce or potentiate disease states in other parts of the body, *often corresponding directly with the acupuncture meridian on which the interference is located.*[430,431,432]

Dr Ernesto Adler, a dental physician with over thirty years' experience in neural focal dentistry, has published an amazing volume of over three hundred pages of case studies, many of which he had followed for over twenty-five years.[433] These cases are described within the volume, some of which are associated with impacted wisdom teeth. Dead teeth and infected foci have been shown to be common neural interferences.

The way that the Neural Medicine doctor will treat these disturbances is to inject a local anaesthetic into the focus. In the case of dental foci, it is also imperative to remove the focus (i.e., extract the dead tooth, remove electrical interferences from metal fillings and/ or clean the cavitation). This local anaesthetic "introduces outside energy into tissues whose voltage level is reduced. It recharges the cells and protects them against renewed premature voltage loss. This repolarization by procaine (Professor Fleckenstein) restores the cell's normal functions and switches off the transmitter of interference signals, at least temporarily. When the injection is repeated at the same site, the organism learns to cope better each time with the restoration and maintenance of the correct potential."[1]

Most Western schools of medicine have a very fixed idea of what the regulatory systems of the body are—principally the brain and nervous system, in conjunction with the endocrine or hormonal system. Till recently we have not moved far beyond this. The German research, on the other hand, gives us a much larger picture of what the regulatory systems of the body are. Thankfully it incorporates explanations of how acupuncture and massage may work. Researchers like Pischinger and Kellner have even dissected the anatomical structure of acupuncture points and shown the physiological relationship of these points to the regulatory systems of the body.[434] No longer is acupuncture some sort of Asian witchcraft, as allopathic medicine has implied.

Basically, the concept of neural interference fields rests on the premise of a completely new and radically different understanding of what the body's regulatory systems are made of. The main features are the

- Extracellular tissue fluid,
- Capillary network,
- Nerve ending network, and
- Autonomic Nervous System [435]

Any area of scar tissue, foreign body, foreign chemicals (vaccinations and bee stings, for example), dead tissue, or chronically infected tissue, can interfere with the body's regulatory systems. Chronically inflamed tissue is included as a cause of neural interference. *All* root-canalled teeth have chronically inflamed tissue surrounding the end of the root. They have also been shown to induce inflammatory changes in other parts of the body by the release of neurotoxins. Consequently, other areas of the body may become weakened and diseased. Usually the diseased tissue (or the referred pain) will be in a part of the body which is distant from the area of the Neural Focus of Interference, and often on the same acupuncture meridian that the focus rests on. This is not the same as a focus of infection, but a focus of infection can, as we will see, act as a Focus of Neural Interference.

"… a (neural) focal disturbance is a chronically altered area of tissue, from which general diseases or focally separate, circumscribed processes in the organism, are initiated and maintained"[436]

If this sounds like hocus-pocus, be aware that in Germany most of the medical profession is trained, to some degree, in Neural Therapy. In Australia, very few doctors have even heard of it. The dental profession still thinks mercury is safe! If we are to understand the bizarre symptoms associated with dental conditions, we must understand the concept of neural medicine and the concepts of the regulatory mechanisms of the body. If we are to understand and treat our patients more correctly, we need to have a good grip on this concept of medicine. From this perspective, I believe that Germany and Switzerland are about twenty years ahead of the rest of the world, and China about three thousand years ahead.

Which area of the body is most interfered with by other people? Which part has the most things done to it—scars, surgery, infection, chronic infection, foreign body implants, and mechanical wear and tear? You guessed it—the mouth. Usually it is the dentists who create this Neural Focus.

Other forms of mass interference come from broad-spectrum vaccinations and additives in the water supply, such as fluoride, but no other area of medicine affects so many people so consistently.

Consequently, we find a large number of primary neural interferences in the mouth.

Dentistry causes this sort of interference on such a mass scale that everyone considers it normal. If you do not personally fit the bill, you will know someone who has in his or her mouth every conceivable form of insult that dentistry can offer. It is common to find mouths with a combination of several root-canalled teeth, amalgam fillings, titanium implants, gold crowns, and chrome-cobalt dentures, combined with routine six-monthly X-rays and fluoride poisoning! Go into any dental surgery any day of the week, and you will see mouths and treatments like this.

Electro-Acupuncture and Energy Medicine

In the 1950s, another German doctor, by the name of Reinholdt Voll, showed that the acupuncture points had a different electrical resistance to the skin on other parts of the body. He used miniscule electric currents to demonstrate the acupuncture meridians and many relationships between different parts of the body. Dr Voll is regarded as the father of Electro-Acupuncture. He was able to electrically map the acupuncture meridians. These were almost identical to Chinese Acupuncture meridians. He was able to map out the meridian that passed through each tooth. He mapped the relationship of each tooth to the rest of the body. Interestingly, the modern equipment that is used for electrodermal testing is completely based on Dr Voll's methods and findings.

As we might expect, his work is also ridiculed by the dental and medical establishments. They refuse to acknowledge that the mouth and body are connected. They refuse to acknowledge that the teeth and areas of the mouth are intimately connected with specific areas of the body. They acknowledge only the mechanical and aesthetic outcome of any particular dental procedure.

This dedication to mechanics is, in reality, a dedication to ignorance.

The following is from a wonderful book called *The Memory of Water*:

> ... it is not only the dominant position of a theory, of a discipline or of a scientific leader that is being threatened; the possibility that orthodox science might be wrong in this instance also threatens each individual's world view.

> Our relationship to knowledge in the West is one of domination. For instance the manner in which the western world has reacted to acupuncture is a case in point. Acupuncture developed empirically in a traditional culture and was used for several thousands of years. Recently scientists have substantiated that acupuncture points are indeed located where the tradition had situated them and that they can be measured by changes in the resistivity of the skin.[437]

Explanation: "resistivity of the skin" in this comment is describing the electrical resistance of acupuncture points as opposed to the rest of the skin. When a weak electrical current of only half a millivolt is passed through the body, one can detect the electrical resistance at different parts of the body. Voll and other researchers found that the acupuncture points had a completely different electrical resistance compared to the skin adjacent to them and the skin on the rest of the body.

The concept of energy flow in the body has been known for thousands of years. The Chinese were able to map these energy "meridians" and found relationships of the different parts of the body. They were able to understand the relationship of points on the skin to various organs and metabolic systems. They also found that these acupuncture meridians and points encompassed all aspects of people, from their physical bodies to their emotional bodies and spiritual bodies. These are all parts of one being.

By using the electrical resistance of the skin with minute electrical currents, Dr Voll found, for example, that the front teeth are on the Bladder meridian and that interference fields here may cause disturbances and disease in the kidneys, knees, and reproductive systems of the body. Wisdom teeth, on the Small Intestine meridian, can affect the heart. The upper molars and lower premolars, being on the Stomach meridian, may cause diseases in the breast. Many such relationships exist.

I used to place silk sutures rather than dissolving ones in most of my surgical cases (except those that came from far away) so that I had a chance to review the patients a week later when I removed them. Many times, after removing the upper molars or lower premolars in women, they would report a week later how the lumps in their breasts had disappeared in that week. Many of these lumps had been there for years, causing great distress to the women and their partners. Many of these patients thought it miraculous, and all were very grateful. Years later, most of these patients did not experience a return of the lumps. Many patients who had breast cancer also had dead teeth in these positions especially, but in other parts of the mouth as well.

The chapter of case studies includes many examples of neural interference and the resolution of the disease states after the interference was removed. Yes, they are anecdotal, and they are true.

If you search for images of 'Dental EAV Charts - images', you will find many on the web. They demonstrate these relationships. If you have a dead tooth, it is worth checking these charts against your own symptoms. (Also at www.realdentalinfo.com.)

Special Note

Many people become attached to these EAV relationships, and if a symptom is not listed on the chart, they believe that there is no relationship between disease and teeth. This may be the furthest thing from the truth, as *these charts are a guide only* and do *not* cover all possibilities. As this is another mechanism only, it must not be regarded as the only correct one. You may also be affected by the toxins from the bacteria and dead tissue that remain in the tooth, as well as the toxic chemicals the dentist seals into the tooth.

The focus can just as easily influence the immune system, the blood, and the hormonal and endocrine systems of the body. Psychological effects are also common outcomes of neural interferences. I have been very privileged to have seen firsthand the results of neural treatments. They can be very dramatic (e.g., when a pain in the knee disappears as the local anaesthetic is being injected into the extraction site). The pain can be stopped completely and long term by a single injection of anaesthetic.

The treatment is to remove the neural interference—take out the dead tooth! What sorts of diseases can we expect from a neural interference field? Anything from pain to cancer, and everything between!

"Secondary diseases can become established not only at individual organs or tissues but can also occur to a general extent as disorders of the autonomic nervous system, and as disorders in a psychosomatic context."[3]

The autonomic nervous system is that part of the nervous system which controls all of the unconscious functions of the body, such as heart rate, breathing rate, blood pressure, digestion, and crying etc. If the respiratory centre is affected, you may have trouble breathing or become asthmatic. One of the most common symptoms I have seen clinically associated with root-canalled teeth is Sinusitis. This is so common that I would suggest that of those with root-canalled teeth, at least 90 per cent have some degree of sinusitis or postnasal drip associated with them. I believe this to be a combination of neural interference and /or direct infection from the dead tooth. Later you will see the connections between sinusitis and Multiple Sclerosis.

The relationship of a neural interference to systemic disease conditions is very hard to demonstrate. Electrodermal Testing can establish the relationships. Often the healing of the disease state is the only thing that, in hindsight, relates the disease to the extracted tooth. However, if the neural interference is causing pain, then it may be possible in many cases to switch the pain off by the use of a little local anaesthetic—Procaine.

If procaine is injected into or around the interference (e.g., a dead tooth) and the pain in a distant part of the body suddenly disappears, then you can estimate fairly accurately that the interference is the cause of the pain. (Make sure the dentist uses local anaesthetic without any vasoconstrictor.) Procaine is best suited to this purpose, if available. The solution may be as simple as applying a local anaesthetic next to the root-canalled teeth, which switches off the Trigeminal Neuralgia. This is, in my opinion, much easier than brain surgery. To all the sceptical dentists out there, try it; you may be amazed at what you find. If that's too much to ask, try reading the published science.[438,439] It's important to understand that procaine can be used as a diagnostic as well as a treatment tool. If the dead tooth is shown to be an interference, however, it must be removed for proper long-term healing. If, as a dentist, this is still too much to ask, then at least let your patients read this information and make their own informed decisions, before dismembering parts of their brains!

Dr Issels says the following:

> ... these manifestations are based on depolarizing processes in the affected tissue. By elimination of the focus, the affected tissues may be repolarised.

> ... any focal surgery must be followed by desensitizing and neural-therapeutic measures. e.g. injection of Procaine.

It is essential that, after removing the dead tooth or cleaning the cavitation, the sockets that remain are washed with local anaesthetic to switch off any residual neural interference.

I don't know how to stress this enough. The variety of disease conditions that may result from a neural interference are as varied as your imagination. The diseases are far from imaginary though. It is critical for all in the healing professions to at least acknowledge the possibility; medicine's and dentistry's potentials are far greater than what our endodontists would have us believe.

From *The Holographic Universe*:

> Another feature that must be a part of the restructuring of science is a broadening of the definition of what constitutes scientific evidence ... when vast numbers of people start reporting the same experiences, their anecdotal accounts should also be viewed as important evidence. They should not be dismissed merely because they cannot be documented as rigorously as other and often less significant features of the same phenomenon can be documented. As Stevenson states, "I believe it is better to learn what is probable about important matters than to be certain about trivial ones."[440]

Professor Otto Neuner gives us a summary of the dental conditions that can and often do act as neural interference and thus cause disease in remote parts of the body:[441]

1. Teeth with dead roots
   a) With root fillings
   b) Without root fillings
   c) With incomplete root fillings
2. Disorders which are consequences of dead teeth
   a) Widening of the periodontal gap
   b) Chronic apical parodontitis
   c) Radicular cysts
   d) Odontogenous disturbance of the maxillary sinus
3. Conditions in sections without teeth
   a) Impacted teeth

b) Odontogenous tumours

c) Impacted remnants of tooth roots

d) Follicular cysts

e) Dermoid cysts

f) Sclerosis

4. Further disorders, such as the following:
   a) Gingivitis
   b) Parodontitis Marginalis
   c) Intra bony pockets
   d) Subgingival tartar
   e) Soft tissue inclusions
   f) Foreign matter of many different kinds
   g) Osteitis manifestations

5. Metallic influences in the oral cavity
   a) Corrosion of metallic materials in the mouth
   b) Release of metallic ions
   c) Charges arising in the metals present
   d) Electric tension and current in the oral cavity

6. Vital or diseased teeth with inflammatory or degenerative alterations in the dental pulp.

Neural interference does exist—in particular from dental foci.

8

Other Dead Tissue Issues

• •

Dentistry has a couple of other exciting treatments for dead teeth, with big dental names, that you should never allow to happen. Endodontics is not just about "saving" an adult tooth. It is about saving any tooth at any age, no matter what the consequences. The "apicectomy" and "pulpotomy" are two procedures that should never happen. "Cavitations" on the other hand, are holes in the bone that dentistry says have no clinical significance. They almost always do need to be treated, especially if you have pain or degenerative diseases like cancer or MS.

Apicectomy

Some years after having the root canal done and the gorgeous crown put on top, you may find that the original symptoms have returned. The tooth just doesn't feel right or the pain itself drives you back to the dentist. And now the dental ping-pong game begins again. You are returned to the endodontist to fix the big abscess visible on the X-ray. The endodontist consults the X-ray and has a look on his face between "there must be something wrong with you, as my work is faultless" and a quiet, detached excitement that you are going to spend a whole lot more money with him or her. Now the problem is so great, though, that the help of a very special oral surgeon is also going to be called for. Only a "great oral surgeon" is able to surgically cut off the end of the root, scrape out the abscess that is in the bone, put a filling in the end of the root, and sew you up again.

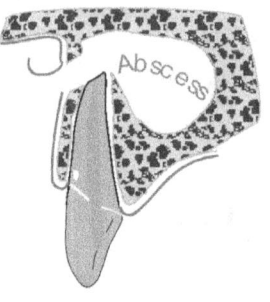

This procedure is called an Apicectomy because it removes the apex (or end) of the root. These days it is sometimes called "Surgical Retreatment". This is usually accompanied by what is called a "Retrograde Root Filling"—a filling in the end of the root. Removing the apex of the root supposedly allows the oral surgeon to reach the abscess and clean out "all of the infection". This completely ignores the fact that the tooth is still loaded with bacteria and will remain so. From here, you will go back to the endodontist to have the root canal redone and then back to the dentist to remake the crown that had to be destroyed. Inevitably, the ping-pong game will start all over again if you let it.

When 66 per cent of an endodontist's work is to redo failed root canal procedures, there must surely be something amiss. Know that when the endodontist redoes the root canal, he or she will be doing *exactly the same or worse* than what was done before. They too cannot sterilise or fill the tooth. There is just the expectation that the specialist can perform miracles. Doing the same thing over and over again and expecting a different result doesn't sound too intelligent to me. The reality is that no matter how much money and how many chemicals you throw at these bugs, they just smile and get on with what they do best. As time goes by and the happy little anaerobes have babies and generations grow older together inside your tooth, then the physiology becomes very unbalanced. There is no such thing as "physiological balance."

With a failure rate of over 30 per cent, as announced by the Australian Dental Association, retreatment or apicectomy are offered to try to fix the problem. Often an endodontist will try to "retreat" the tooth non-surgically, as this is more readily accepted by the patient and is more lucrative for the specialist. If this approach fails again (which it has to), then the surgical approach will be offered.

Apicectomy procedures are based on the belief that the only way the bugs and their toxins can get out of a tooth is through the hole at the end of the root. There is no acknowledgement that the bacteria and their toxins escape from the whole length of the root all the time. In this surgical procedure, the gum is lifted back off the bone and a hole is drilled into the bone to gain access to the end of the root and expose the abscess. The end of the root (the apex of the root) is cut off (apicectomy) and the abscess curetted out in an attempt at cleaning away whatever infection is in the bone—the supposed source of the problem.

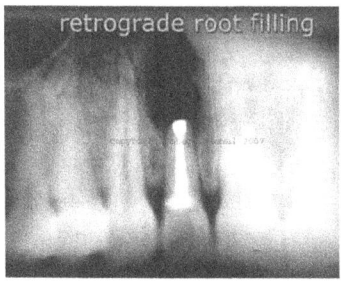

When the surgeon decides that all is clean, (on what basis no one knows), a filling is placed in the end of the root, with the aim of sealing the canal (and thus the tooth) so that nothing can escape in the future. This is called a "retrograde root filling," as it is put into the cut end of the root, deep in the bone.

Dentists don't acknowledge that the bacteria coming out of the tooth shouldn't have been there in the first place. It must be the patient's fault for not healing. "Do you smoke? Do you drink alcohol? How much? Do you take medications? Which type? Oh, you already have an illness that compromises your immune system. Did you pray enough? Perhaps you need a sleeping device." There are so many ways that it can be your fault. I have heard these delusional comments for over forty years from both specialists and GP dentists. My sarcasm rides on the backs of those who become sicker and sicker and spend more and more money on useless "treatments" that even the published science calls useless. Even the professors who teach this lunacy know that it is useless. It must be an ethical dilemma for them—or not.

Patients are usually *not* offered a choice of materials which will be implanted into the body. To date, the most common material used for this retrograde root filling has been mercury amalgam. That's right, your treatment is to have mercury amalgam implanted into the end of your tooth, deep in the bone. The mercury escapes from that amalgam filling 24/7. It travels to every cell in the body. The mercury will pass directly into your brain, as it passes through the bones of your nose and skull. It is a cumulative toxin. It is severely neurotoxic and cardiotoxic. It will travel across the placenta and breast milk and store preferentially in the foetus and newborn baby. This process has been associated with the development of autism.

This practice is against the advice of the manufacturers, who state clearly that their mercury amalgam should not be implanted into bone as a retrograde filling.[442]

Amalgam at the end of the root is an *implant of mercury directly into the brain*. Mercury has been shown to move through the bones of the palate and base of the skull and enter the brain directly.[443] Only arsenic and lead are more toxic than mercury. This malpractice is still legal in most countries.

The Australian Dental Association also agreed in 1996, that this is a useless procedure, but only on mechanical grounds: "Amalgam does not satisfy the conditions required of a root canal filling and its use must now be questioned ... although no studies have demonstrated which material would be ideal."[444]

"... no studies have demonstrated which material would be ideal" is pure Double-Speak, as there are no studies which have ever found a material that does seal the canals. Neither mercury amalgam nor any other filling material can effectively seal the end of the root canal.[445,446,447,448,449,450,451,452,453,454,455,456,457, 458,459, 460, 461, 462, 463,464,465!!!]

Nothing works. The whole procedure is based on illusion from beginning to end. If it were possible to sterilize the tooth, then this problem would not exist. There is a blanket denial that bacteria and toxins escape from the tooth the whole way down the length of the root, and not just through the apex. It would therefore make more sense to take the whole root out and not just the end of it. Fantasy and illusion reign in the minds of endodontists.

More recently, another material, ProRoot MTA, has been assigned the task of sealing the end of the root of a failed root canal procedure. Sealing the end of the root *always* means that the material is placed directly into, and in contact with, the bone, blood, lymphatic tissue, and nerve endings. Transport to the rest of the body via all these routes has been demonstrated. I apologize for repeating a section from the earlier part, but it's too important to turn back the pages. ProRoot MTA is accompanied by the following warning by the manufacturer on the Material Safety Data Sheet for this product:

> **This product contains chemicals (trace metals) known to the state of California to cause cancer, birth defects or other reproductive harm.**
>
> **INCOMPATIBILITY:**
>
> Wet ProRoot MTA Root Canal Repair Material is alkaline (caustic/basic). It is incompatible with acids, ammonia, ammonia nitrate, ammonium salts, aluminum metal and chlorine.
>
> Although small quantities of dust are not known to be harmful, ill effects are possible if larger quantities are consumed. Take care not to eat any of this product.
>
> **Carcinogenic potential:**
>
> The ingredients used to manufacture ProRoot MTA Root Canal Repair Material are not listed as carcinogens by NTP, OSHA or IARC. It may, however, contain trace amounts of substances listed as carcinogens by these organizations.

> **Crystalline silica**, a potential trace level contaminant, is now classified by IARC as a **known human carcinogen** (Group I). NTP has characterized respirable silica as "reasonably anticipated to be a carcinogen.

Considering the warnings, would you really care if it sealed the end of a root or not? Would you have this material implanted into your bone, within inches of your brain, after being misinformed that it will be implanted into your tooth? Believe it or not, this same material is now beginning to be used in children's teeth for pulpotomy treatments (covered in the next section). It is spun down the centre of the canal and is left in place for years. This *is prolonged exposure.*

Following are the words of Professor Abbott and the Australian Dental Association 1996, on the practice of apicectomy (with my emphasis added):[24]

> ... the problem of bacteria contained deep within the dentine or in areas of the canal beyond the apical three to four millimetres cannot be addressed ...

> ... there appears to be *little point in doing the above procedures in the apical few millimetres of the canal while still leaving bacteria in the rest of the tooth.*

> ... *after a period of some years the tooth will again eventually become associated with a periapical radiolucency indicating root canal infection.*

> ... *endodontic surgery per se* **will not provide the long term solutions** *required for an infected root canal system* **unless all bacteria are destroyed** *and the pathway of entry of the invading bacteria is identified and rectified.*

I agree with most of what he says till we get to the last few words: "... and the pathway of entry of these invading bacteria ..." This sets the implication that the bacteria only come into the tooth from the rest of the body. There is no acknowledgement that the bacteria were in the tooth in the first place. If you are confused by this, then join the club. I often shake my head in disbelief when I read the official dental literature.

It begs the question of whether complete sterility is critical to the success of the treatment or whether it is an elusive goal. The British Dental Association claims that it is not necessary to completely sterilize, because we know that we cannot do it. They admit that bacteria remain in the tooth and claim that they present no harm to health. The American dental trade organization says that focal infection is not relevant for endodontically treated teeth. As a dentist, who are you going to believe? Most dentists just put their heads in the sand and carry on regardless, hence the term "physiological balance". These specialists are associated with Psychological Imbalance. As a patient, would you believe any of them?

Professor Abbott continues: "In conclusion, one could say that the main concepts, aims and procedures in endodontics have changed little during the last 300 years ... Elimination or destruction of all organisms within the entire tooth is essential for long term success ..."[3]

> "Come here," said the mad hatter. I'll teach you how to do a treatment that's impossible to achieve and doesn't work but will return you a great financial rewardand a respectable place in our mad hatter club."

Pulpotomy—Do You Love Your Child?

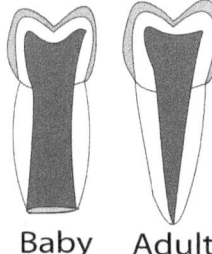

Baby   Adult

A baby tooth is a bit different to a fully formed adult tooth. The end of the root of an adult tooth forms a conical apex. This allows for the preparation of the root canal into a shape which mimics the end of the root and supposedly limits the possibility of pushing the root filling materials through the end of the root. This limits but does not seem to stop this bad end result. A baby tooth differs in that the ends of the roots are wide open. If you push a gutta percha point down such a canal, it just keeps going. So, what to do? Well, instead of going to the other side of the jawbone with files and things, some genius decided that one could "mummify" the pulp of the tooth without mummifying the rest of the kid. Perhaps the ancient Egyptians were consulted, because not only is there a mummy, but there is also a sarcophagus in the form of a stainless-steel crown. Is it a wonder that the genius in question was a past president of the American Dental Association?

To "save" such a baby tooth which has died (usually because of decay), the specialist kid's dentist, the paedo-file-dontist, will perform the next miracle that dentistry offers. It is called a pulpotomy. To achieve this, the pedodontist will drill out a huge hole in the top of the tooth to remove the dental pulp from the crown section of the tooth. This will of course weaken the tooth, which is the argument for the placement of a stainless-steel crown over it, to protect it and keep it working for chewing. As the ends of the roots are wide open, there is no attempt to remove any of the dead tissue from the roots. There is also no attempt at sterilization.

Instead, the stumps of the nerves of the tooth, at the top of the roots, are bathed in solutions that are intended to "Mummify" the tissue. The material of choice for this has, for many years, been Buckley's Formocresol, which, as the name implies, is a mixture of formaldehyde and cresol (19% formaldehyde, 35% cresol, 17.5% glycerine.) This material is still used today in some dental practices, and as mentioned before, there is a whole society of endodontists in America that still promote the use of formaldehyde.

"Because of its long history and lasting popularity, formocresol has been the most widely studied of the many pulpotomy medicaments. Although other techniques have been proposed and studied, the vast majority of pediatric dental practitioners in Canada (92.4 %) and dental schools worldwide (76.8 %) utilize either the full-strength or the 1:5

dilution of formocresol as the preferred pulpotomy medicament for vital primary teeth."[466]

The "long history and lasting popularity" are the argument for its supposed safety and efficacy. This is not a scientific approach. In fact, it has never been a scientific approach. This material was introduced into the world of dentistry around 1925 by a man called John Peter Buckley (1873–1942). This is the same Dr Buckley who was president of the American Dental Association in 1922. This is the same Dr Buckley who had the famous debate with Dr Price in 1925. This is the same Dr Buckley who concluded the debate with the following: (Shakman Quotes)

"God giving me the strength, I will spend the remainder of my life, if need be, correcting this damnable and criminal practice for which you sir, Dr. Price, whether you realize it or not, are in large measure responsible."[467]

It has never been shown to be safe or effective. There are precious few published peer-reviewed scientific papers that say it could be used as a treatment in children. Most pedodontists spread this poison far and wide without a care because it is popular and has been used for one hundred years. Precisely the same argument is still used to justify the use of mercury amalgam to demonstrate the safety of the material. It makes no difference to these criminals how much real science is thrown against their arguments; they always resort to how long we dentists have been doing it, because "only we dentists have dental knowledge." Sadly, we dentists have *no* medical, oncological, toxicological, embryological, psychological, or neurological knowledge. I also don't apologize for my name-calling. A paedophile is someone who abuses children. There would be few abuses worse than implanting these carcinogenic materials into children's bodies.

Formocresol was touted as the best mummifying paste, and stupidly, the dentists assumed that it did not mummify the child as well as the dental pulp. There is no science, only presumption, including the presumption that the material will stay in the root of the tooth and not spread to every other organ and tissue in the body. Dr Buckley was the person who promoted the use of a known carcinogen in a child's body and was fully supported by the American Dental Association. When I went to university, we were taught the fine art of using Buckley's Formocresol, and stupidly, for a short while, I also contributed to the ongoing abuse of children. Dentists are instructed on how to do something and are also instructed not to think. This "not thinking process" is enhanced by the student's exposure to massive levels of mercury throughout their course, and in the great lands of Australia and America, our brains are further impeded by exposure to fluoride in the drinking water.

The MSDS information for formaldehyde was given earlier. This horror is matched with Cresol, the other active component of "Buckley's Children's Poison." It, too, has some rather concerning effects on health. The EPA has classified Cresol as a human carcinogen. It causes cancer. It, like formaldehyde, is sealed into baby teeth for several years. This constitutes a long-term chronic exposure. The following is from an MSDS for Cresol:

Potential Health Effects

Cresol is toxic via ingestion and skin absorption. Cresol is similar to phenol in its action on the body, but is less severe in its effects.

Inhalation: Breathing vapor, dust or mist results in digestive disturbances (vomiting, difficulty in swallowing, diarrhea, loss of appetite). Will irritate, possibly burn respiratory tract. Other symptoms listed under ingestion may also occur.

Ingestion:

Poison. Symptoms may include burning pain in mouth and throat, abdominal pain, headache, dizziness, muscular weakness, irregular breathing, weak pulse, lung damage, liver damage, pancreas damage, kidney damage, coma, and possibly death from circulatory or cardiac failure.

Skin Contact:

Corrosive. Causes severe pain followed by numbness. May be absorbed through the skin with systemic poisoning effects to follow. Discoloration and severe burns may occur.

Eye Contact:

Corrosive! Vapors are irritating and may cause damage to the eyes. Contact may cause severe burns and permanent eye damage.

Chronic Exposure:

Repeated exposure may cause symptoms described for acute poisoning as well as liver damage.

Aggravation of Pre-existing Conditions:

Persons with pre-existing skin disorders or eye problems or impaired liver or kidney function may be more susceptible to the effects of the substance.

Label Hazard Warning:

POISON! DANGER! MAY BE FATAL IF SWALLOWED, INHALED OR ABSORBED THROUGH SKIN. CORROSIVE. CAUSES SEVERE BURNS TO EVERY AREA OF CONTACT. AFFECTS CENTRAL NERVOUS SYSTEM, LIVER, KIDNEYS, PANCREAS AND CARDIOVASCULAR SYSTEM. VAPOR IS IRRITATING TO EYES AND RESPIRATORY TRACT. COMBUSTIBLE LIQUID AND VAPOR.

A 1985 study demonstrated the spread of formaldehyde from a tooth that had been "treated" with a pulpotomy. Radioisotope-labelled formaldehyde was applied to the nerve stumps at the top of the root, in the crown of the tooth, for only five minutes. About 30 per cent of the formaldehyde was transported systemically throughout the body.[468] Cresol in the Buckley's Poison will of course, also be transported throughout the body!

More recently a different substance, called **Ferric Sulphate**, is being used to replace Formocresol because it is supposedly not as toxic. The manufacturer of Ferric Sulphate gives the following advice about its product:

WARNING! HARMFUL IF SWALLOWED OR INHALED. CAUSES IRRITATION TO SKIN, EYES AND RESPIRATORY TRACT. AFFECTS THE LIVER.

Inhalation:

Causes irritation to the respiratory tract. Symptoms may include coughing, shortness of breath.

Ingestion:

Low toxicity in small quantities but larger dosages may cause nausea, vomiting, diarrhea, and black stool. Pink urine discoloration is a strong indicator of iron poisoning. Liver damage, coma, and death from iron poisoning has been recorded.

Skin Contact:

Causes irritation to skin. Symptoms include redness, itching, and pain. May cause skin discoloration with irritation.

Eye Contact:

Causes irritation, redness, and pain.

Chronic Exposure:

Prolonged exposure of the eyes may cause discoloration. Repeated high exposure could cause too much iron to build up in the body. Symptoms of upset stomach, nausea, constipation and black bowel movements may occur. Chronic exposure may cause liver effects.

Aggravation of Pre-existing Conditions:

Persons with pre-existing skin disorders or eye problems, or impaired liver, kidney or respiratory function may be more susceptible to the effects of the substance."

These toxins are easily transported into the brain. Remember that injury to the dental pulp of the tooth may be seen as far away as the Gasserian (Trigeminal) Ganglion in the brain.[469,470,471] Is it really a wonder that brain cancers and other neurological diseases are associated with root-canalled teeth?

Both formocresol and ferric sulphate are embryotoxic and teratogenic (cause malformation of embryos).[472,473,474,475]

This institutionalized abuse continues to this day. As a parent, you have done what the specialist has advised and believe that because it came from a specialist, then it must be correct. It becomes more and more confusing and heartbreaking as you go from doctor to doctor to try to find out why your child is sick or has suddenly started bed-wetting at twelve years of age or went from a healthy kid to one with leukaemia. The specialist advised the Stainless- Steel crown, and therefore it must be good. There is no need to worry that the SS crown is releasing nickel all the time, which is a known carcinogen. Not to worry that EMF radiation from telephones will increase the release of nickel from those crowns.[476,477,478] Not to worry that the leukaemia has no known cause. Not to worry that the mercury and aluminium injected into your child from birth have sensitized your child to other metals, such as iron or nickel. These are just a few of the patients that I have seen. The patients' disease states resolved when the dead teeth came out. I don't care how much you paid the "really good specialist pedo ..." The treatment that your child has received is potentially going to kill him/her. The argument for doing this is that the alternative is to extract the teeth, which will stop the kid eating and lead to major problems of tooth crowding when the permanent teeth come through.

So, I guess that as the parent, it is your choice to treat the cancer if possible or to straighten the teeth when the child is a bit older but still alive. This is not to mention the psychological effect of these treatments, which sadly has led many down the path of schizophrenia, depression, and suicide. No, I am not being over dramatic—these things have happened to people I have seen as patients. I am not surprised that most people are afraid of the dentist.

One of the most memorable experiences I have had in dentistry involved a bright eight-year-old girl. The little girl was not my patient, but that of Dr Hall Huggins. When I went to his clinic in Colorado to register for the course I had booked, I was delighted by this young girl, who was having a great time playing in the waiting room. I made a comment to the receptionist about what a gorgeous, happy kid she was. The receptionist said, "Take a good look, as she is part of your course." By the time she had come to see Dr Huggins a year earlier, she had been sent home to die because her leukaemia was untreatable. Dr Huggins was very thorough. He had blood tests and biomarkers from the time he saw her, throughout her treatment, and follow-ups a month, six months, and a year later. What was the treatment? Dr Huggins removed a tooth that had been "treated" with a pulpotomy and covered with a stainless-steel crown. The pulpotomy had been performed about a year earlier, and she was diagnosed with leukaemia a month after the dental treatment. Within a week of this tooth being removed, her white cell count returned to normal. A month later, she was told that the leukaemia had disappeared. One year later, there was still no trace of cancer.

The number of pulpotomies that are done every year
is only an indication of the madness of dentistry
and is *NOT* an indicator of their safety.

Cavitations

Dentists are taught to take out teeth with the equivalent of specially designed pliers, called "forceps." If you get the right shaped pliers, you can remove just about any tooth. The patient tries to demolish the armrests of the dental chair, and the nurse looks on supportively. Supportive, that is, for the poor dentist who is working so hard! When it is finally out, you will get a piece of gauze put over the hole in your jawbone and you will be told to close down on it. Preferably you will have paid the bill, left quickly, and been halfway home before the bleeding starts. There is nothing quite as barbaric in medicine or dentistry as taking a tooth out in this way. Perhaps electric shock therapy? Then we barber/barbaric/dentists expect that this bony socket will heal by filling in the hole with bone and the gum healing over the top. Occasionally this does happen, even when the tooth is removed with such brutality.

One of the common outcomes of this type of technique is that very often the tip of the root will break off in the deepest part of the socket. By now you will probably have guessed that the teachers of oral surgery will claim that it is OK to leave it there, as the body tolerates it well—as determined by the look on an X-ray. Patients are told this every day and sent from the surgery with a little disaster festering in the jawbone. Of course, the dentist will expect you to pay the bill for the disaster. I doubt that many patients would have the knowledge or courage to take the dentist to court for this stuff-up. Of course, even with the best technique, there will be root tips that fracture. It's not a problem as long as this root tip is removed and the bone cleaned. All it takes is a little more time and some skill that most dentists are *not* taught.

With forceps extractions, there is a massive amount of force applied to the bone. These areas of bone, which are so severely compressed, will die. This is called "Compression Necrosis." Dead bone does not heal. This is one of the most common causes of dry sockets. The other is the root filling that was put into the tooth. Materials like formaldehyde will kill the surrounding bone. This bone cannot heal properly either.

Dentists are generally taught to *not remove the periodontal ligament* after the tooth is out. This is the ligament that holds the tooth to the bone and surrounds the root of the tooth. As long as this ligament is left in the socket, it will be impossible for the bone to heal properly. X-rays can be unreliable to diagnose the cavitations that are thus produced. This hole in the bone is lined by dead tissue. It cannot fill in and heal, as there are no living, bone-producing cells anywhere to be found and no blood to supply them.

These holes have been given many names over the years;

- Jawbone Cavities
- Osteocavitation Lesions
- Pathologic Bone Cavities
- Odontogenic Trigeminal Neuralgias
- Alveolar Cavitational Osteopathies
- Trigger Point Bone Cavities
- Ratner Bone Cavities
- Roberts Bone Cavities

Most current dentistry regards cavitations as inconsequential. Most dentists and even oral surgeons have never heard of them. The professors either prefer not to talk about them or are in complete ignorance themselves. This is remarkable, considering that they were described by G. V. Black, the father of modern dentistry, in 1920. He gave us what is probably the first textbook description of jawbone osteonecrosis. He called it "chronic osteitis" to distinguish it from osteomyelitis. He mentions "cavity" formation and slow death of bone "cell by cell."[479]

Black also comments on his treatment approach:

> The treatment of chronic osteitis is surgical and should be radical. The area should be opened freely, and every particle of the softened bone removed until good, sound bone forms all of the walls of the cavity.
>
> … Generally when all of the softened bone is removed, the case makes a good recovery. … When several teeth were involved, I have generally extracted them.[480]

Dr Black was not alone in his research, just as Dr Price' was not alone in his. There is a plethora of published research describing these lesions and their effects on the body.[481,482,483,484,485,486,487,488,489,490,491,492,493,494,495,496]

Dr Jerry Bouquot is one of the world's leading oral pathologists, who himself has taken much flack for making cavitations official. He answered one of Australia's leading oral surgeons, who made the claim that cavitations were nonsense and had no clinical significance. Dr Bouquot replied,

> I initially thought that this disease occurred only in persons with trigeminal neuralgia. This is far from true. Many cases, perhaps most, are completely pain free, even though great marrow destruction occurs … this is also the case for osteonecrosis of other parts of the body. Also, for those patients with pain, it can follow a wide variety of pain patterns, including classic trigeminal neuralgia … And, of course, we have no idea how many TN patients have a bone disease as an underlying association. To the best of my understanding, however, surgeons

treating maxillofacial osteonecrosis or NICO are simply treating a BONE disease, which may or may not be painful or to refer pain elsewhere ... just as might occur with a periapical infection. I cannot explain the TN connection, but there have been far too many cases reported and seen by myself to deny that some sort of connection exists. The atypical facial neuralgia/pain connection is much more readily explained. If you read any detailed discussion of ischemic osteonecrosis (avascular necrosis) of the hip, you will find a remarkable similarity between the pain symptoms and referral patterns of hip lesions as compared to maxillofacial lesions.

These holes in the bone are the cavitations that have been discussed in the section on neural therapy and by Dr Issels. These holes are another source of endotoxins, just as the dead tooth is. Of course, they and their bacterial manufacturers will spread through the body, acting as a source of focal infection. They will also act as foci of neural interference and in this way also produce disease states in distant parts of the body. Very often these neural pathways will follow the acupuncture meridian that passes through the cavitation. Sometimes they can be very large and cover a few meridians.

Lower wisdom teeth are a very important source of cavitations, as they are often removed with a great deal of force and the surrounding necrosis will be set firmly in place. Why is this an issue? Firstly, this is the most common area to find a cavitation in any part of the mouth. (See the EAV charts.) Thus, it becomes the most common neural interference of dental origin. The Small Intestine meridian is the meridian which passes through this area. It is related to conditions like eczema, dystonia, migraine, tinnitus, epilepsy, arthritis, and facial neuralgia. Oh! Did I forget to mention that it is *the area that mostly affects the heart* and that cardiovascular disease is often associated with cavitations in the wisdom tooth area? This is *heart attack land.*

As one might expect, the PTOs are very concerned that the cavitation issue is given little credence, as they would then have to acknowledge that dead root-canalled teeth may cause some serious health issues. Here is what the American Association of Endodontists have to say in their position statement: "… the concept of NICO gained notoriety decades later when it was used to describe bony lesions associated with symptoms characteristic of trigeminal neuralgia like facial pain."[497]

(Their reference - Bouquot JE, Roberts AM, Person P, Christian J. Neuralgia inducing cavitational osteonecrosis (NICO). Osteomyelitis in 224 jawbone samples from patients with facial neuralgia. Oral Surg Oral Med Oral Pathol. 1992;73:307-19)

Since when does a serious medical condition "gain notoriety"? It is a reality, whether the AAE wish to discredit it or not! Dr Bouquot was not the person who brought notoriety to this issue. He was just the easy target.

Most of the research demonstrating the connection of Trigeminal Neuralgia (TN) to cavitations came through the well-published work of Dr Eugene Ratner.[498,499,500] He demonstrated the link by surgically cleaning out the cavitations and noting the disappearance of TN in most cases. His work is ground-breaking and is ignored by current dental teaching.

Dr Ratner was able to map the areas of pain referral from cavitations in various parts of the mouth to various parts of the body. These pains were all over the body, not just the head and neck. The disappearance of the pain after surgery was how he was able to do this mapping. For example, some lesions in the upper jawbone referred pain to the front of the legs, to the big toe, and also down the spine. Lesions in the mandible may refer pain to the groin and insides of the arms and the three fingers from the little finger. Many other relationships exist.

Dr Ratner also examined the contents of many of these lesions. He found that various bacterial colonies existed in them, both aerobic and anaerobic, and one third of the organisms had not yet been identified. "... *a unique microbiotic spectrum.*"[501,502,503,504]

Dr Ratner published his research in the 1960s and 1970s. Fifty years later, oral surgeons are still ignoring his work in favour of the acceptable treatment for Trigeminal Neuralgia, which is *BRAIN SURGERY.*

The AAE continue as follows in their position statement: "In addition, the practice of recommending the extraction of endodontically treated teeth for the prevention of NICO, or any other disease, is unethical and should be reported immediately to the appropriate state board of dentistry."

So much for a scientific approach and clinical integrity. Ethics in this industry is a joke!

Although the PTOs find it unethical to clean a socket and remove the periodontal ligament and infected bone from an extraction socket, it is clearly shown that this is the best way of preventing cavitations and allowing the bone to heal properly. They also claim that cavitations are rare because they cannot be seen easily on X-rays. They also claim that it is unethical to clean out these cavitations for the benefit of improving health. They also claim that root-canalled teeth are completely safe and are not related to the production of cavitations.

The dental trade talks about good healing as observed on X-ray to demonstrate that cleaning the cavity properly is not necessary. "Complete radiographic healing occurs without post extraction curettage in teeth with periapical raidiolucencies and without preoperative or postoperative antibiotic therapy in most cases."[505]

I was told once, by a colleague who I went to university with, that mercury amalgam was safe because it was "well tolerated on an X-ray"!

A study published in 1996 ("Routine Dental Extractions Routinely Produce Cavitations"), revisited extraction sites from 112 patients.[506] Those conducting the study were looking only for the numbers of cavitations found, rather than any disease relationships. The extraction technique was critically analysed.

That there were 691 extraction sites in 112 patients (from 1991 to 1995, in patients from nineteen to eighty-three years of age, forty male and seventy-two female), clearly shows that cavitations are more the norm than a rarity. Third molar (wisdom teeth) areas were the most common. Remember that these are the areas associated with heart attacks in acupuncture relationships.

Area	Number of Extraction Sites	No of CVs	%
3rd molars (wisdom teeth)	354	313	88
2nd molars	50	35	70
1st molars	73	60	82
Total Molar sites	517	441	85
Mandibular non-molars	51	23	45
All non-molars	174	95	55
Overall, regardless of site	691	536	77

The researchers made the following comments: (Note that "CV" is an abbreviation for "cavitation.")

> … the most obvious reason for not finding a CV is not looking for it.

> A CV, obvious on radiological examination of the jaw, is definitely the exception rather than the rule.

> Taking at least one millimeter of good bone insures removal of both periodontal ligament and most of the bone directly bathed with the toxins produced by the mutant streptococcus in the dentin tubules.

> It is theorized that the use of antibiotics may convert the osteoblasts back into osteocytes, impeding a full healing of bone in the socket area.

> Simple manual curettage is discouraged, for the scraping required in the process can "push" much of the toxic products into the adjacent, good, cancellous bone, resulting in a greater chance of persistent or recurrent CVs, or simply a lack of primary healing after a tooth extraction.

Regarding the periodontal ligament being allowed to remain in an extraction socket, they stated the following:

> ... its continued presence in the extraction site effectively prevents the adjacent bone from biologically recognizing that the tooth has been extracted. Bone cells are not going to proliferate spontaneously and migrate through a membrane intended by nature to define their growth limits.

> At the upper portion of the extraction site, however, where there is no periodontal ligament, osteoblastic bone activity does initiate, and a thin cortex of bone will heal across the hole. This cap of bone is rarely more than several millimeters thick.

> Similarly, the mouth flora undergo metabolic transformations when oxygen deprived, and exotoxin production can be anticipated.

> ... the only successful treatment for necrotic tissue is debridement.

> Pathologically, CVs are focal pockets of gangrene in the jawbone, since gangrene is defined as necrosis due to obstruction of blood supply which may be localized or widespread, as in an entire extremity.

The following diseases and disorders have been reported to be associated with osteonecrosis:

- Heart Disease
- Trigeminal Neuralgia
- Other atypical facial pains
- Referred pains anywhere on the body
- Cirrhosis
- Pancreatitis
- Arthritis
- Blood dyscrasias
- Disseminated intravascular coagulation
- Leukemia
- Sickle cell anemia
- Cancer
- Hyperlipidemia & embolic fat
- Hypertension
- Osteoporosis
- Atherosclerosis
- Anorexia nervosa

Wisdom Teeth Extractions

A word of warning to anyone about to have his or her wisdom teeth removed—*DO NOT* have a general anaesthetic (GA) for this. Use local anaesthetic for pain control. The only reason that surgeons want to do it in hospital instead of under local anaesthetic is financial. Why not take four of the suckers out in one hour instead of just the one that needs to come out in half an hour? You are charged by the number of extractions. Apart from the dangers of general anaesthetic and the extra cost of hospitals and anaesthetists, etc., you will be subjected to four times the amount of pain and discomfort. This will be on both sides of your mouth and will make for a very unhappy camper. The GA will also lower your immune response to the trauma and the bacteremia, and your face might start to resemble a chipmunk. Most people take much longer to recover from this approach than removing only the wisdom teeth on one side at a time, under local anaesthetic.

Another important reason to not have a GA is that when you are conscious you can resist the forces that will be applied to your jaw. You can work with the dentist. Under a GA, this is not possible, and you are then dependent on the surgeon being so gentle as to not compromise your jaw joint. This is a common cause of damage to this joint. Many TMJ problems are caused by extraction of lower wisdom teeth under general anaesthetic. They can take many painful years to resolve.

Fatty Osteo Necrosis

More often than not, after extracting a dead tooth or cleaning out a cavitation, the dentist may observe a layer of shiny fat globules on top of the blood which is oozing from the socket. This fat is released from cells in the dead bone and should be allowed to bleed out if possible. Allow the bleeding to continue till the visibility of fat has stopped. Most dentists are not aware of this, as they almost always cover an extraction socket with gauze before the bleeding has stopped. They don't clean out the socket or periodontal ligament and therefore never spend the time to observe this.

Confidence, Ignorance, and "General Knowledge"

Dental associations worldwide refuse to acknowledge that dead, infected, gangrenous teeth and cavitations are a danger to health. "The British Dental Association … is satisfied that there are no grounds for believing that endodontic treatment could cause general health problems … It would also be unethical of a dentist to promote extraction of root-filled teeth as a means of alleviating illness."[507]

Dr Price made a comment on this sort of attitude one hundred years before the BDA made their announcement. He wrote, "… this point of view is not based upon any great truth but, is confidence inspired by ignorance …"

Anecdotal stories include the numerous cases in which breast lumps have disappeared within a week of extracting dead teeth. I lost count of the number of women who had this experience. I'm not surprised that specialist endodontists have never seen this in their "clinical observational" practices. After all, they put the root therapies in rather than take them out. If you don't look, you don't see! Very few women would go back to the endodontist or dentist to have their breast lumps checked.

Jacques Benveniste, one of the greatest scientific thinkers of the twentieth century, makes a relevant comment: "… why are scientists so opposed to the evolution of science? Is it to defend their piece of turf? Why, in the name of intangible dogmas, which the history of science has shown to be so often ephemeral, do they reject advances, which represent progress for their discipline?"[508]

Why are dentists so opposed to the idea that their treatments may be killing people? Surely there is some sense of altruism, which desires to help others rather than kill them. Are we all so terrified of opposing the dogma of the institution?

In 2003, the Superior Court of California passed legislation requiring dentists in that state to display the following warnings in their surgeries:[509]

> Warning on dental amalgam, used in many dental fillings, causes exposure to mercury, a chemical known to the state of California to cause birth defects or other reproductive harm.

> Root canal treatments and restorations including fillings, crowns and bridges, use chemicals known to the state of California to cause cancer.

By 1923, Dr Price had demonstrated that every belief about root canal therapy held by the dental community at the time was based on a complete lack of scientific research.[510] These beliefs, based in hope and myth, were later set in concrete by the incomes of current dental specialists! These "beliefs" form the bases of their clinical observation and "general knowledge."

Professor Daunderer, in a 1998 interview, said,

> The dental work we get from dentists is not something biological or medical. I'd say it is a technical thing, and the technique gives the dentists a number of very strong poisons to be implanted in the mouth.
>
> If you kill the tooth and then fill its root canal with mercury, formaldehyde, cortisone, streptomycin, arsenic, … you are not doing a healthy thing.
>
> All this dentistry is just a sin against the biology of the body and a sin against the 'real' medicine.

In Summary

- Dead teeth cause the largest number of diseases ever traced to a single source.
- There have been very few advances in root canal procedures in the last three hundred years!
- This practice is based in anecdotal evidence which supports general knowledge.
- The dangers of Root Therapy have been known for over one hundred years.
- A root-canalled tooth *is* a dead tooth.
- Dead, gangrenous material always remains in the tooth.
- It is *not* possible to sterilize a tooth.
- It is not possible to completely fill and seal a root canal.
- All root canal filling cements are toxic. Some are carcinogenic. Some cause irreversible nerve damage.
- All toxins and *all* substances placed in a tooth are transported to the rest of the body.

- Amalgam implanted into the end of the root of a tooth is an implant of mercury directly into the brain.
- Teeth may affect the energy flow in acupuncture meridians and thus affect the health of distant tissue.
- Root therapy has a 33 per cent failure rate.
- Teeth are an integral part of the body!

9

Cancer—The Unmentionable Taboo

. . . .

As mentioned earlier, there are many diseases that can be caused by and associated with the presence of dead teeth in the body. The association with cancer predates 1900, and even though it is well reported in the dental literature, it still remains the single greatest taboo in dentistry. Very simply, root-canalled teeth are not allowed to cause cancer. They're not even allowed to be dead! There is a blanket denial that these teeth can cause any disease, but cancer is the big one that causes every PTO to freak out.

I was honoured once by the president of the Austrian Society of Oncology, Dr Wolfgang Köstler of the Medical University of Vienna. We were both speakers at a cancer conference in Darwin, Australia. Over drinks one night, he came and congratulated me for the talk I had given that afternoon. I thanked him, but I felt it was too great a compliment, as I was the only dentist, and the rest of the presenters were all professors of medicine, and half were themselves oncologists. I said something along these lines to him, and he laughed out loud, followed by, "We are all trying to treat the cancers we see in our patients. You are the only one talking about one of the biggest causes. This is most important." Sadly, not one Australian oncologist attended this international conference; neither did the AMA nor the ADA.

Endotoxins

Endotoxins are the toxins produced by anaerobic bacteria. Endotoxins are mostly found in the outer membrane of Gram-negative bacteria. They are an integral part of the outer cell membrane and are responsible for the organization and stability of the bacteria. They are also called Lipopolysacharides", or "LPs". Many are deadly. Many can cause cancer. It is well known that endotoxins are found throughout the depth of the dentine tubules and that they leak easily from the tooth.[511,512]

The dental research is full of studies that have looked at every conceivable method to eliminate these highly poisonous substances from a dead tooth, all to no avail. To date it remains an unsolved problem. A study from 2014 shows that even though the root canal procedure reduced the levels of endotoxin in all teeth studied, the fact remains that no matter what procedures were done, all of the teeth were still loaded with endotoxins.[513] Even though the levels may be reduced by some of these procedures, the bacteria that produce these toxins remain in the dentine tubules. There they continue to live happily and keep making more of the same toxins as before. There is no way to eliminate or contain the bacteria that produce these substances.[514,515,516,517]

All root-canalled teeth will contain levels of endotoxin that *will* affect your health. There is a world of difference between reducing some of the endotoxins and removing them all. Even at low concentrations, these endotoxins have profound effects on the immune system.[518,519,520]

"This molecule is recognized by the human host as a foreign, eliciting a potent immune response that results in the release of different pro-inflammatory cytokines …"[126] Root fillings do *not* block the passage of these toxins. They escape readily through the accessory canals, dentine tubules, and the apex of the tooth (no matter what the tooth has been filled with) and will then be transported through the body.[521,522,523,524]

Dr Weston Price stated in 1923, "… soluble poisons may pass from the infected teeth to the lymph or blood circulation, and produce systemic disturbances entirely out of proportion to the quantity of poison involved."

In 1975 the *Journal of Endodontics* published that endotoxins are potent biological agents capable of initiating a variety of biological responses: "Pyrogenicity, Schwartzman's reactions, inflammation of skin, vascular and hemodynamic effects, abortion, immunotolerance"[525]

The toxicity of the endotoxins has been demonstrated by injecting them into experimental animals. After repeated injections, there was severe liver damage, and the animals died within weeks. Inflammatory and degenerative changes were found in *all other organs*, especially in the *joints, muscles, and blood vessels*. This is precisely what Dr Price was finding in the 1920s. Unlike the modern claims that Price's work has been proven to be false, the more recent research completely supports these earlier findings.

"… transformation of a normal cell into a malignant cell requires a certain quantity of a carcinogen—the carcinogenic minimum dose. It does not matter whether this quantity is supplied in a single dose or in a number of smaller doses, because the toxic effects of each dose are stored, and accumulate without loss."[55]

Endotoxins escape more readily from teeth than do the bacteria producing them.[526] They pass easily through the dentine tubules.[527] Endotoxin is found in dead teeth, with or without pain.[528] This flies in the face of endodontic teaching that claims there is bacterial presence only if pain is present, just as they claim a lack of infection if the bone looks normal on an X-ray.

Endotoxins have a wide variety of effects in the human body:

- They interfere with blood clotting.[529] I have seen many patients who were regarded by their doctors as "bleeders", until the dead tooth was removed. Then, miraculously and almost suddenly, they stopped being bleeders.

- They alter the development of nerve tissue in the brain, and they also damage nerve tissue in both the developing and adult brain.[530,531,532,533,534 535]
- Endotoxins are Neurotoxic. They kill nerve cells.[536,537,538,539]
- They alter transmission within nerve fibres and may have other far-reaching and varied effects including headaches, nausea, vomiting, depression, personality changes, nosebleeds, and breathing difficulties.[540,541]
- They're associated with miscarriage and low birth weight children.[542]
- They're associated with Coronary Heart disease, Stroke, and atherosclerosis.[543,544,545]
- They cause allergic sensitivities.[546]
- They cause bad breath.[547,548]
- They're cytotoxic (they kill cells).[549,550,551,552,553]
- They reduce the ability to breathe and will affect lung function severely. Asthmatics are at greater risk.[554,555,556,557]
- They cause cancer.

The list of diseases from dead teeth that Dr Price found in the 1920s is remarkably similar to the one above and included Diabetes, Hay Fever, Periodontal disease, Asthma, Rhinitis, Skin Conditions, Neuritis, Degenerative arthritis, Nervous Breakdown, Stroke, Kidney diseases, Rheumatism, Arthritis, Heart disease and Cancer.

Recent literature emphasizes the role of nerve transmission of these substances for the spread of inflammation. "… thus an endotoxic stimulation of a couple of nerve endings could induce a _widespread inflammatory reaction_."[558]

There are many studies demonstrating this.[559,560,561,562,563,564] This could be an explanation for Trigeminal Neuralgia. These toxins can diffuse and circulate through the body. (References demonstrating the extreme toxicity of endotoxins can be found in Appendix 9 on www.realdentalinfo.com)

The most dangerous of these endotoxins are the thio-ethers, such as dimethylsulfide.[565] Thioethers and Methyl Mercaptans have devastating effects on the body and are produced by the bacteria in dead teeth and periodontal pockets.[566,567,568,569,570,571,572].

> **Thio-ethers** are strongly related, both in their structure and their effect, to <u>mustard gas and other poison gasses used in the First World War</u>. They are amongst the **most potent of all carcinogens**. They **paralyze the aerobic action of cells.**[55]

> **Methyl Mercaptans** may cause fever, cough, shortness of breath, a feeling of tightness and burning in the chest, pulmonary edema, respiratory failure and collapse. Headache, loss of smell, dizziness, staggering gait, and heightened emotions may occur. Memory loss, damage to the central and peripheral nervous system, tremor, convulsions, and coma may also result. People exposed to high concentrations may develop acute hemolytic anemia and methemoglobinemia. Individuals with pre-existing conditions of the heart, lungs, blood, and nervous system may have increased susceptibility to the toxic effects of methyl mercaptan.[573]

> Methyl mercaptan is a central nervous system depressant that acts on the respiratory center to produce death by respiratory paralysis. Methyl mercaptan **inhibits mitochondrial respiration by interfering with cytochrome c oxidase**. Restlessness, headache, staggering, and dizziness may develop; severe exposure may lead to convulsions and coma. Irritation of the mouth, throat, and esophagus are possible. Dermatitis can occur with chronic exposure to methyl mercaptan.[574]

Thio-ethers **almost exclusively target the mitochondria** in the cells. The mitochondria are the energy power supplies for all cells. It stands to reason, then, that the tissues which have the most need for energy and the largest numbers of mitochondria in them will be the tissues most affected by these poisons.

> Therefore, it is the vital organs—the liver, nervous system, endocrine glands, heart, and reticuloendothelial system—whose cells may consist of up to one-fifth mitochondria, that are primarily affected.
>
> The nervous system is thus doubly affected by focal intoxication. **Psychological effects are a part of the symptomology of thio-ether poisoning.**[575] Dr Joseph Issels 'Cancer a Second Opinion'

The carcinogens that are primarily responsible for the development of cancer are those which inhibit the aerobic function of cells, even in minimal quantities, without destroying the cell, and which are constantly present. Eventually a level will build up which will cause overt cancer. As Dr Issels states, "There is hardly a carcinogen which so completely fulfils these conditions as do thio-ethers. Incessantly, from the moment the pulp is removed, hour by hour, year by year, minimal amounts of these most virulent of all the odontogenous toxins will be released into the circulation—minimal doses, but nevertheless sufficient to more or less totally paralyse the aerobic action of the cell."

Miniscule amounts of these toxins are able to have profound effects on the tissues of the body. These toxins cause cancer and many other conditions. They may also be the reason we see so many depressed people in our society. I have personally seen several patients who, after having just one root-canalled tooth removed, went home and tore up their suicide notes. What a tragedy it is when young people take their lives, and it is so much worse if that psychological state is caused by chemicals emanating from a "root-therapied" dead tooth.

Suicide is a permanent solution to a temporary problem. When a doctor tells you that it is all in your head, you should know that he or she may be partly correct. More specifically, get the root-canalled tooth and the amalgam out of your head and you may find that life really is beautiful.

As an aside, Fluoride in drinking water causes an increase in cancer rates. Mercury significantly depresses the function of the immune system, and there is an accompanying increase in cancer.

Dr Issels makes the following points;

> The head *foci* therefore seem not only to contribute to the development of secondary lesions, to the origin of cancer disease, but also to exert a direct influence on tumour growth by stimulating it. Many tumours seem to respond to immune therapy only when *foci* have been removed.

> In the vast majority of the patients I have treated, it was quite clear that foci treatment should have been carried out years before - and certainly long before the manifestation of the tumours.

> That this was not done is a sad reminder that far too many doctors and dentists fail to recognise a fundamental truism: untreated foci can be linked to the development of cancer.

Dentistry is clear about the idea of fixing up your teeth before any chemotherapy or radiotherapy to the head and neck. Get rid of decay and gum disease. After radiotherapy in the head and neck region, the blood supply to the jawbone will be affected, and future healing after extraction may be a problem. The "god" oral surgeons are all advocating filling the teeth with mercury amalgam and retaining any dead teeth with a root canal. They claim ignorance when confronted with the information that these two procedures will quite effectively wipe out the immune system almost totally. My response is that they do not have the right or the luxury of claiming ignorance when holding such important roles. They should not be doing their jobs if this ignorance is real.

Dentistry's Contribution to the Creation of Diseases

Clearly there are several ways that a dead tooth can affect health, and there are always more than one of these aspects operating at the same time. As well there is the individual's response to these causative factors, which underlies how your body will respond. As Dr Price showed, the responses of individuals to a given stimulus vary widely. It is not just the odd dental researcher who thinks this way.

Dr Issels was a German oncologist with one of the most respected cancer clinics in Germany. He succeeded in *curing* many patients. It may be of interest that in Australia, Canada, America, Britain, and New Zealand, it is illegal for anyone but an oncologist to claim a *cure* for cancer. This is written in the law! If anyone but an oncologist cures cancer, he or she will be jailed immediately. The oncologists in these countries even have the power to remove children with cancer from their families if the parents refuse chemotherapy or radiotherapy for their children. There are many families travelling around in camper vans to avoid the persecution of medical and government institutions while treating a child's cancer with other methods. With such a powerful cancer industry, do you think they would want to advertise one of the causes of their income? There are great profits to be made from "controlling" cancer rather than curing it.

Before starting any of his treatments, Dr Issels first instructed the patient to rid the mouth of all toxic material, including amalgam fillings, dead or root-canalled teeth, and cavitations. He was fully aware of the devastation these dental conditions and implants could create. Dr Issels was also well aware that leaving these dental disasters in the mouth would interfere with any of his treatments in a negative way. He attempted to teach both the dental and medical worlds of his findings, which again supported those of Dr Price. His work was supported by a huge amount of German research which has never seen an English translation. Today there are many cancer clinics that acknowledge his work and use his concepts in their treatments, including getting rid of amalgams and dead teeth. Mercury, silver, copper, and zinc are in amalgam, and they release deadly amounts of mercury all the time. All metals in the mouth will generate electrical currents of one thousand times that at which your brain is operating. Titanium implants will also generate these electrical currents. The dead teeth and cavitations will generate toxins that even the military would be envious of.

Quoting Professor Daunderer,

> If we take Multiple Sclerosis patients who removed amalgam but refused both extraction of root canals and treatment of infected maxillary bone, we observe a cure rate from MS of 16%

> But when we consider multiple sclerosis patients that beside amalgam removal accepted our full treatment (root canal extraction and cleaning of alveolar bone), the percentage of cures increases to 86.[576]

This is a vastly different approach to the "one treatment fits all" concept, where radiation and chemotherapy are all that are on offer, even though they generally do not work. In his book *Cancer: A Second Opinion*, Dr Issels devotes a whole chapter to dental foci.[577] This is a profoundly important concept to understand if we are to start treating cancer or any other degenerative, neurological, or cardiac disease properly. If you or your friend has cancer or any other degenerative condition, I would strongly suggest you purchase and read Dr Issels's book. It is available at www.issels.com and is an easy read.

In my limited exposure in one tiny dental practice, I have seen too often how tumours disappear after the removal of root-canalled teeth. Most disappeared in about three to four months. Not on any of these occasions were the oncologists interested in what had happened. The patients did try to tell them, but not even a glimmer of interest was expressed. Can you believe it? Not one of them said, "Wow that's great. I need to look into that." Not one. I find that staggeringly depressing. "Spontaneous remission" is the term medical people use to describe this seemingly miraculous way that diseases can just disappear all by themselves without any known reason. If they were to accept that there is a reason (i.e., a dead tooth being extracted), they would have to acknowledge that this same dead tooth might have been the cause of the cancer. This falls into the taboo area, the no-man's land, of never condemning the dental (or medical) trade organizations. They are a cartel that works to maintain disease. Health and well-being are not on the agenda. The last thing that the medical profession wants to do is take any responsibility for dental "treatments". Besides, it would probably be seen as unethical for the mouth to be regarded as a part of the body by either the medical or dental merchants.

Dr Issels, Daunderer and many others have rated their treatments as only average, unless the dental work is done first. Then their success rates increased to about 80 per cent. This is a far cry from the miserable cure rates of chemotherapy and radiotherapy. According to a 2004 report by Morgan, Ward, and Barton, "The contribution of cytotoxic chemotherapy to 5-year survival in adult malignancies … survival in adults was estimated to be 2.3% in Australia and 2.1% in the USA."[578]

Try looking up the success rate of radiation therapy and you will find a never-ending array of articles claiming a 95 per cent success rate for Prostate Cancer *ONLY*. No other type of cancer is mentioned. Also, no mention is made that radiation is itself carcinogenic. The use of radiation started as a bad experiment in the 1920s but proved to be too profitable to discard.

The only time in forty years of practice that I have seen just one root-canalled tooth in an otherwise healthy mouth is when it was caused by trauma (e.g., a front tooth being hit in a sporting or fighting scenario). Occasionally it will be caused by a tooth being moved too quickly by a specialist orthodontist. Few of these specialists would admit to having killed the tooth and would blame it on bad luck. Yep, it is bad luck to be "treated" by such a specialist. If a tooth is moved too quickly, the blood supply will be compromised or severed, and the tooth dies. Without taking responsibility, this unsuspecting patient will be shuffled off to the endodontist mate, who will quietly do a root canal on this tooth and praise himself or herself for saving the tooth. A pituitary tumour that quietly develops over the next five years or so could not possibly be related!

Usually, a single root-canalled tooth is only a part of a mouthful of issues. There may be multiple metals in the mouth, creating all sorts of electrical interference. There may be amalgam in the mouth, constantly releasing mercury into your body. There may be missing teeth that hide a cavitation just below the gum. Titanium implants are common, and there is no consideration of what else is in the mouth. Often there will be more than one root-canalled tooth. Two, three, and even four root canals are common. Do these teeth have one, two, or three roots with the increased toxic disaster? Are there three miles of dentinal tubules, or twelve or twenty? This is at least four times the number of anaerobes, and there could be four times the amount of endotoxins floating around in your system. This could represent a neural interference on four different acupuncture meridians at the same time.

What if most, if not all, of the teeth are root-canalled? Thankfully this is not common, but it does happen, with horrifying consequences. Each time we dentists add insults to the immune system or load the body with more and more toxins, the ability to stay healthy is reduced. You may start off as healthy as an ox and slowly but surely see your health degrading over time. Those who have poor immune systems go down first. Permanent exposure to the assaults of environmental toxins, electromagnetic radiation, poisoned and genetically engineered foods, and toxins that are injected into the majority of the population in the form of vaccines will see your chances of reaching old age criminally compromised. Why else would we need to mandate "herd vaccination" if it were not to create an amazingly long-term financial benefit to the medical merchants? Yes, I know I sound too cynical, but it may be worth doing a bit of reading about vaccines, their contents, and the effects that they have on your body and those of your loved ones, especially your children. There is a lot of information out there, but not in the mainstream media.

Mercury is the third most toxic element known. Arsenic is the first and lead the second. Mercury from amalgam is one of the most serious neurotoxins on the planet. It has both physical and psychological effects. Mercury will make you as mad as a hatter! Endotoxins also have strong physical and psychological effects. They modify the way we think. Depression and suicidal thoughts are high in these groups of people. Often their health is also so compromised that it can be seen that the depression is secondary to the ill health. As you read this, remember to multiply the outcomes by the number of dead teeth and the amount of metal in your mouth. I have no idea whether the maths equation is 1+1=2 or whether the constant increase means that 1+1=100, as in other synergistic models. For example, when adding mercury and fluoride in the same body, the toxicity is not doubled; it is literally increased one hundredfold. This is called the synergistic effect. That which causes suicidal thoughts in one person may have to be multiplied many times over to cause the motor neuron disease in later life in another person. We are all different physiologically, and our personal responses to these assaults will be unique. The more toxins you are exposed to, the greater the chances of serious disease.

Dr Issels describes the dental foci as

> ... the most lethal of all foci.
>
> The emphasis I place on the removal of devitalized teeth and chronically-diseased tonsils is one of the better-known aspects of my work, but also one of the most criticized and misunderstood ... if they are diseased, they cause the body's natural resistance to be lowered, thus acting as an important contributory

factor to tumour development. In these cases, I insist on their removal.

When the body's resistance has been reduced or broken down, it will be easier to create effects distant from the foci. There will be an increase in generalized intoxication of the body, with a generalized breakdown of the body's defences. This will cause a concomitant increase in malignant growths.

> For decades, the erroneous belief was held that, after such treatment, (root canal procedure) the tooth is an isolated, lifeless thing, no longer involved in any of the body's processes. This assumption was originally based on the premise that the pulp cavity had only one orifice to the apex of the root below, and by filling, this opening was sealed. However, the dentinal canal does not end in just one opening; instead, it resembles a tree with many branches which penetrate the tooth's body in all directions … there is a lively metabolic interchange between the interior and exterior milieu of the tooth, and this two-way process takes place along many thousands of hyperfine, capillary canals joining the pulp cavity to the exterior surface of the tooth. In fact, the conservation treatment may literally convert a tooth into a toxin producing factory.[55]

X-Ray Appearance

Dr Issels also noted, as did Dr Price in 1920, that if the body's defences are strong, they will create an encapsulated fibrous area around the end of the root in an attempt to quarantine the toxins from the rest of the body. Dentistry calls this a "granuloma" or, more recently, "periapical periodontitis"—or, in lay terms, an "abscess". (Just a bit of nit-picking here, as Dr Price noted: this is an incorrect term, as the abscess at the end of the root is not cancerous, and consequently the term "granuloma" is incorrect.)

As the body's defences are compromised, this abscess loses its fibrous capsule and toxins are more easily able to enter the body. On an X-ray, the abscess is still visible, but the edges of it are less defined. It becomes harder to tell where the abscess starts and stops. As the immune system is even more compromised, the abscess disappears, and the toxins will spread through the rest of the body, causing greater harm. The X-rays which showed a well-defined abscess he termed "X-ray positive", and those where the bone looked more normal were "X-ray negative".

He noted that the cancer patients he treated who had root-canalled teeth mainly showed as X-ray negative. This is exactly what Dr Price found in 1920 and what Dr Rosenow found in the 1930s. This is exactly opposite to what modern dentistry teaches. Incredible as it sounds, the teachers of current endodontics will look at an X-ray with an abscess visible and tell you that there is infection around the tooth. After the procedure, when the abscess has disappeared, they will tell you how successful their treatment was, and that the infection is gone. This will be repeated in twelve months when the X-ray shows very dense white bone on the X-ray, which is called "condensing osteitis." Instead of realizing that the patient is rapidly heading down a path towards cancer, they pat themselves on the back for a job well done. If you cannot see the abscess, it is assumed that there is no more infection.

In 1940, Rosenow stated,

> Roentgenographically positive are usually, but not always, infected teeth … however, … roentgenographically Negative teeth are still nearly always considered sterile and harmless and are allowed to remain, despite the fact that they have been shown by methods to be infected by streptococci having elective localizing powers in most instances in which

patients are suffering from mild or severe systemic disease ...

Streptococci isolated from roentgenographically negative pulpless teeth in my experience have been more specifically virulent than those isolated from roentgenographically positive teeth ... Improvement, often permanent, following removal of foci from which the causative streptococci were isolated in my experiences, have occurred with such regularity that I have come to consider the lack of improvement as evidence that the removal was faulty, that the focus did not contain the causative microorganisms or that other foci were overlooked.[579]

Rosenow was head of bacteriology research at the Mayo clinic for over forty years and was one of the most respected scientists and doctors of the time.

Thus, one of the main markers of success of the root canal procedure, the disappearance of the abscess on the X-ray, is really a sign that the body's defences are ruined. Endodontists will never admit this but instead will tell you that this thinking is insane. They are not cancer specialists. They are not scientists or medical researchers. They are only myopic idiots who preach to the converted. They claim to have all the answers in their "clinical observations" at the other end of a microscope, that can look down the centre of a root canal!

No Pain, No Brain

The only other marker of success of this treatment, by the specialist endodontist, is a lack of pain. The tooth has stopped hurting. Of course, the patient is happy! The problem is that pain happens in a tooth only when there is pressure either inside the tooth or in the abscess around the end of the root. As soon as the pressure is gone, there is no more pain. Thus, the infected dead tooth that no longer hurts is still a toxin factory, no matter which way you turn it. Usually, the pain should have been stopped at that very first appointment when the root canal was started. If it was done according to the teaching, the nerve of the tooth will have been removed and the abscess drained through the tooth. It is always dramatic for both dentist and patient when the pulp chamber is opened and pus starts to pour out. The patient's pain usually disappears immediately. The pressure is relieved. By the way, if a tooth like this is sealed up again, the pain usually returns in a day or two as pressure slowly increases again. Do not allow the dentist to seal it up again. The reality is that it is not going to get more infected, and you have already decided to remove this tooth.

Lack of pain is what we all want. In this case, though, it may be a sinister sign. Dr Price's comments in this regard are most pertinent: "Local comfort … may constitute both what is probably one of the greatest paradoxes and one of the costliest diagnostic mistakes through injury to health, that exists in dental and medical practice … the absence of this local reaction and the consequent destruction by the infection products, permits them to pass through the body to irritate and break down that patient's most susceptible tissue."

Dr Issels states, "In my cancer patients, I have found that such non-encapsulated foci—that is those who show X-ray negative—were particularly common, as one would expect from people whose body resistance has been lowered … It is therefore the most dangerous of all dental foci which most frequently prove X-ray negative."

Dentistry has only a couple of tools at its disposal to test whether there is a problem with a tooth. Can we cause pain or not? If I put ice on a tooth and it hurts, it is assumed to be alive. Otherwise, the assumption is that it is dead. What if we had a tool that could tell us not only that the tooth is dead but also that it correlates to the disease in your body? These tools exist and are called Electrodermal Testing machines. The TGA and FDA have done their homework and have seriously restricted the use of this sort of equipment that can be used for diagnosis and treatment. We are not allowed to use electrodermal or infrared screening, as it may show the direct relationship of the dead tooth to the cancer. This would be bad for both industries.

Inflamed tissue is hotter than the surrounding tissue, and this can be seen with infrared photography over both the dental foci and the cancer. "After treatment, a decrease in the infra-red activity of dental foci was as a rule accompanied by a decrease in infra-red emission over the tumour areas."[66] Dr Issels found that 98 per cent of his cancer patients had between two and ten dead teeth. "The diagnosis of foci in teeth had been greatly improved by electro-acupuncture. It is now possible to differentiate foci not only with regard to their type and position, but also to their virulence and pathogenic efficacy. The result of focus treatment can consequently be observed and improved, before, during, and after dentistry, to an extent never known before (Kramer)."[580]

I once had a twenty-two-year-young lady come to see me who had developed severe and acute mastitis, with her breasts swelling to twice their size in just a couple of weeks. The doctor she saw was at a loss and referred her to a gynaecologist. None of the dental tools showed anything. Ice on all teeth evoked pain. It was only testing with Electro Dermal equipment that allowed us to determine that the upper left first molar was the culprit. Although the ice caused a pain reaction when applied to the outer roots, it was the palatal root that was dead. We tested this in every conceivable way with this equipment. I wanted to check this before taking the tooth out and drilled down to check. Sure enough, it was only the one root that was dead. This tooth is on the stomach meridian, which passes through the breast. Within two weeks of the tooth coming out, her breasts returned to their normal size. Four months later, she came in to tell me that since then she also had not had any period pain, a great improvement after spending weeks on her bed prior to this. I have not found any other equipment that can make such a diagnosis. Incredible as it sounds, the TGA and FDA have ruled that these machines are only as good as snake oil, and their use is now very limited.

There are many claims made by dentists of all persuasions. Anyone offering a root canal as part of their services is to be avoided. The ones that have the latest and greatest equipment and claim sterility are also to be avoided, because even if they were able to achieve sterility, they are still ignorant of the other major effects. Ask them for the scientific references that support their claims, and then read them. Any dentist who claims to assess each individual on his or her particular case is worth questioning and then running from. They also do not understand the complexity of these issues, and the assessment is always to do with money. Many "holistic" dentists have found the great profits to be had by doing implants. They offer to take the root-canalled tooth out, for lots of money, to put a new tooth or implant back in its place. They will tell you that if you do not do this, your whole face will collapse into a little space, like a bad 3D cartoon, or that the other teeth will move and fill that space in a bad way. You might be told that it is the best aesthetic solution. Many will try to convince you to take out the tooth and replace it with an implant at the same appointment. This lunacy is purely a money-making exercise, as is the one-treatment root canal procedure that puts formaldehyde into your tooth and body. I have many reasons to oppose using implants, but inserting one into a socket that is still infected is a recipe for disaster. They forget to tell you about the infection that resides around most of them, whether titanium or zirconium. Intelligence and good motives often give way to financial considerations.

Yes, I sound scathing because I am. The criminals who taught me made *me* responsible for creating an unknown quantity of disease. I have no idea how many people I have poisoned and killed. This is one of the greatest burdens for any dentist who takes on this new paradigm. There is no exaggeration in what I am saying. As a good, conscientious dentist, I looked after my family and friends. I did what I was told, going by what the great professors and deans taught at university. I had a chance with some of these people to undo the damage I had caused. Others died of all sorts of medical conditions caused by my "treatments". Did I really cause these deaths? Do I feel differently about the patients who are not my inner circle? No! I became a very good "sick-making" machine. I was the perfect dentist because I did everything that I was taught to do at university. Everyone suffered. It is time for the paradigm to change. As Joseph Campbell stated,

> There are many gods,
> Choose your gods wisely.
> The god you choose
> Is the one you deserve.

10

No Known Causes!

● ●

Our greatest freedom
is the freedom to choose our attitude.

—Victor Frankl

Most of the degenerative diseases of our times are regarded as having "no known causes". Potential causes are linked to genetic and environmental conditions when you ask the doctor the why, what, and how. Many of these diseases have "societies" attached to them for the support of patients and research. For as long as I can remember, the evening news has carried regular stories of trial treatments for cancer, which are always in their research stage. The level of depression in our society has gone through the roof. Behavioural problems in children are also increasing at alarming rates. There seems to be a potential vaccine for just about any disease, even including those that are not infectious like the human papillomaviruses that cause cervical cancer.

Medicine is fantastic at fixing acute damage. I am thankful to have been put back together several times, and I am very appreciative. Things that were once life-threatening are now often reparable. Unfortunately, medicine is not very good at treating many of the degenerative conditions of our times. Treatments are mainly geared towards relief of symptoms and rely on picking the correct drug that may fit the diagnostic label. Sometimes they work for a while.

When there's no known cause, there can never be a cure. Gradually the "no known cause" becomes a part of the language and the thinking of both doctor and patient. There is an acceptance amongst most people that if there is 'no known cause', then it is just bad luck. Perhaps it is your genetic makeup? The genetic argument never states as much but strongly implies that if you have a particular genetic weakness in some area, then that's what's going to kill you. We all have a genetic weakness, as well as genetic strengths. To a point, this totally explains the variety of diseases found by both Price and Rosenow. Many of these conditions may not kill you but will certainly reduce your quality of life.[581] Perhaps it is time to look in other directions for a cause.

Trigeminal Neuralgia and Other Horrible Pains

An adult human incisor (a single-rooted front tooth) has about 500 myelinated nerve fibres and 40–150 unmyelinated fibres. Each nerve fibre has eight terminal filaments that go to the outer surface of the pulp, which is about 40 mm^2. That's about *120 nerve filaments per square millimetre*. This is vastly more than the cornea in your eye, which has only 70–80 nerve fibres for its entire surface area of 20 mm^2.

Areas of the brain which control motor function and sensations like pain have now been well mapped. There is a specific area of the brain which recognizes pain and other sensations. We can trace various parts of the body to various parts of this region of the brain. It's called a "somatotopic projection" of the body onto the outer surface of the brain, which is called the cortex. When this is done, we see that the face is large compared to the back of the head and indeed the rest of the body. The legs take about 15 per cent of this area. The arms and hands get about 25 per cent, and the trunk of the body a whole 8 per cent. The mouth, teeth, face, and neck get about 50 per cent of this area. This is true for the motor areas also.

In the sensory somatotopic projection, the *Trigeminal nerve takes up 28 percent*, compared to the rest of the body. This is the nerve which supplies sensation to the teeth, mouth, lips, skin, and the rest of the face. The *Trigeminal* nerve has the largest innervation zone of all the cranial nerves and has the largest ganglion. The nerves in the tooth are a part of the total area innervated by the *Trigeminal* nerve.

The nerves in the tooth form a massive surface area which feeds directly back to the brain. Organic toxins are transported back to the brain along the nerve fibres at a rate of 250 mm per day.[582] Remember that these toxins are also transported throughout the body.

I imagine it like a massive net, with the fibres of the net being like nerves—sponges—that absorb, from a massive surface area, all toxins produced in the mouth and teeth and then carry them back down a channel called the Trigeminal nerve to the brain.

All of these factors would support the hypothesis that relatively minor, low-grade inflammation or infection in a tooth could have profound effects on the whole nervous system. This research was published in 1980. "Virtually any irritation of the dental pulp or 'amputation stump' has the potential of transporting alergesic toxins throughout the Trigeminal system whether they be of chemical or bacterial origin"[583]

Way back in 1976 it was demonstrated that there is "evidence of demyelenation of the Gasserian (Trigeminal) Ganglion after damage as far away as a tooth pulp."[584]

Demyelenation of the nerve means that the myelin sheath around the nerve has been damaged or removed. This has a profound impact on nerve transmission. Demyelenation of the Trigeminal Ganglion is a massive concern. This could cause pain to be referred to any part of the body. A tooth can be a major cause of Trigeminal Neuralgia or severe pains *anywhere* else.

In the 1970s, an American dentist, Dr Eugene Ratner, published research which clearly demonstrated a strong causal link between cavitations in the jawbone and Trigeminal Neuralgia (TN). He was able to show that these holes in the bone, which were then known as Ratner's Bone Lesions, now just called cavitations, were causative for not only trigeminal neuralgia but also indeed many other forms of intractable pain in many other parts of the body. The relatively simple process of cleaning out these holes led, in most cases, to a complete remission of the pain. His research is vast and spans many years and is well-published in both medical and dental journals.[585,586,587,588,589,590]

The "relatively simple" surgery is, of course, relative to doing irreparable brain surgery. I went through university in the 1970s, and this research was *never* discussed. It was ground breaking and saved so much suffering, yet our oral surgeons at Sydney University never spoke of it. The "no known cause" flag was always dragged out with the "hypochondriacally bad nut case" flag. I didn't learn about cavitations and Dr Ratner for another twenty years. Today dental students are still refused this knowledge. I don't understand why the dental profession totally refuses to acknowledge the relationship of cavitations to TN. Nothing is allowed to even hint that a root canal may cause a cavitation and that both may be linked causally to cancer. It is sacrilege to suggest that the root-filling cements, forced through the tooth and into the bone, might be a cause of the cavitation that follows the extraction. Needless to say, there are many other reports of treating trigeminal neuralgia being caused by cleaning out the cavitations in the jaw bones.[591,592,593,594,595]

Bacteria do not need to spread all over the affected tissue to induce extensive inflammatory reactions. They may be located in foci, such as an infected dental root. Recent literature emphasizes the role of nerve transmission of vasoactive substances (those which cause a contraction or expansion of blood vessels) for the spread of inflammation. These substances can be released at all of the nerve junctions when the nerve is stimulated. Thus, an endotoxic stimulation of just a couple of nerve endings could induce a *widespread inflammatory reaction*.[596,597,598,599,600] Remember the power that comes from splitting just one atom. It is a similar analogy.

This relationship should not be surprising when we remember that all toxins in the tooth are transported back to the trigeminal ganglion and can sensitize the whole of the trigeminal and other nerve systems.

The reason I am making such a big deal of it is that the pains that are associated with this condition are usually of short duration but intense. They are usually triggered by something as simple as a breath of wind over the sensitized area on the skin (e.g., the face). This is not an ordinary toothache or a pain that an aspirin will resolve. The intensity of the pain, when it hits, will completely immobilize anyone. The pain is so intense that many have suicided because of it.

Dr Ratner found that by cleaning out the cavitations and restoring health to this part of the bone, many of the Trigeminal Neuralgias disappeared. Every patient with this condition improved after jawbone surgery and most – around 90 per cent—were free of pain completely. These were the first reports of a solid dental cause and treatment for Trigeminal Neuralgia.

Most people who are suffering so severely are usually referred by their doctor or dentist to one of the pain clinics associated with major teaching hospitals. Before being accepted into these units, the patients are almost always referred for psychiatric assessment just to make sure they're not "imagining" it. Anything to do with the mouth or face is seen by an oral surgeon. I have seen many such people who attended the pain clinic and were prescribed a sedative or an antidepressant. All reported the same treatment. Not once were the mouth or teeth examined. Not once was an X-ray of the mouth looked at. Not once was there any intervention, such as injecting local anaesthetic next to a root-canalled tooth to see whether it switched the pain off. Never once was any electrodermal screening undertaken. Medical histories were almost insulting in their brevity.

When the antidepressants have not cured the condition and the pain has still not gone, the patient is referred to the brain surgeon. A brain surgeon's point of view is that "There are several possible causes of trigeminal neuralgia, including ordinary aging. In many cases, trigeminal neuralgia is caused by an abnormal blood vessel or tumor pressing on the trigeminal nerve; the pain can also be a result of ..."

Cavitations and dead teeth are not in the realm of consciousness for the brain surgeon.

A time is made for the hospital visit, and the surgeon proceeds to cut the trigeminal nerve from the base of the brain or a variety of other more modern techniques, thus producing complete or partial numbness on that side of the face, head, and neck. This is definitely a preferable outcome to suicide, but sadly, this treatment usually does not stop the pain. The patient is left with the same pain in a numb face. There is no attempt in any of their procedures to address the dental causes of TN. All are aimed at interrupting the messages from the Trigeminal ganglion to the rest of the brain. It's like using an atomic bomb instead of insect spray to get rid of a cockroach. And still the cockroaches return with either.

I've never understood why it's preferable to do brain surgery instead of cleaning out a hole in the bone.

Searching for and finding the dental cause can sometimes be a bit time-consuming. Sometimes we get lucky and find the cause quickly. Many times, the cause is in a cavitation, and an injection of procaine (local anaesthetic) turns off the switch for long enough to see that the pain is either reduced or gone. Many times, the dead, root-canalled tooth is the direct cause of TN. This is so unacceptable to the dental community that it is never discussed. It's really simple! Remove the dead tooth and save your brain.

Teeth don't need to be dead to act as a trigger for TN. For example, I had a case in which the root of a patient's upper molar was exposed by a bit of gum recession. By scratching at the root with a probe, I was able to cause an immediate TN attack. I was then able to turn it off for days by injecting Procaine around and onto the root. The other exposed roots on this tooth did not induce the pain. By injecting a little Procaine into the gum around the root (and bathing the root in it), I caused the pain to disappear as fast as it came. The injections were repeated every few days for two weeks, and the pain did not return in this period. This was an interesting case referred by another dentist. I advised removing the offending tooth. The other dentist advised a crown, which the patient chose to go with. Needless to say, she suffered for another six months before losing the tooth and the $2,000 for the useless crown. I instead received hugs from a very appreciative patient and a huge bottle of my favourite whisky. To my knowledge, the TN never did return.

Diagnosis of these cavitations can sometimes be difficult. They may be visible on an X-ray but often are not. Even when they are clearly visible to the trained eye, the untrained dentist may not have a clue what they are looking at. My first day of education by Dr Horst Poehlman was a little frustrating for both of us. It took me a couple of hours of being shown one X-ray after another before I began to see what he was showing me. I'm a very slow learner, so it took me a year or so before I felt comfortable with what I was seeing. This all came about after reading a short paper by Dr Hal Huggins, who spoke of a German doctor in Adelaide who taught him to read X-rays after twenty-five years of looking at them himself. I figured that if this doctor was good enough to teach Dr Huggins, then he might see fit to also teach me. Crossing the threshold of his front door was, in reality, stepping into the abyss of realization that my dental training was about to begin. It did. I am forever grateful to Dr Poehlman, who was one of my gentle teachers.

Some cavitations will be found that still have a hole at the top of the bony ridge, merely filled in with soft tissue. If a Procaine injection can be put down into this hole, the most amazing things can happen. Simply injecting procaine into the gum around these holes can have a similar effect. The Procaine repolarizes the disturbed tissue, and its return to a healthier state can be diagnostic for a cavitation that is acting as a neural interference, especially if the pain is switched off. To me this seems an easier approach than any form of brain surgery! This speaks volumes for treating the causes rather than the symptoms.

Three-dimensional "cone beam scans" are reasonably good at seeing holes in the bone. These scans are not foolproof, but only a trained dentist will look for and see the holes. One of the best tools, though, is the Cavitat machine, which uses ultrasound to demonstrate holes in the bone. It is genuinely both safe and effective, which could also be the reason why it is no longer on the market. It works! It's also possible to demonstrate these holes using Electro Dermal Screening. This is a brilliant energy medicine system which is also being attacked by the medical profession. The efficacy of many of these instruments can and should be confirmed by the use of local anaesthetic around the suspected area. This technique is simple and far less invasive than brain surgery and CT scans.

Other excellent sources of information can be found at https://www.biodentistalabama.com/research/windham-cavitations.pdf.

Multiple Sclerosis

MS and other brain diseases deserve special mention, if for no other reason than the horrifying increase in the number of cases over the last twenty years. Dentistry is not the only cause. It is only one of the most overlooked of causes. Following is information which I hope will be of help. It is a brief summary of a huge wealth of knowledge in this area. The MS diagnosis does not have to be a diagnosis without hope. Many can recover.

Quoting Professor Daunderer,

> If we take Multiple Sclerosis patients who removed amalgam but refused both extraction of root canals and treatment of infected maxillary bone, we observe a cure rate from MS of 16%.

> But when we consider multiple sclerosis patients that beside amalgam removal accepted our full treatment

> (root canal extraction and cleaning of alveolar bone),
> the percentage of cures increases to 86%.[601]

In the1970s and 1980s, Professor Patrick Stortebecker, who was then the Professor of Neural Surgery at the Karolinska Institute in Sweden, demonstrated that the primary lesion in Multiple Sclerosis is *not* demyelenation but instead is an infected plaque around the venous side of the blood supply to the brain. Cerebral MS plaques showed the same organisms as found in dead teeth, periodontal disease, and other oral infections. Spinal MS lesions showed the same organisms that are found in the bowel and vagina. Stortebecker described the pathway of transmission through the non-valved venous plexus for both areas. By injecting dyes into the angle of the mandible (therefore not a bony connection to the rest of the skull), he was able to fill the whole of the intra-cranial blood vessels. This demonstrated that the non-valved veinous plexus below the skull allows movement of blood in both directions. This is critical to the understanding of how the microorganisms from the mouth could enter the brain.[602,603,604,605] (One purpose of the veinous plexus is to regulate the pressure within the skull. Additionally, deoxygenated blood is emptied from the skull through this venous plexus.)

This research is ignored by not only the whole of the medical world but also by the Australian MS Society itself. A clever doctor once told me that we will never find a cure for any disease that has a society or organization associated with it. I tend to agree!

Apart from nerve transmission of toxins, there are several ways that teeth may be related to brain conditions. The ends of the roots of upper molars and premolars are either very close to, or sit within, the floor of the maxillary sinuses. (The sinus spaces in your cheek bones). At best there is a millimetre of bone or less around the end of these roots. Infection or abscess at the end of these roots will cause infection and inflammation in the lining of the sinuses—otherwise known as sinusitis.[606,607,608,609,610,611,612,613,614,615,616,617,618,619,620,621] Remarkably, this one millimetre of bone also separates the medical and dental worlds. It separates the domain of the "Dentist" and the domains of the "Ear, Nose and Throat" specialists, and also the domain of the "Neurologists." Since when were our bodies divided into states and countries to be ruled over by separate dominions?

Research as recent as 2007 indicates that the development of a "fungus ball" in the maxillary sinus is directly associated with root treatment of the upper teeth.[622]

Even the American Association of Endodontists recognizes the relationship of dead teeth and sinusitis.

> … failure to identify and properly manage the endodontic source pathology will result in the persistence of sinus disease, the failure of medical sinus therapies, and the potential advancement to more serious or even life-threatening cranio-facial infections.

> Out of 85 sinusitis guidelines, published between 1998 and 2010, only eleven mentioned an odontogenic cause for sinusitis and only three gave a recommendation for a dental examination [623]

So what does sinusitis have to do with the brain? Ask any Ear, Nose & Throat specialist, and they will likely tell you, "Not much." Ask these same people about the association of dead teeth and sinusitis, and most likely they will also say, "Not much." They treat the repercussions at the other end of the roots, without ever seeing a causal association. I once had a lady come to see me who had been treated for breast cancer. The X-ray of her teeth showed that the upper first molar was root-canalled, and at the end of one of the roots, lying on the floor of the sinus, was a huge abscess that looked like a sea cucumber. She freaked out and was scared that this was cancer too. I assured her that it was not and explained what it was and how this may be associated with the cancer that she'd had. I suggested she have a second opinion from an ENT specialist who was a friend of hers. He assured her that there was no abscess and that there was no association to her cancer. (The upper molars sit on the stomach meridian, which passes directly through the breast area.)

There is a strong and well-published association between Sinusitis and Multiple Sclerosis and other brain diseases.[624,625,626,627,628]

The epidemiologic studies of the incidence of Sinusitis and MS are directly linearly related. More sinusitis equals more MS [629,630]

"In an analysis of general practice records the rate of chronic sinusitis was significantly greater in 92 patients with multiple sclerosis (MS) than in matched controls. MS and chronic sinus infection were also significantly associated in the timing of attacks, in the age at which patients suffered their attacks, and in the seasonal pattern of attacks."[631]

There is a *linear relationship*
Between the *incidence of MS* and that of *dental decay.*

This has been known since 1978, and yet the link between dental decay rates and the incidence of MS is blindly ignored by the dental and medical professions and the Australian MS society.

Causal comparison of the WHO map of dental caries incidences throughout the world reveals a striking parallel in general trend. Comparison of decayed, missing and filled teeth with the MS death rates results in a correlation coefficient of 0.97, and the probability of a chance occurrence is less than 0.002. This represents a nearly perfect linear relationship between dental disease rates and MS death rates.

The geographical distribution and other epidemiological characteristics of multiple sclerosis are compared with those of dental caries. The rates of death due to MS in Australian states are linearly related to the numbers of decayed, missing, and filled (DMF) teeth found in individuals from those states. In the United States of America, a strong positive correlation also exists between MS death rates and dental caries indices. The prevalence of MS in 45 counties or areas correlates well with the frequencies of DMF teeth among children of school age in those locations ... The prevalence of MS also correlates well with the percentage of edentulous individuals in certain countries."[632]

It's a good fit, like holding your two hands together; they match perfectly.

The relationship is clear, strong, and well published. There is no room for denial at the expense of so many lives.

There is a strong and well-published association between

Sinusitis and Dental Infections.

Sinusitis and Multiple Sclerosis.

Optic Neuritis and Dental Infections.

Optic Neuritis and Multiple Sclerosis.

Autoimmune

Multiple Sclerosis is more than just dead teeth. There also appears to be a relationship via autoimmune reactions to heavy metals as well. From the work of Professor Vera Stejskal in Europe, it is clear that all metals must be avoided in Multiple Sclerosis patients. This includes the metals in composite resins that are used to colour the filling materials. Porcelains should be the filling material of choice and should be cemented into place with old-fashioned, but safer, zinc phosphate cement. For all those with an autoimmune disease, I strongly recommend you read the information at www.melisa.org.

As Professor Störtebecker states, "Can our society really afford to take care of all these 'dental diseases', generated from infectious foci of the teeth and jaws, involving a spread of highly pathogenic agents out into the human body, even to the cranial cavity and the brain, with all the gruesome consequences being reflected in various symptoms from the nervous system, only to mention disorders like epileptic fits, hallucinations in schizophrenia, and moreover multiple sclerosis and malignant brain tumors."

Bill was another patient who came to see me in desperation because, at the age of thirty-two, he figured that he was too young for an MS diagnosis. The treatment he received was the removal of a single root-canalled tooth. Of course, our surgical procedure involved removing the periodontal ligament and unhealthy bone from the cavity. Bill stated the following:

> In September 2003, I went along to my dentist and had a root canal treatment performed. Months later in January 2004, I started to experience problems with my balance, tingling sensations and numbness in my hands and feet. Subsequently I was referred to a neurologist and after many tests – C.T. scans, lumbar puncture etc, – I was told that the probable cause of my problems was Multiple Sclerosis.
>
> The amazing thing for me was I had this root canal filled tooth pulled out in September 2004 and a week later, literally a week later, my balance started to improve, and the sensations that I had been experiencing for 9 months, started to abate. The numbness & tingling – and basically things have just improved from there. It is now December 2005![633]:

Although anecdotal, I would like to present just one case study out of several. A lady in her forties—Helen, for want of a name—came to see me after being diagnosed with MS She had a few young children and a great relationship with her husband. She was very happy but felt that she was too young to be sent home with a death sentence and no hope of treatment. On examining her mouth, I found one root-canalled tooth on the upper left and a small metal-and-porcelain bridge to replace a missing front tooth. There wasn't any amalgam in her mouth. Technically, the bridge was very well made, but we had no idea which metals were used. The root canal looked like a job that any endodontist would be proud of, and there was no abscess visible on the X-ray. No matter what the tooth looks like on an X-ray, *all* dead teeth remain infected, as it is impossible to sterilize them. She'd had great mechanical dentistry done.

She also brought in her MRI scan, which showed two large lesions in her brain.

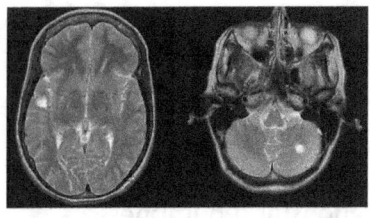

She had done her research and requested that I take out the bridge and the dead tooth. I told her there was no promise it would affect her health, as I always did, and she accepted this completely. I also agreed with her that there was a good likelihood the MS could be related to these. At this first appointment, she decided to remove both the tooth and the bridge immediately. She was not interested in proving which was a cause. She just wanted to eliminate *all* possible causes. She was quite happy to go home with a "gappy" smile.

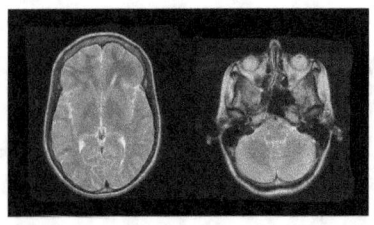

Three months later, Helen came back in to see me with a new MRI. All of her symptoms had resolved, and the MRI scan was clear of any lesions. Her neurologist had declared her free of MS and *did not want to know what she had done to make such a radical change.*

It's important to understand that this does not happen in all cases, but for Helen it was a fantastic outcome. She remained free of MS for several years before I retired. It's also important to understand that *it can happen* and that we should always be hopeful and try everything to heal, even though it may sound radical to the dental authorities. Dental associations and endodontic societies worldwide condemn the idea that a dead tooth could cause any problems, in particular things like MS and A.L.S., let alone cancer. I believe that *if it can happen for one, then it can happen for others*. Never give up hope.

Yes, I did contact the Australian MS Society, who were very polite but totally disinterested in this information. I was told clearly that MS had nothing to do with dentistry and that as a mere dentist I would not be able to understand the medical significance of this disease.

Mercury and Amalgam

There is another and important confounding aspect of Multiple Sclerosis which must be mentioned at this point. The symptoms of mercury poisoning and those of multiple sclerosis are identical. The main source of mercury to the general population is, of course, dental amalgam. In fact, mercury exposure occurs at a rate ten times higher through this source than through all other sources combined, including seafood.[634]

Studies have found mercury-related mental effects to be indistinguishable from those of MS.[17,635,636,637]

Does mercury from amalgam play a part in the development of, or long-term outcome of, MS? Unfortunately, there is still too much that we do not know. There are a few things, however, that we do know, which are worth mentioning here.

Elemental mercury vapour is converted to methyl mercury in the body. This is forty-five times more fat-soluble than ionic mercury, making it that much more dangerous to nerve cells. The nerve cells are covered in a myelin sheath, which is a highly lipid material. Methyl mercury destroys these myelin proteins.

The following is from *The Invisible Rainbow*: "This disrupts the myelin sheath and changes their conductivity which, in turn, alters the excitability of the nerves they surround. The entire nervous system becomes hyperactive to stimuli of all kinds, including electromagnetic fields."

It is well known that the cerebrospinal fluid of MS patients has substantially higher levels of mercury than in people without MS MS patients also usually have a higher body burden of mercury.[176,211,638,639,138,]

A study from 1994 looked at a variety of effects in MS patients with and without amalgam fillings and a non-MS control group. "Hair mercury was significantly higher in the MS subjects compared to the non-MS control group. A health questionnaire found that MS subjects with amalgams had significantly more (33.7%) exacerbations during the past 12 months compared to the MS volunteers with amalgam removal."[640]

MS displays characteristics of autoimmune disease as well. Mercury can cause autoimmune diseases.

A study from 2016 shows that repeated exposure to mercury accelerates progression of MS through mitochondrial damage related to oxidative stress and, finally, apoptosis (cell death).[641]

Many MS patients have been helped by reducing their mercury loads. This can be achieved only if the source of the mercury is removed. Thus, all amalgam fillings need to go, as well as all other sources of mercury, including amalgam tattoos. Several published studies have clearly demonstrated an improvement of symptoms after the amalgams are removed. Not all recover, but many do. Amalgam may be an important risk factor for patients with autoimmune diseases.[642,643,644]

Dr Huggins noted that the incidence of both ALS and MS started going through the roof after 1976, with the introduction of high-copper amalgams, which release about fifty times more mercury than the older formulations of amalgam with less copper. Dr Hal Huggins, the person who brought mercury from amalgam to the attention of the world, continued to research the health effects of dentistry till his death. In 2010 he published some findings in relation to these high-copper state-of-the-art amalgams. In his words,

> My attention was drawn to the increase in autoimmune disease after the high-copper amalgams of 1975 were initiated as "state of the art" fillings, which ADA claimed released no mercury. On the contrary, studies from Europe found that the high-copper amalgams released fifty times more mercury than previous amalgam!
>
> In watching these changes regarding the onset of autoimmune disease, I noticed a blip in the statistics— an increase in amyotrophic lateral sclerosis (ALS or Lou Gehrig's disease) in 1976.

Hal Huggins stated the following: "The actual number of cases of multiple sclerosis increased tremendously, from an average of 8,800 per year during the period 1970 to 1975, to an increase of up to 123,000 in one year. That year being 1976, the birth date of high-copper amalgams."[645] June 25, 2010 by Hal Huggins, DDS.

Multiple Sclerosis was not known before *1830*, when *mercury amalgam* became a worldwide phenomenon!

Dr Hal Huggins is by far the leading expert in the field of mercury poisoning and the effects of dead teeth. As a dentist, he has helped thousands of people to get well, many of whom had been given *no* hope from the medical profession. His knowledge in this area and in relation to the effects of dead teeth on the human system is second to none.

Dr Huggins has written the single most comprehensive book on this subject. It is *essential* reading for anyone who has or knows of someone with MS It is called *Solving The M.S. Mystery: Help, Hope and*

Recovery by Dr Hal Huggins. You can order it from his website at http://www.hugginsappliedhealing.com/ (ISBN 0-9724611-1-6). I believe that this book is so important that every doctor, dentist, and patient should read it.

Many times, I have seen patients who were diagnosed with MS from their clinical symptoms only. I, too, was diagnosed with MS when in 1986 I had an attack of Acute Optic Neuritis. The optic nerve in my left eye became severely inflamed, and overnight my vision in that eye became a peripheral blur. The neurologist immediately proclaimed MS because optic neuritis is often one of the earlier symptoms of this disease. I asked what else it could be, and all I got was "a list as long as your arm." I asked why he would immediately choose MS when other causes could also be considered. He did not reply. Sadly, this scenario is all too common, and many people become misdiagnosed and mistreated. I believe that neurologists should have a responsibility to include dead teeth and mercury from amalgam fillings, in their arsenal of diagnostic tools. I finally worked out what was wrong with me when, several years later, I read Dr Huggins' book *It's All In Your Head.* As a dentist still using amalgam, I had been exposed to astronomical levels of mercury vapour. I was mercury poisoned. Thankfully the diagnosis of MS was wrong.

Often the removal of the dead tooth results in complete resolution of the disease state. There are unfortunately also times when it does not. A stone is thrown through my window. The window breaks. I pick up the stone and throw it back out. It hits the person who threw it through my window. I have addressed the cause, but the window is still broken. So too with dental and systemic diseases. We may remove the cause of the problem, but if there is too much damage, it may be difficult to repair this damage just by removing the cause. Very few of my patients used dentistry as the only means of healing. The range of approaches is as diverse as the number of people seeking treatment. What works for one person may not work for another. Many medical and non-medical modalities can help. It is important to understand that there may be other contributing causes of any disease. Dentistry is *not* the only cause of disease. It is the *most neglected cause* and, I believe, one of the greatest causes of degenerative diseases in our society.

People with MS and other neurological diseases are advised to remove all amalgam fillings and any other metals in the mouth—including implants and, of course, dead teeth, whether root-canalled or not. It is also imperative to locate and treat any cavitations in the jaw bones.

Find a dentist or oral surgeon who is trained in these techniques. Most dentists are *not*.

Crazy or Poisoned?

Just as dead teeth can create disease states in the brain, which manifest as either pain or physical changes like MS or cancer, so too do these toxins affect psychological states. Our modern conditioning is to separate psychological and physical, even though they may have the same cause but express differently in different people. Thus, the drugs given for psychological manifestations will differ from the ones used to treat the brain tumour. Both treat only the most superficial of symptoms and manifestations because the cause often remains undetected and untreated.

The hatters of old used to cure rabbit fur with mercuric nitrate. They had profound psychiatric manifestations—they went quite bonkers. They became as "mad as a hatter", as clearly demonstrated in *Alice's Adventures in Wonderland*! Many patients who have amalgam implanted into their mouths also become mad, from the mercury they're exposed to. Any dentist who uses or drills out amalgam will also be mercury poisoned and often will also become as mad as a hatter. Should we wonder why dentists have the highest suicide rate of all professions? Fluoride in the drinking water also has profound psychological effects. Fluoride will lower IQs across a whole population.[646,647] It was put in drinking water in German concentration camps to keep the inmates more apathetic. It is used in our water supply for the same reason. Both mercury and fluoride act as inhibitors of brain growth and maturity when foetuses are exposed in utero. Neither is in any way beneficial.

Why, then, should we wonder about the toxins coming from a dead tooth having psychological effects? They, too, can have profound psychological effects, from total psychosis to dementia to a bit of depression. I have personally seen six patients who each had one dead tooth removed and went home and tore up the suicide note that night. It usually took less than a week for them to find that their sanity had returned, and the blackness had departed. The youngest was sixteen, and the eldest forty-eight years old. These were the obvious and successful cases. I lost count of the patients who reported a lift in their depression. This was always accompanied by a much more positive approach to the rest of their lives. Everyone is shocked to experience the changes that can be caused by toxins in dead teeth. As Price and Rosenow found, there really is no limit to the variety of effects these toxins can have.

The literature is full of research linking psychological effects with infections in the teeth, gums, and tonsils. Hydrogen Sulphide (H_2S) is principally a neurotoxin. It poisons nerve tissues and will seriously interfere with brain development. In fact, the central nervous system appears to be the major target organ.[648] "The consequence of one or a combination of such alterations may lead to behavioral and structural abnormalities."[649] Hydrogen Sulphide is an endotoxin produced by the bacteria in dead teeth.

Of course, this is regarded as anecdotal evidence and of no clinical significance. As long as the patient's endodontic bill is paid, there's no drama about a few suicides. Besides, once the person has died, there are rarely any complaints by the family. It is a far leap of knowledge to blame the endodontist for the child's suicide. Very few would support this link. Endodontists, who see a patient only to carry out a root canal procedure, would never even know that the patient went mad or killed themselves. The general dentist, who referred the patient, also wouldn't have a clue. If we don't see it, there can be no association. It's very convenient to rely on our non-existent clinical observation rather than on the published research! If the patient has died or gone mad, they will not be attending the dentist or endodontist to let him or her know. There is *no* association with systemic affects! Lack of evidence is not evidence of any clinical observation. As Carl Sagan said, "Absence of evidence is not evidence of absence".

Typically, both the medical and dental worlds have continually ignored the research and reports not just of the last 20 years but of the last 120 years. In 1908, Dr Henry Upson MD., published his research on the association between "Insomnia, Nervous Disorders and Dental Infections." In 1919, Dr Henry Cotton published in the *Journal of Dental Research* (1919) the association of "Oral Infection and Mental Disease." Their research was voluminous. (Both of these men's work was brought to us by Dr S. H. Shakman in 1998.[650]) The research conducted over many years was the result of watching patients in mental institutions improving and then re-entering normal society after oral infections were removed. Prior to tooth removal, the patients' conditions worsened, as was evidenced by them being institutionalized. This research was, of course, fully supported by that of Drs Price, Rosenow, Billings, and Mayo. The more recent work of Professor Patrick Stortebecker, published in the 1980s, is also strenuously ignored.[651] All found the same effects from the dead teeth. If the brain is affected, then the psychological makeup is affected. It is really that simple. How profound these effects are will vary amongst individuals. It makes me wonder how many frontal lobotomies and electric shock treatments could have been avoided by taking out dead teeth? It's a bit like our current approach to trigeminal neuralgia, with brain surgery being favoured over tooth extraction or cavitation cleaning. Currently, if it cannot be fixed with a drug from a "reputable" drug maker, then it cannot be fixed. How many people are today suffering with their psychiatrist and therapist, or just quietly committing suicide, because dentists and doctors are too myopic to accept the published science?

Many people still have amalgam mercury fillings in their heads. "Mercury causes a suppression of our total immune defence mechanism; hence people suffering from chronic mercury poisoning, are highly susceptible to all kinds of infections, may be even indirectly disposed to an increased risk of getting some types of cancer, whose origin is infectious."[28]

11

How to Fix the Problem

• •

Faith, Ethics, and Dogma

For health to be regained, the toxin factory must be removed. Unfortunately, there is *no* definitive test which shows that the dead tooth or teeth may be causing a particular disease. Usually, the relationship is seen only after the tooth is removed and the disease state disappears. We do need to weigh up the risks and benefits of any particular approach, treatment, medication, and the like. When enough information is given, we can make an informed decision. When no information is given other than the word of the practitioner, then we are making an uninformed decision based on blind faith. I hope I have presented enough information that faith is unnecessary and *informed* consent or dissent is available.

As a practitioner who, for thirteen years, performed thousands of root canal procedures, it came as quite a shock to realize that I may have been poisoning my patients instead of helping them. My training and brainwashing meant that if I were to take this new information seriously, I had better learn all about it. So I read and read and read, and studied with some very knowledgeable doctors, such as Dr Hal Huggins and Dr Horst Poehlman, till I was ready to offer a different service to my patients. No matter how much theory, it was still a leap into the unknown to move from doing root canals to taking them out. It was not only regarded as unethical to extract a "perfectly good root-canalled tooth", but it was a heresy against all the dental religious dogmas. There was not one specialist in any area of dentistry that would have supported such a treatment. If a patient complained to the dental board about me doing this, there would have been total demolition from this group, who support the high ethical standards espoused by the dental association. If, on the other hand, the patient's health improved, this would have made me an even larger target. Neither dentistry nor medicine want a treatment that makes the patient healthy.

I gave Dr Price's information to the first person to whom I suggested taking out root canals before I would accept her consent to remove the teeth. I was not prepared for the results. I was hopeful that taking out the dead teeth would help, but I was shocked to see the speed at which the body can heal when the rubbish is removed. It was terrifying to see my patients come back a week later to have the stitches removed and report that the symptoms they had suffered with, sometimes for years, had disappeared within a matter of days. This single event of resolution of disease in days, which was repeated time and again, really drove home to me the dangers of dead, infected, gangrenous teeth. It's similar to the dangers of mercury, where the smallest levels can produce profound physiological and psychological effects. The value of honest scientific research is clear. When the anecdotal evidence supports the scientific findings, then these anecdotes should be acknowledged.

One of the most common stories that I heard was that of breast lumps. I lost count of the number of women who told me their breast lumps had disappeared after a root-canalled tooth was removed. This often happened within a week of the tooth coming out. The psychological stress of living with lumps in the breast is one thing. The very real rise in the incidence of breast cancer is another. Many other factors are, of course, involved in the cancer process, but this is an association that has been reported many times over. Anecdotal reports, when repeated over and over again, must be given credence of clinical observation, to be at least listened to by the rest of the profession.

In contrast, the denial by the dental profession that this is even a possibility is nothing short of criminal negligence. They have themselves published that formaldehyde, MTA, phenol, and many other substances routinely placed in dead teeth cause cancer. They know it and yet still do it. Perhaps their clinical observation is carried out with eyes wide shut, and their ethics with a heart which is only interested in money!

There is now more than sufficient published research which demonstrates the role of oral infections as a cause of heart disease, diabetes, kidney disease, Multiple Sclerosis, and other neurological diseases, to call for an immediate ban on the practice of keeping dead teeth in the body. It is certainly time for the dental profession to take responsibility for the disasters they cause.

The Process

The extractions clinic in a dental hospital is where you get to understand the barbaric mindset that dentistry has arisen from. As a student, I once watched a professor of oral surgery show a few of us how to take out a lower molar that none of us were able to move. He held the jaw with one hand, grabbed the forceps in the other and almost lifted the patient out of the chair to get the tooth out. He hurriedly disappeared, as the patient's fist was bigger than both his hands together. True story. This is how dentists are "taught". The words "gentle and caring" do not fit in these extractions clinics. Pulling teeth with forceps only, is an ancient barbaric practice that should be banned. If not, then it should be compulsory for the patient to be given a big bottle of whisky (and a baseball bat) before the extraction begins. There is a much better way.

271

As with other aspects of dentistry, the extraction of teeth is still done as was taught by the barbers of old: grab the bloody thing and rip it out. Unfortunately, apart from being mind-blowingly brutal, this approach has some serious problems, which I will describe before discussing a much better way of doing it. The intent is not for the sake of a horror story, although it would be hard to beat. It is to give you, the patient, some knowledge of what to look for and ask about *when you are interviewing the dentist* who might do the job. If you can be informed before you go into the surgery, then you will be in a position to conduct the interview, rather than being told what you need to do by the well-meaning dentist. I also hope the information will show dentists how to not stuff up the process. While on this point there are a few stuff ups that should be discussed.

The Holy Sinus—Don't Stuff It Up – No1

Very often the roots of the upper teeth are close to or within the maxillary sinus. There is only a millimetre or so of bone between the end of the root and the floor of the sinus. If there is an abscess at the end of these roots, then the floor of the sinus will most likely be involved. This knowledge produces brain-numbing fear in dentists, who are taught that we must never expose the sinus. This could, they believe, lead to all sorts of dramas, such as your head falling off. The reality is that over 90 per cent of extractions of the upper back teeth will damage the floor of the sinus to some degree. This is the reality, whether noticed or not. Very few ever present any long-term issues.

I mention this as I have heard often that this is the reason to leave the dead tooth in place or even to do a root canal instead of taking it out. Of course, it is not a good idea to try to make holes in places that should be protected, but it is still better to get the tooth and abscess out and let the sinus floor heal than to leave it for the sake of not perforating the sinus floor. I have always thought that it would be easier to close a sinus floor than treat MS

The Fractured Root—Another Stuff-Up – Stuff Up 2

Dead teeth are brittle, especially if they have had a root canal procedure. Many root-canalled teeth already have a fractured root. Often the bone around such teeth is quite dense and hard. The combination can result in a broken root even when great care is taken. Again, this is not such a big deal. It just means taking a bit more time to get the root tip out. (The procedure I describe below for the extraction really minimizes the incidence of such fractures.)

Because most dentists are not trained to properly do this, we are now faced with a situation where the status quo actually condones the practice of leaving a broken root tip in the socket. In dental speak this is called "decoronation". If your dentist claims that this is okay and that it is safe to do so, my advice is to run. Do *not* pay the bill that they will charge for a botched job. Instead issue a letter of complaint to the dental board for a job badly done.

It is imperative for your health to remove the entire tooth—root tips also—and of course the infection that remains in the bone and the periodontal ligament. If the dentist does not understand the seriousness of this issue, find another dentist. Do not get bullied into thinking that lousy work is acceptable. If it is your regular dentist who is doing this, you might be grateful to know in advance and change your regular dentist. Remember that your dentist does not own you. Be loyal to yourself and your knowledge. Also remember that most dentists simply do not know because they have not been trained correctly. Be gentle with them.

Dead Bone—The "Ethical" Way

Dentists are taught to take teeth out with pliers, otherwise called "forceps". The tooth is gripped tightly, rocked from side to side until it loosens and is eventually pulled out of the jaw. Often, great force is applied and will be the main thing that the patient is aware of, if not pain as well. When lower teeth are removed in this way, it is easy to damage or at least inflame the jaw joint. Hence the warning about not taking out wisdom teeth under general anaesthetic. Damage to this joint can take a long time to resolve. When upper teeth are removed with this amount of force, it will often cause a compression of the bones at the base of the skull and palate. This will then cause an imbalance in the whole of the cranio-sacral system, which in turn may create an imbalance in your autonomic nervous system. This is not a problem for dentistry, as there is no concept of cranio-sacral involvement. None of these associations are taught in dental school. Neither medicine nor dentistry even acknowledges the cranio-sacral system, as this is a chiropractic concept, and very simply chiropractic treatments are not allowed to be seen to work. It is common when these forces are applied to also cause some strain and possible damage to the neck muscles, which are fighting the force applied to one small part of your head. If you complain to such a dentist, you will often be told that you are being neurotic or just mad and that you should not dare to tell the dentist how to do it. Often, nurse Ratchet will be in attendance to support the dentist against you. She will also be holding you in some type of headlock so that the dentist doesn't need to work so hard. FACT. This is what we are taught in dental school! If the times have changed, I would be very happy to be proven wrong.

"Compression Necrosis" is the term used to describe the death of the bone which has had too much pressure applied to it. Although the dental profession is aware of this result, they do nothing about it and instead keep teaching students to repeat the insanity. Dead bone cannot heal. This can be and often is the beginning of a dry socket and/or a cavitation.

A dry socket is one that has not healed properly. The way a socket should heal is to fill with blood, which will clot and then becomes "organized", with blood vessels growing through it. Collagen fibres are laid down, and then these are converted to bone. As this happens, the gum grows over the top of the socket. A dry socket, on the other hand, is one where the blood clot either does not form or is washed out of the socket before it can get locked in with blood vessels. Of course, most dentists will claim that you rinsed your mouth too soon and washed out the clot. It's a great way to put the responsibility back onto the patient instead of modifying their own practice. When the bone around the root is dead, it will not form a proper blood clot. Thus, the bone is exposed to the mouth, becomes infected, and is usually very painful. This is usually the beginning of a cavitation and should be treated by the dentist to stop the pain and help the healing. The common dry socket rate is about one in ten. In my clinic, the rate was closer to one in a hundred. That is quite a dramatic difference. Your health will be potentially a hundred times less affected if the bone heals properly.

Root-filling materials themselves are also a common cause of dry sockets. Materials such as formaldehyde and those that break down to release formaldehyde will literally mummify the bone around the root. It cannot heal properly. Research demonstrates the spread of these materials from the tooth to the rest of the body. The highest concentrations will initially be found in the bone around the root. It isn't rocket science.

Treatment of this condition may be fairly straightforward. If the socket is dry, then make it wet again. This means that under local anaesthetic, the socket should be cleaned out again, dead bone removed, the socket washed with Procaine (local anaesthetic), and healthy bleeding reinstated. Not only will the healing be much faster, but the pain is usually gone by the time the anaesthetic has stopped working.

Most dentists will consider their job finished when the tooth is on the bracket table or the floor. They will put a piece of gauze over the socket and get you to bite down on it to apply pressure to stop the bleeding. A gift of pain killers and more gauze is offered as you are led to the receptionist to pay the bill. Make sure you are given a written quote before anything is done. The hidden extras could send you broke.

Healthy Bone—A Less Ethical Way!

For a socket to heal fully, it must be cleaned down to healthy bone.

Many PTOs and dental boards consider the use of a surgical approach for extractions to be overservicing. Cleaning out the abscess is also considered overservicing. Health funds and governments pay out more for a "surgical" extraction than a "simple" extraction. It therefore becomes unethical to do the job properly—particularly so in countries that run a national health scheme, such as the UK.

Root-canalled teeth need to be extracted carefully. Especially when there is more than one root, it is wiser and easier to take a surgical approach to the removal. In this way, the roots can be sectioned and removed separately. Rather than using forceps, the dentist should learn to use an instrument called a luxator. This is a delicate tool that the oral surgeons like to keep for themselves. By placing it between the root and the bone, the root can start to be moved with the slightest rotation movement of the luxator—slight finger pressure rather than arm and shoulder pressure. The dentist can work their way around the root from all sides of the tooth. Usually as the root loosens, the luxator can slip further towards the apex of the tooth and will often pop the root out without any pulling. In this way, there is very little pressure on the bone.

Dentistry teaches that the cells of the immune system will clean up the abscess tissue that is left in the depths of the socket. This is one of the greatest of clinical mistakes, as it rarely happens. If the abscess remains at the end of the socket, the bone will usually heal around it and leave the abscess, to create a cavitation. When the socket is open and the roots are out, it is a relatively easy procedure to then remove the abscess tissue and the periodontal ligament, both of which inhibit healing. It is imperative that the abscess tissue be removed. If the floor of the sinus comes with it, then this can be addressed later, if necessary, without any danger.

There is another good reason to remove all dead tissue from the socket. Many of the toxins produced by the bacteria in these teeth stop the blood from clotting. They are the most common cause of a tooth socket continuing to bleed after extractions. When we do as we are taught and just cover the socket with gauze, the risk of severe bleeding will skyrocket. I don't remember one patient calling to say the bleeding would not stop after I had taken this on board. If the socket is cleaned down to healthy bone, the bleeding will only be a gentle ooze, which tends to stop as the blood fills the socket to the top. All dentists who follow these principles are aware of this phenomenon. The rest of the dental world has no teaching in this regard. The surface bone should also be gently drilled away to about one millimetre, into the healthy bone. This is to remove any layers of infected or mummified bone. Although it may sound horrible, it really is easy and painless. Before suturing the wound, it is recommended to wash the socket with Procaine, which should switch off any remaining neural interference by repolarizing the nerves in this area. German research has shown this to enhance the healing process. Other local anaesthetics may be used, so long as they do not have any vasoconstrictor, such as adrenalin or Octapressin, but procaine gives consistently good results.

Please understand that there are many technical steps which I have left out here, as they are relevant only to a dentist who is taking on this healthier paradigm. I have created training videos to help dentists understand what we are doing, and these are all available. There is a special page for dentists on www.realdentalinfo.com which explains in detail the steps taken.

Since following these protocols, I have never had a patient complain of excessive bleeding. Yes, it costs more to do a surgical extraction than a forceps pull. Yes, it takes longer. Yes, it heals better. No, there is *not* more pain. Most patients undergoing this treatment told me that they took a painkiller because I recommended it, rather than needing to.

Remember that the aim of doing all this work is to lighten your body's toxic load. There cannot be any promise of improvement of any medical condition, as there are many possible causes for any condition. In saying this, though, there are too many serious degenerative diseases that are only being treated superficially if the dead teeth remain in the mouth. The evidence for the support of what I am saying is largely anecdotal clinical observation. The clinical observation in this case is repeated all over the world by people who have practised in this way, including dentists, cancer specialists, and neurosurgeons. Yes, it is a leap of faith to take teeth out without any promise for the improvement you may be searching for. At the same time, has anyone else been able to really treat the condition? If not, then what have you got to lose?

I saw a patient about thirty years ago in my Sydney practice who was horrified by my suggestion that she have all her teeth removed. She was only in her thirties and, as a model, had paid thousands to get root canals and crowns *on every tooth*. Her health had suffered badly in the five years that followed all this dental "treatment". She left unconvinced of anything I was saying. By chance, she came to see me again about fifteen years later. To say that she was a mess would be an understatement. She had become fairly psychotic and depressed, and had tried suicide on several occasions. By this stage both she and her partner had started reading some of the alternative literature about root canals and sought me out. Her partner was one of the most supportive people I have ever met. He watched her progress carefully and reported to me often. She could not wait to remove the dead teeth, even though she was terrified of the whole idea. As the teeth came out over several appointments—with various lengths of time between appointments to allow her to recover at her own pace—her partner would fill me in on her progress. A year later, a happy, fulfilled, competent person came in to give me a hug as she was passing by. Sometimes it is a big leap of faith.

Filling the Gap

Taking teeth out can create a bio-mechanical problem in the jaw joint and therefore the spine. The position of the first few vertebrae in your neck is determined in part by the position and function of the jaw joint. This will have a ripple effect all the way down the spine. The jaw joint can be moved into an unbalanced position if the teeth move too much or if there is no support from the back teeth. This can affect the position of the vertebrae in the neck and then the rest of the spine. It can cause all sorts of TMJ (temporomandibular joint) problems. This is the reason I was often accused of creating dental cripples. It is, of course, important, for a host of reasons, to maintain what is called a well-balanced occlusion—or bite.

The question, then, is, which disease state would you prefer to risk? It's usually much simpler to fix a bite problem and fill a gap than to treat a disease like cancer. Aesthetics may also be a major consideration if you are losing a front tooth. Teeth are also useful for chewing and thus digestion. It's amazing how much good food can be eaten without any teeth! For most situations, it's a relatively simple matter to replace missing teeth. Here are some thoughts about what to do with the spaces.

Bridgework

This involves cutting down the teeth on either side of the space to place crowns over them. The crowns are joined together with the false tooth, thus creating a bridge.

If the teeth on either side of the space are themselves heavily filled and need crowns anyway to support their mechanical integrity, then I would consider a bridge as an option. Always make this bridge from porcelain rather than metal and porcelain (as shown). The porcelains that are available now (e.g., Zirconia), are comparable in strength to metal bridges and lack the electrical interference and the potential for heavy metal immune responses caused by metal in the mouth. Another aspect to be considered before preparing a bridge is the state of the occlusion—the way the bottom and top teeth meet. Certain situations make a bridge preferable, and others make it not so.

If the teeth on either side of the space are lightly filled or not filled at all, I would strongly recommend against the use of a bridge, because it damages the healthy tooth unnecessarily. To place a crown on a tooth requires the removal of about 1.5 mm all the way around and about 2 mm off the top of the tooth. In other words, it means removing almost the whole of the enamel of the tooth. As I said, if this has already been lost to decay, then you are removing only filling material, not tooth structure.

It is commonly thought in dental circles that 60 per cent of all crowns will need root therapy. I believe this is an excuse for sloppy dentistry, the same type that claims that mercury from amalgam is safe. The removal of tooth structure for a crown does *not* necessitate a root therapy at any time in the future. Provided the tooth is drilled carefully with copious amounts of water and cooling, there should be very little inflammation of the pulp.

Partial Dentures

Dentures are another option. No, not the kind granny had, all pink and teeth and bits of metal. Some recent advances are actually good. We now make very small unilateral dentures from injection-moulded plastics. There is no metal, and the pink clasps disappear into the gum. There is usually no need to do any drilling on any teeth to make them fit. They are a bit like the new magic bullet, especially as they are only about one third the cost of a bridge, require no tooth removal, are aesthetic and functional, and are about the most biologically compatible denture material on the market. They can also be made so small that they take little room in your mouth.

The best part about filling the gap with a denture is that you can take it out at any time. Comfort and function can thus be balanced.

Implants

At present, implants are the ultimate state-of-the-art replacements for missing teeth. Every dentist and his dog claims to be fantastic at placing and working with implants. The profit margin is hard to pass up if you need to have that overseas ski holiday with the family or mistress.

Most implants are made from titanium alloys. Titanium implants release small amounts of titanium all the time. These titanium atoms are carried throughout the body.[652,653,654,655,656] Even the *Australian Dental Journal* discusses the release of titanium from implants to the rest of the body.[657] As mentioned previously, the presence of fluoride dramatically increases the corrosion of titanium. It is also known that titanium can interfere with cell function and promote inflammation.[658] The immune system very often creates a reaction to these atoms, and this can easily lead to a range of autoimmune diseases.[659]

Dr Carlson considers there to be two ways that implants fail and possibly cause disease. The first biological factor is that of microbial infection within the soft tissues and bone around the implant. The second biological factor is that of the direct currents (DC electrical currents) generated by the implant fixtures, post, abutment, and replacement crown. "In over 50% of implants that were removed and sent for pathological testing, actinomyces were present and associated with the pathological picture."[660]

Many autoimmune diseases are related to titanium. "Like all metals, titanium releases particles through normal corrosion. These metals ions enter the body and then bind to body proteins. For those who react, the body will try to attack this structure. This starts a chain reaction which can lead to many symptoms including Chronic Fatigue Syndrome (CFS) or, in the most severe cases, Multiple Sclerosis (MS). The MELISA® test is the only scientifically-proven test which can diagnose titanium allergy and measure its severity."[11]

It is worth noting that there are many other sources of titanium. Some are from the diet, in desserts which are decorated with shiny colours. Nanoparticle-sized titanium dioxide is increasingly being used in our food to make it prettier! It's also an active constituent in cosmetics, such as shiny lipstick and mascara. Titanium dioxide can supposedly be made in "food grade" form, which is considered safe by the food and advertising industries! It is in many pharmaceutical drugs also. The number code is E171. Avoid all foods with this additive. Believe it or not, the purpose for adding TiO$_2$ is aesthetic. Icings on cakes and lipstick on lips can shine. Other products are made whiter to look better. Health is not a consideration. A Sydney University study published in 2019 looked at the effects of E171 on the health of mice.

> There is increasing evidence that continuous exposure to nanoparticles has an impact on gut microbiota composition, and since gut microbiota is a gate keeper of our health, any changes to its function have an influence on overall health.

> This study presents pivotal evidence that consumption of food containing food additive E171 (titanium dioxide) affects gut microbiota as well as inflammation in the gut, which could lead to diseases such as inflammatory bowel diseases and colorectal cancer.661

An earlier paper from 2017 demonstrated that titanium dioxide crosses the intestinal barrier and passes into the bloodstream. Their findings demonstrated that TiO$_2$ causes and promotes colorectal cancer and alters intestinal and systemic immune response.[662] If you have titanium implanted into your body, you will have titanium atoms floating around the whole of your body. Increasing rates of dementia, autoimmune diseases, cancer metastasis, eczema, asthma, and autism are among a growing list of diseases that have been linked to soaring exposure to nanoparticles.

Titanium is *not* inert. (By the way, neither is gold.) Titanium is released from any source implanted into the body. Titanium can have profound effects in the body, especially when in nanoparticle size:

- damage to human bronchial cells [663]
- stimulation of bone resorption, which is one of the main reasons for these implants getting loose and falling out[664] (That's right, the titanium causes the bone to resorb away. It causes the failure of the implant all by itself.)
- antibody-mediated immune responses [665]

- excessive corrosion of titanium caused by exposure to fluoride[666,667,668] (In Australia most of our drinking water contains fluoride and most dentists like to slop it around your mouth every six months. Income and efficacy are not necessarily related.
- generalized allergic reactions[669,670]
- (when amalgam and titanium are in the same mouth) increased corrosion of the amalgam and thus the increased release of mercury, copper, and tin[671]
- Titanium and amalgam together, produce dramatic pH changes and a change in taste sensation[672]
- Some are carcinogenic[673] (It is possible that NiTiSMA particles are directly carcinogenic.)

Electrically Charged

Apart from the direct effects of titanium, there is also an electrical interference created by any metals in the mouth, including titanium implants. Titanium implants are routinely used in the mouth with other metals, which creates a battery. This is called a galvanic reaction and happens when two or more different metals are put together in an electrolyte, in this case the saliva. High electrical currents are generated between titanium implants and other metals in the mouth.[674,675] Levels of over one hundred micro amps have been routinely mentioned in research and in my own clinical findings. These currents, although only in the range of microamps, are in reality, one thousand times higher than what the brain operates at (i.e., nanoamps). These currents will have a profound effect on the whole organism and in particular on the brain and the heart. "Human cellular structures operate electrically in all actions in pico-ampers ... currents greater than pico-amps (in the direction of nanoamps and micro amps) will cause cell destruction while currents smaller than pico amps stimulate cellular growth."[676]

As well, all metal fillings and implants in the mouth can act as antennae for microwave transmissions and will increase the 'Specific Absorption Rate' (SAR) of this radiation into the body and, especially, the head.[677]

The presence of metal in or near the body can significantly increase a person's wireless exposure. Metal can reflect and refocus wireless radiation, resulting in much higher SAR absorption rates into the body. "Electrically conductive objects in or on the body may interact with sources of Radio Frequency energy in ways that are not easily predicted. Examples of conductive objects in the body include braces, orthodontics, and implanted metallic objects. Examples of conductive objects on the body include eyeglasses, jewellery, or metallic accessories."[678,679,680]

Metal piercings have a similar effect of increasing the radiation into the tissues, and if made from stainless steel, they will also influence the release of nickel from these implants.[681,682] Metal-framed eye-glasses will increase the Specific Absorption Rate into the eye and the brain up to 29 per cent.[683]

You might remember Jaws, the character from some of the old James Bond movies. His metal mouth is only a bit less subtle than what is done daily in dentistry. The main difference is that nowadays the metal is hidden under porcelain and plastic. Dentistry will happily combine all sorts of metals in crowns with amalgam fillings and titanium implants and chrome cobalt dentures, all in the same mouth. The perfect metal mouth is also the perfect antenna for microwave radiation. This radiation is focused within a couple of centimetres from your brain. Of course, it will affect the central nervous system and associated functions of the body. This has been linked to such symptoms as inexplicable fatigue, constant headaches, and mental confusion.[684] With metal dental work, your electrosensitivity is heightened, and consequently the potential health risks of EMFs are much higher.

Metals in the mouth will act as antennae and collect EMR which causes a reduction in the flow of blood inside your head.[685] Symptoms that have been reported include balance difficulty, lumbago, shoulder stiffness, neck pain, hip joint pain, and facial pain.[686,687] Cell phone radiation was also found to have dangerous effects on the salivary glands, facial nerves, and cells of the tissue that lines the mouth (oral mucosa).[688] Other reports indicate sleep disturbances, anxiety and other neurological problems, thyroid dysfunction, digestive problems, heart problems, and other chronic symptoms.[689] Keep your phone away from your head. Do *not* sleep with it anywhere near your body. Use it hands-free or not at all.

Because the symptoms of EMF exposure are often psychological and varied, the psychiatric conclusion is often that people suffering from them are "delusional" and "paranoid". It seems to never occur to these highly trained drug-pushing doctors that the complaint may be real, and thus they would have an explanation as to why their antipsychotic drugs don't work. Heaven forbid that the patient might actually have something wrong. Even in the dark ages, when I was a student, we heard about the occasional people who heard the radio in their heads. The voices were real, and the people were laughed at. No one understood that the amalgam fillings were acting as antennae for AM radio waves.

There is another reason to worry about cell phone use mixed with metals in the body. It has now been verified that Electro Magnetic Radiation alone can cause cancer.[690] 2018 saw the publication of a study conducted by "National Institutes of Environmental Health Sciences - National Toxicology Program Study on Cell Phone Radiofequency Radiation, Cancers and DNA Damage" which

> … found statistically significant increases in DNA damage, heart damage, malignant glioma tumors of the brain, and malignant schwannomas of the heart. The increased incidence of heart tumors were considered by the expert peer-reviewers and staff of the NTP to demonstrate "**clear evidence of carcinogenic activity**" of modulated cell phone radiofrequency radiation.'

> This is the latest of a series of studies linking cell phone radiation to acoustic neuromas, gliomas and Schwannomas of the heart.

> The malignant schwannomas of the heart seen in the Italian study are the same as those described by the U.S. National Toxicology Program (NTP) earlier this month as the basis for their concern that cell phone radiation, both GSM and CDMA, can lead to cancer.[691]

The Italian study comes from the Ramazzini Institute in Italy and was published in August 2018. It concludes with the following: "These tumors are of the same histotype of those observed in some epidemiological studies on cell phone users. These experimental studies provide sufficient evidence to call for the re-evaluation of IARC conclusions regarding the carcinogenic potential of RFR in humans."[692]

We are all living in a new environment that just forty years ago did not exist. The quantity and intensity of Electro Magnetic Radiation has affected everything on the planet. Our bodies are still trying to catch up. All these effects are being compounded with the metals that dentistry calls state-of-the-art treatments. These devices go deep into the bone. All this extra radiation is taken deep into the body. Is dentistry inadvertently adding to the increase in brain cancers by using implants which act as antennae and focus this radiation deeper into the body?

The titanium implant will usually have a gold and porcelain crown screwed to it; this constitutes a permanent galvanic cell. In other words, it is a charged battery implanted into bone on top of acupuncture meridians. Such implants act like lightning rods. For over twenty years, orthopaedic surgeons have known that it is dangerous to place dissimilar metals in the body. Dentistry obviously knows more than the bone surgeon specialists.

To put it simply, there is no such thing as a good implant. I would never have one in my mouth, and I have personally lost many teeth over the years.

A Few other thoughts about implants

Where the post protrudes through the gum to get into the mouth is another area causing serious consequences. The gum does not form a fibrous seal with the titanium post, as it does with the root of a tooth. Instead there is a very tight inflammatory reaction in the gum. This leaves a space, which to bacteria is like the Champs Elysees. The gum around the implant will be permanently inflamed; dentistry cannot control this reaction, so instead they have given it the name of "peri-implantitis". There will always be a high likelihood of infection in the bone around the implant. Osteomyelitis is not pretty or comfortable. It will be present no matter how good your oral hygiene is. This inflammation is the key to most implant failures and is a major source of systemic infection and disease. Remember that fluoride in the drinking water will cause an increased release of titanium from the implant. It is also known that there are higher concentrations of titanium in the tissue which makes up this inflammation.[9]

There is now evidence that the titanium released by the implant is *causative* of peri-implantitis.[693] In other words, the titanium implant itself is responsible for the inflammation and bone loss, which is one of the main causes of failure of implants. Yep, you read it right! One of the main causes of implant failure is the implant itself. Titanium is far from inert.

The periodontal ligament that surrounds a tooth and attaches it to the bone does not exist with an implant. Therefore, there is no cushioning of the forces that are applied to it. Any forces that are applied to the implant are transferred directly to the bone. This can then have an effect on the whole of the craniosacral system. It can also feel like a strange, weird pressure when you bite on it.[694]

The Last Option

Which is not necessarily a bad option for many people is just leaving a space. This may not be appropriate for everyone. By the way, your face will not collapse into the space left by one or two extractions. It is very different to a whole mouth full of missing teeth.

12

Case Studies

● ●

If you are meditating and the devil appears,
make the devil meditate too.

—G. I. Gurdjieff—Advice to his daughter.

Following are a series of case studies that I have personally witnessed. I do not make excuses for what I have had the pleasure to witness.

Case studies are, by their very nature, anecdotal. This is the story of some of the people I have had the honour to treat and have then witnessed the dramatic improvements in their health.[695] These stories are repeated hundreds of times in the writings of other researchers, including Dr Price and Dr Eugine Ratner. They are the stories that many of my colleagues also witness when they take out dead teeth.

When we take the garbage out, the body has a chance to heal. This can happen so quickly it can make your head spin. If there is no improvement, keep looking for the cause.

A Note on Overfilled Root Canals

As mentioned earlier, at least 17 per cent of all root canals are overfilled. Extrapolating that, 17 per cent of 2.3 million is 391,000 teeth that are overfilled and accompanied by liquefaction necrosis of the bone. When a dentist thinks about this situation, they are usually talking about Gutta Percha points that protrude through the end of the root. More often though, it is the root-filling cements that are forced through the ends of the roots and also through the accessory canals. These materials are all cytotoxic, and some are carcinogenic. They will kill the surrounding bone, cause inflammation of the nerves around these areas, and cause inflammation of the sinuses when they end up in there. The inflammation of the nerves can translate into Trigeminal Neuralgia. There is evidence of damage to the Trigeminal ganglion at the base of the brain caused by damage to the nerves from the tooth.

The Itch from Hell

I will never forget the first patient who had decided to have her dead root-canalled teeth removed. Although I was well prepared intellectually for what came about, I had not yet put into practice what I was learning. At that stage, I was still concerned by what the dental board might think of me! They considered it unethical to remove "sound and good root-canalled teeth". Ann was a fifty-five-year-old lady and had a fifteen-year history of eczema all over her body. She would wake every night to walk around naked to cool her body down while she would scratch herself raw—literally. She had not had a full night's sleep for over fifteen years. She presented with a medical history about two inches thick, outlining every conceivable treatment that she had tried. She'd had her amalgams removed about ten years earlier. She had two upper front teeth, an upper premolar and a lower left premolar, that were root-canalled. I was so nervous that I made her read some of Weston Price's work before making the decision. This was also my introduction to Dr Price's work in the form of a book that

Hal Huggins had compiled from his writings. It's called *The Price of Root Canals* and is definitely worth reading if you can get hold of a copy.

We first took out the three upper teeth. One week later, she returned for the final extraction and reported that in the past week there had been no change in her condition, which she regarded as a positive sign. Previously any medical interventions had brought only exaggerated misery. One week after the final tooth was removed, she reported that all the itching had stopped two days after the extraction.

I saw her again three months later, and she was hardly recognizable. She was sleeping through the night, which meant that for the first time in fifteen years she was having unbroken sleep and was dreaming again. Her spiritual life was returning. All of her scars were healed. Sixteen years later, there are no signs of itching. Four root therapies had produced fifteen years of living hell.

Eczema is one of the common symptoms from root-canalled teeth. The neurotoxins that spread from these teeth have profound effects, and although eczema is not going to kill you, it can make your life totally miserable. If the cause is the dead tooth, then no number of creams, balms, or medicines are going to make a difference. If the tooth is already dead, then what do you have to lose by getting rid of it?

Multiple Sclerosis

Jane was a forty-three-year-old woman with three children living a life of country sustainability with a love of nature. She was incredibly sporty and active till she was struck with the diagnosis of Multiple Sclerosis. The MRI showed two massive lesions in her brain. Her symptoms were becoming increasingly difficult, although she was not yet in a wheelchair. The medical specialists sent her home to die slowly, as they claimed there was nothing they could do for her. This was not a prospect that filled her with joy. Jane was a very intelligent fighter. She started the journey of self-education and tried a few things before reading some of what I had written about root canals and then the actual research that I referenced it with. She sought me out and came from Victoria to NSW for treatment.

She showed me her MRIs and the dead tooth and the single Maryland's bridge that replaced her upper lateral incisor. No one knew what metal the bridge was made from. The MRI scan showed two distinct MS lesions.

She needed no convincing. She knew exactly what she wanted and had prepped herself perfectly. On that first appointment, we removed the bridge and the dead root-canalled premolar. As we parted, I wished her well on the rest of her journey.

Three months later, she made the effort to travel about five hundred kilometres to come and see me again. She brought new MRI scans of her brain that had been done a week earlier. All symptoms of MS had vanished. The MRI was completely clear; the lesions had gone. Jane was ecstatic. As so often happens, her neurologist had no interest in what she had done.

We removed the cause of the MS, and she healed herself. I did not cure the MS, and this distinction is important for everyone. Watching disease states resolve when the dead tooth is removed is why I used to call myself the garbage collector. "I take the rubbish out and you heal yourself" was the agreement I made with all of my patients.

Local Anaesthetic "In the Stars"

Bill was a physicist who lectured at Sydney University. He had many diverse interests and was certainly one of the more entertaining people that have graced my life. I had done a great deal of work for him, as we were removing amalgam, dead teeth, root canals and a few other bits. His treatment was mainly uneventful and straightforward. That is till we came to remove his lower left first molar, which had been root-canalled many years prior. There was simply no way that I could anaesthetize this tooth. I had given him a couple of block injections, intraosseous injections and intra-periodontal injections. *Nothing* worked. I suggested that he come back another day so I could try to work out a solution. He had other ideas that involved me taking the tooth out with him holding the armrests of the chair. He was far stronger than I would have been. Needless to say, this was one of my worst experiences as a dentist. The tooth came out, and he went on his way.

A week later, he came to have the stitches out and reported the following. The night of the extraction, he went to a meeting of astrologers and other like-minded people. Being a bit upset, he voiced his distress to some of his friends there. Four of them went off with his birth time and date, and in a short while each came back and told him the same story. The time of his extraction appointment was exactly the worst time of the month and day for the moon cycle to interfere with anaesthetic. I asked a few astrologers who were patients, and they all confirmed that this is actually possible. Whether or not you believe in astrology, the experience was very real. I had not had any problems with making him numb before or after this day.

Fungal Infection Under Fingernails

This is the story of a forty-six-year-old male restaurant owner. For many years he had suffered with chronic fungal infections in and around his fingernails. He had, like most of the patients I see, tried everything to get rid of this, as it had a profound effect on his ability to work with food. Within one month of removing a dead tooth and doing some periodontal cleaning, all of the troublesome infections had gone.

In his words: "it is now time that I should say that I am breathing a lot easier. I can breathe in without opening my mouth all day long. The same at night – I can breathe in without breathing through my mouth. Whereas before was completely the opposite …" He told me his story while showing me how he could use his fingers as drumsticks on the table. This was impossible before because of the excruciating pain.

Chronic Headache and Migraine

The patient is a man of thirty-two years. He had some fillings and one root therapy in his upper front tooth. It was, of course, quite a decision to remove his front tooth. Again, in his words: "… Robert looked at it and told me that it was pretty bad. And it did actually look pretty horrible. I took away some literature on root canal therapy and looked it up on the net and considered the choices that I had. I decided that I should have it out. The headaches had completely stopped – it took about two weeks for them to decrease and two weeks till they were completely gone. And they haven't returned since."

Pituitary Tumour

Jeff was thirty-nine with a young family and lots to live for. He was getting all sorts of weird neurological symptoms and was finally diagnosed with a pituitary tumour. Surgery was proposed. As most people do, he tried to put it off for as long as possible by using all sorts of other remedies which managed to stop the tumour from growing too quickly. Then he saw a video about root canals and decided to check it out. He arrived with his OPG, which showed not only a root canal on the lower right first molar but also a mouth full of amalgam and a metal crown on the root-canalled tooth. Many of his symptoms had started within a year of the root canal being finished. Six years later, he was in my surgery.

The X-ray is interesting, as it demonstrates the condensing osteitis of a completely depleted immune system, as was shown by Dr Price in the 1920s, and a still rarefying abscess at the end of the roots. To modern endodontists, the condensing osteitis is nothing to worry about and is, in fact, seen as a good thing. The tooth was removed, along with as much as possible of the condensed bone. It felt like drilling on steel. Within two months, many of the symptoms had abated. A follow-up MRI scan six months later showed that the tumour had disappeared. All symptoms were gone as well, and the need for brain surgery was no longer necessary.

I wish that all brain tumours would respond so wonderfully, but sadly this is not the case. I have been fortunate to have seen some that do respond to removal of the cause only. From what I have seen, and this is purely anecdotal as a dentist, the two main causes of brain cancers are dentistry and mobile phone usage.

Headaches and Sinusitis

A fifty-three year old male patient with multiple fillings and two root-canalled front teeth (central incisors), one of which showed a large area on the X-ray. He stated, "… could I put up with the two dark teeth, and the headaches, or do I take the quantum leap and thinking I am going to lose two of my old friends, and it's going to be a fairly major change. I thought It's got to be better than this beforehand, and straight away it has been …"

All headaches went within a week, and the sinuses cleared almost immediately. The next day, he was breathing through his left nostril, which he had not been able to do for more years than he could remember. His energy levels returned, and now he tells me that he is happy to mow the lawn, whereas previously he could only watch his wife do it. I'm still not sure whether I did him a favour or not!

Painful Knee

The patient was a fifty-seven year old man who came for a routine examination and discussion about his fillings and his very sore lower right premolar tooth. This tooth had lots of decay and a small abscess.

Being a medical man himself, he needed very little information to understand the danger of leaving a dead tooth in his body and decided to have the tooth removed there and then.

One week later, he came in to have the sutures removed. Although the socket was pain free and showed excellent healing, he complained loudly that I had caused his right knee to become so painful that he could hardly walk. Never before had there been an issue with either of his knees.

I assumed that this was a neural interference rather than an infection and offered a diagnostic injection of procaine to see if it would make a difference. I injected the local anaesthetic directly into the socket, as deep as it would go. To his utter astonishment, I asked him to walk to the front desk as soon as I had injected the procaine. Insulted by my request, he told me this would be impossible but he would try. To his total astonishment, he found that he was able to walk without any pain in his knee, immediately after the Procaine injection. Eight years later, there is still no pain in his knee. As dentists, we can be creating neural interferences every working day without ever knowing it. The patient would not have returned to see me but would be taking a whole other course of treatment.

Multiple Allergic Sensitivity

A forty three year old female had one root treatment performed about seven years before seeing me. She had been in excellent health. For the past couple of years, however, she had started to become allergic to everything. She found that she was constantly sniffling, and changes in weather, as well as perfumes and many other substances, would send her into fits of sneezing and wheezing, although she had never been asthmatic. The doctors, not being able to treat her symptoms, suggested that she was hysterical and should have antidepressants. Her energy levels were seriously depleted. The patient was a close friend and I had watched her health deteriorate for a few months.

The root-canalled lower left first molar looked perfect on the X-ray. These sorts of teeth I always found easiest to section and then take each root out separately. I was thus able to take an X-ray of the roots from ninety degrees to the normal view. This is a perfect example of how deceptive X-rays can be. In normal view the root filling looks very good. Looking sideways, though, we could see that the root filling did not even fill half of the main canal. Yes, of course it was done by a very good endodontist. This is also an example of how long it can take before symptoms become clinical and really hard for any medical person to diagnose.

Within one week of this tooth coming out, she started to feel better. Within a month, there were no more allergic symptoms and all medications had stopped. Ten years later, she still does not have any allergic reactions, sinusitis, headaches, or listlessness.

Post-Cancer Depression and Fatigue

A sixty-two year old lady had beaten breast cancer and was trying to rebuild her life. She had little money and even less energy. She had been fighting hard for years to get healthy. A month or two later, she reported that "a couple of teeth removed, and the abscesses are gone, and the amalgam is gone, and I feel like I've got a new lease on life. I feel like a different person. And it's all fantastic." It took only a few weeks for her body to start healing after all the toxins were taken out of her mouth. Several years later, her health and income had improved so much that she was able to pay me for the treatment that had happened so much earlier. Some people are truly wonderful.

Arthritis and Nightmares

This patient was forty years old but looked as if he was seventy. Up till his first couple of root therapies, he had been an athlete and runner. For the past seven years, he had been barely able to walk a hundred yards before the pain in his knees was so great that he needed to sit. He had three completed root therapies and one that was halfway through treatment. As they were his four front teeth, he was loath to take them out. He decided to remove all the amalgam and see what would happen. Although his energy levels improved following the amalgam removal, the knee pain was, in fact, worsening. He was having nightmares every night, and the heart palpitations he'd had for the past five years were also getting worse. The doctors had given up.

In desperation, he decided to bite-the-bullet so to speak, and have these four front teeth removed. The procedure was simple, and a small immediate denture was placed at the time of the extractions so that he could go out smiling. He returned a week later to have the sutures removed and reported that the nightmares stopped the night after the extraction and that the palpitations had ended the next day. What surprised him most though, was that the knee pain had stopped on his way back to his car. This is a great demonstration of the influence of neural interferences. The front teeth lie on the Bladder meridian and influence the reproductive system, the kidneys and the knees. Removing the teeth removed the interference, and the effect was immediate. Twelve years later, he is still running five kilometres per day and has never had another palpitation or nightmare.

Arthritis

Dr Price gave many examples of the relationships between arthritis and tooth infections. Arthritic changes are common with dead teeth, whether the tooth has been root treated or not. Two cases follow:

1. A woman of 67 years attended for a check-up and to see whether I could find any problems in her teeth. The lower left first molar had been root treated about ten years prior,

and for the past eight years the arthritis in her right shoulder had stopped her from swimming and exercising. Her rheumatologist had prescribed medication for this a week before coming to see me. There was a huge abscess on one of the roots. After lengthy discussion, she decided to take away all of my written material and do her own research. Another consultation appointment followed, and I answered another half hour's worth of questions. She had certainly done her homework. I felt honoured that she decided to try taking the tooth out. Two weeks after the extraction, she went back to the rheumatologist to show her how easily she was able to move her fingers and shoulder. The doctor said, "See, I told you the medicine would work." The patient responded by giving the doctor the unopened bottle of pills and told her that the only treatment she'd had was the removal of the one dead tooth. Within three months, she was so pain free that she could return to her passion of swimming. Eight months later, the arthritic changes in her fingers were barely noticeable. The rheumatologist was not interested!

2. This next patient qualifies as my oldest success. She is ninety years old and the mother of a dear friend of mine. For more years than she can remember, she has suffered with crippling arthritis in her hands, feet, and spine. Her fingers are so badly affected that she needs to use both hands to pick up her cup of tea. She has been in constant pain. Within two weeks of removing the one root-canalled tooth, she rang me with a heart full of gratitude, as she no longer had pain in her hands. The fingers have not magically straightened or become mobile, but even this she does not mind now that she is pain-free. Even at such an advanced age, the body has the ability to repair. There are people who bring tears to my eyes and hope to my heart; she is one of them.

The relationship of arthritic changes to dead teeth is one of the more common associations. Infections in the mouth produce arthritis. This can be from gums or teeth.

Mastitis and Period Pain

A young woman first attended my surgery when she was fifteen years old. An associate working with me at the time treated her. A number of fillings were placed to repair decay in some of her back teeth. Several years prior to this, when she was about thirteen, she damaged her two right front teeth on the handle-bars of her bicycle. Her dentist "saved" the teeth with root therapies. Her mother was sure that the worsening depression was more than just teenage neurosis and was trying to get to the bottom of it. They decided to remove the dead teeth.

That night, the patient went home and tore up the suicide note she had tucked away in her room two months earlier. A week later, when she returned for her follow-up appointment, she was no longer depressed.

This teenager grew into a beautiful young woman, though she still had some health problems. When she was twenty, she came to see me again. This time she was desperate and worried. She thought that perhaps a tooth was the cause of sudden acute mastitis. In the previous two weeks her breasts had become so inflamed that they had swollen to almost twice their normal size. She had also developed large lumps in the left breast. She also reported that for the past five years, she had struggled with constant cystitis and period pains every month that laid her out screaming for three days.

Her treatment notes revealed that the decay in the first upper left molar had caused an exposure of the pulp of the tooth at the time of filling it. The tooth reacted normally to cold; it could feel pain. The palatal root, though, did not respond as strongly. I felt that this tooth was a strong candidate, as it is positioned on the Stomach meridian which not only passes through the breast but also has a strong influence on it. Further examination using computerized bio-electric machinery confirmed that the palatal root of this tooth was, in fact, dead, although the two buccal (outer) roots were still alive.

Within two weeks of this tooth being removed, the breasts had come back to their normal size and the lumps were almost gone. Three months later, she came in to tell me that the cystitis had gone and she no longer had any period pains at all. The PMT had also disappeared. Two years later, her health has maintained.

This case highlights both the reality of Neural interferences and also the reality of the susceptible individual. She also highlights the dramatic psychological effects that toxins from dead teeth can have. I have seen five other patients who have similarly decided *not* to commit suicide after the dead teeth were removed. How many people have missed this opportunity? If you believe that you may be similarly afflicted, I would like to pass on some wisdom from a very old friend of mine: "… suicide is a permanent solution to a temporary problem." Before taking any radical action, consider that your teeth may be the root of the problem. There may be a chemical cause for how you are feeling.

This case also highlights the value of electrodermal screening. The only test that dentistry has to decide whether a tooth is alive or dead is to try to hurt it. Thus, the dentist will tap the tooth with the end of a mirror or will apply ice to the root. In this case the false positive was achieved; applying cold to the root caused pain, and thus the assumption normally would be that the tooth is alive. This was a three-rooted tooth, and there are no tests in dentistry to check each root individually. The only way I know to achieve this is with electrodermal screening, which will not only show a dead or alive tooth but will also show whether the pulp in one of the roots is inflamed or necrotic and whether it is acting as a neural interference. Sadly, this equipment is "contraindicated" as a witchcraft machine by the TGA in Australia and the FDA in America. In Germany and other European countries, it forms the basic routine equipment of most doctors. The fact that homoeopathy does work and that there is reliability in measuring the body's electrical interferences reduces the income of the drug manufacturers who run the TGA and the FDA.

A.D.H.D.

While on the subject of psychological effects, the case of a sixteen-year old boy is worth mentioning. His mother dragged him in to see me as she was concerned that the doctor wanted to put him on medication for his worsening ADHD behaviour. Mum just happened to be a teacher for children with special needs and knew the symptoms all too well.

The boy had a dead front tooth which he had damaged in a fall at a swimming pool a year earlier. The X-ray revealed that the tooth had undergone severe internal resorption. That is the jargon way of saying that the inside of the tooth was being slowly eaten away. All that I could get out of him was the typical teenage grunt, which I think means "Yes, no, and I really don't care." With this attitude and a signed consent form, we decided to take the tooth out. It was full of pus and had a huge abscess on the end of it which was not visible on the X-ray. The patient seemed to be completely absent after the tooth came out, and his mother, who watched the whole procedure, was in shock at what she saw.

One week after the surgery, a bright-faced young man came in and thanked me for taking out his front tooth and giving him back his life. His mother told me that she drove home from the surgery with a different boy than the one she came with. He had already seemed to be coming back. He was talking quietly and seemed happy and relaxed. She said that within a couple more days he was back to his earlier happy state. Three years later, he is still not on any medication and doing very well at school. There is no more depression or ADHD. In fact, he became so well that he was chosen for a school cricket team, playing internationally.

Blind Eye

A forty year old man came in to see my partner. He was frail and weak and very pale. He thought that his condition may be due to the amalgam in his teeth and came to discuss this option. He went off to get an OPG

X-ray of his mouth and lined up another appointment to start the treatment. When he returned, the X-ray showed a great big lump of amalgam (possibly a whole filling), in the socket of the lower right second premolar, which had been extracted twenty years prior. It also showed a number of other disasters, including a very dead molar on the right side.

He and my partner decided that this was the first bit of amalgam that should come out, and surgery was commenced. I was lucky enough to take photos of the procedure. About one centimetre of bone around this old amalgam filling was completely black and was also removed. The surgery was extensive. One week later, he came to have the sutures removed and reported a 50 per cent increase in energy levels.

Three weeks later, he rang my partner to tell him the rest of the story. What he had not told at the first appointment was that he had been blind in his right eye for eighteen years and that fifteen years ago an ophthalmic surgeon recommended the removal of the blind eye and the placement of a glass prosthetic eye. Two months later, when I saw him, he could clearly see all the wrinkles around my eyes with this same right eye. Three months after the amalgam had been removed, he was reading the newspaper with his now normal right eye. Ten years later, his vision is still perfect.

I am sure that by now you are thinking that I have lost the plot and I am making up some great medical fiction for a new TV series. I can only say that I am telling you what our experiences have been.

The work of Eugine Ratner is worth mentioning again at this point.[696,697,698,699,700,701] One of the things he found when working on cavitations was that both dead teeth and cavitations in the upper molar region seem to induce a sort of veil effect over the eye on the same side of the face. He found that cleaning the cavitations or removing the dead teeth often resolved this effect and the sight returned to normal. I have personally experienced this when I had my upper left second molar removed. My vision normalized on my return to my car. It had been getting more difficult for the past few years before this.

Serendipitously, I happened to read this part of his research the night after my extraction and experience of my sight improving.

Anal Itch

It may sound silly, but this fifty two year old lady had tried every form of medication to try to stop an itch around her most embarrassing sphincter muscle which had been continuous for eighteen months. Her front tooth was dead. It was not root treated but instead had been calcified for most of her life. For some unknown reason, it had become a problem only in the previous year and a half. Injecting procaine around this tooth made the itch feel much better. Repeating the neural injections over a couple more appointments, a few days apart, convinced us both that the tooth was related to the itch. Removing this tooth saw the resolution of her frustrating end that night. Years later, the problem had not returned.

Heart Attack

This patient was a doctor in her mid-forties. For the past five years, she had avoided taking her swollen gum to a dentist. She had a terror of dentists from childhood so had decided to treat the swelling in the gum with everything from antibiotics to various herbal medications. Although she seemed healthy in all other ways, she ended up in hospital with a heart attack. She was not a smoker and had no other indications that she was at risk of any cardiac disease. A few months after recovering from this, she eventually was referred in to see me. The X-ray revealed an abscess around her lower right first molar which extended from the tooth behind to the tooth in front of the first molar. It was massive. All of her cardiac symptoms and ECGs returned to normal after the tooth was removed and the abscess cleaned. There was no return of the symptoms, and there was nothing wrong with her heart by the time I had retired.

Robert Gammal BDS., FACNEM(dent)

The Bleeder

Jane was in her mid-forties and had been diagnosed by several medicos as a "bleeder"; thus she was very worried about having any dental work done, let alone several extractions. The slightest knock on her skin and she bruised for weeks. If she cut herself, she would need to go to hospital to stop the bleeding. She was exhausted and weak and had not been able to work for several years. On the lower right of her mouth was a molar that was floating in an abscess; there was no bony socket, just a huge gap. Halfway through taking out the tooth, I thought that I would be ringing for an emergency blood transfusion. I have never before or since seen so much bleeding with an extraction. She was one of my great teachers.

I proceeded to remove the abscess and about one millimetre of bone. The bleeding was already easing. I injected some Procaine into the socket. The bleeding reduced to a slight ooze. As the socket filled, the bleeding stopped all by itself. The sutures were placed without any problem. The patient, the nurse, and I were exhausted. After a minute or so, I gave her a little mirror to have a look at the socket herself. She could hardly believe that there was no bleeding.

She decided that since she did not die from this extraction, she would go ahead and remove all dead teeth and all amalgam fillings. Each time we did some work for her, there was an improvement in her overall strength and well-being.

Three months later, she reported that her health had returned, that she was back in full-time employment, and that she was also renovating her home by herself. Hammers, nails, and saws were all her friends now. Years later, her health has not deteriorated but in fact has become stronger. She is no longer a bleeder. The fact is that she was *never* a bleeder. The toxins that poured from her dead teeth simply stopped her blood from clotting.

Fortunately, most people who bleed for long periods after an extraction bleed nowhere near as severely as this patient. The way to prevent this is to remove all the stuff that prevents the blood clotting (i.e., all of the toxins in the abscess and surrounding bone. It is not magic or hocus pocus. Many of the toxins that remain in the abscess will inhibit normal blood clotting. No amount of gauze will control this, and the poor staff at the local hospital will run screaming with their inability and lack of dental knowledge. In practice, it is so simple to prevent this from happening. Simply clean out the socket completely. As this is done and healthy bone is approached, the bleeding will ease of its own accord. Most dentists will find it intriguing that the bleeding will almost stop at the top of the socket all by itself. I have seen this too often to ignore it.

Asthma

A twenty three year old patient had asthma so severely that she had puffers in every pocket and a nebulizer that she used at nights, from the time she got home from work. She had several amalgam fillings and one root therapy in the upper left first molar. After this tooth was removed, all of her respiratory problems started to ease. After a couple of months, she forgot to take her puffers with her to work. She has not had an asthma attack for the past six years and has not used any other medications. Her health is fabulous, and she now enters triathlon competitions.

Triathlon Again

This time the patient was a twenty-nine year old man who had trained for years for triathlons and other fitness competitions. Within five months of having one tooth root-canalled, he had become a chronic fatigue case who could barely walk from the waiting room to my surgery. All other interventions had failed. Needless to say, we took the tooth out. Within a month he was back to work as a gardener and also back into physical training. When a dead tooth is sealed up enough, the infection and toxins can no longer be released into the gut with minimal systemic effects. These toxins then release into the bone and blood stream, and they can have the most dramatic systemic effects. The toxins go directly to the brain via the lymph and the blood vessels, as well as along nerves.

The speed at which people can crash is as incredible as the speed with which people can heal.

Diabetes

A patient seen by my partner was a twenty one year old man who was a fitness buff until six months prior to coming to see my partner. His health crashed suddenly after the root treatment of an upper premolar. Interestingly, we could see the end of the root well within the sinus. Soon after, he was diagnosed with diabetes, which was so severe that he needed to control it with both diet and daily insulin injections.

One month after the extraction, he reduced and finally stopped the insulin treatment and his doctor declared him free of diabetes. Diabetes is not something that normally just turns up and then disappears again. This is not a common medical scenario, yet his doctor had no interest in what had happened to reverse this condition. Eight months later, the diabetes had not returned. He is back on his fitness programme.

Latex Allergy

A woman in her mid-thirties came to see me to discuss her root-canalled tooth. Since the final appointment, she had become very ill and had, in the following two and a half years, found herself becoming increasingly allergic to more and more things. She also reported in her medical history that she had a latex sensitivity. When I told her that the Gutta Percha in her root-filled tooth was the same as latex or any other rubber, she became angry and cursed her dentist. She had informed him of her latex sensitivity, as she had learnt the hard way of what it could do to her. This was basic information to be given to any medical practitioner. That the dentist had ignored this and still filled the tooth with gutta percha was beyond our comprehension. Education often gets in the way of intelligence and caring.

She was a very interesting lady, as she decided to not have the tooth out. She wanted to use herself as a guinea pig and see whether the info I had given was correct. She instead, opted to only remove the root filling—the gutta percha—and see what happened. One month later, when all of her symptoms had subsided, she came in to have the tooth removed. All sensitivities vanished in the next couple of months, as did her fatigue and generalized body pains.

Dentists must remember that Gutta Percha is not inert, it is toxic and can create many immune mediated reactions. To ignore the warning of latex allergy is criminal negligence.

Sinusitis

The case of sinusitis in relation to dead teeth involves more than one or two patients. Literally over one hundred patients that I have removed dead teeth for have reported that their sinuses cleared within days of the removal of the teeth. This has involved upper, lower, front, and back teeth. The relationship is so high, that we could almost say that having a root therapy will offer a 90 per cent chance of getting sinusitis. Yes, this is my estimate from my *clinical observation*. Remember that there is a linear relationship between the incidence of sinusitis and that of Multiple Sclerosis. There is a strong relationship between the incidence of other neurological diseases and toxins from dead teeth.

It is worth remembering that the ends of the roots of upper molars and premolars are often in the maxillary sinuses. Infection and inflammation at the ends of the roots of these teeth will always cause a sinusitis, whether the teeth are root treated or not.

This is particularly important when the specialist endodontist considers it okay to place the root filling about one centimetre beyond the apex of the tooth and into the sinus itself. When I spoke to this patient's endodontist, the only concern that he had was that there was no pain associated with the tooth. He became seriously offended when I suggested that his treatment may have been the cause of this patient's chronic sinus infection and headaches. He also became seriously offended when I suggested that overfilling the root canal is always (100 per cent of the time) associated with necrosis of the surrounding bone. I found that it is quite easy to seriously offend a specialist endodontist who does not even know the literature of his own trade! These symptoms cleared within a week of having the tooth removed. He did receive a full financial refund from the endodontist but first had to sign a document that he would not take any further legal action against the endodontist.

Neck Spasm

A thirty-seven-year-old woman with a great set of teeth suffered from involuntary neck flicking. This was worse when it was cold. This was not an ordinary neck flick. At random times, the muscles of her neck would spasm so violently that her head would swing to the left suddenly and violently, to the point that audible cracks could be heard. It would always leave her disoriented and upset. When the weather was cold, this could happen every two to three minutes. Neurologists, osteopaths, and all other medicos could not find anything wrong with her.

The upper right first molar had been sensitive for years, and finally she came in to see me with a raging toothache in this abscessed tooth. The neck flicking had become worse. The tooth was removed, and within a couple of days her neck flick disappeared completely. Personally, I think this is a better approach than injecting botulism toxin into the muscle.

Over the next couple of years, she remained in comfort, with none of the disturbing symptoms. She came back to see me two and a half years later, as for the previous few months the neck flicking had been coming back with increasing severity but less frequency than previously. I discovered that there was a *cavitation* in the area of the tooth that had been extracted previously. Cleaning out this cavitation led to an almost complete resolution of the neck problem. Minor surgery was all that was necessary to correct this affliction.

It is worth reading about the cases presented by Dr Price about involvement of neck muscles. He had similar experiences even with longstanding torticollis, which is a severe spam of the neck muscles on one side so that the head is pulled to that side. Interestingly, when he injected the toxins from the dead tooth into rabbits, they all developed paralysis from the mid-thoracic region down and died within six weeks. Rosenow and Billings found the same relationships in their research.

It's so easy to *not* see these relationships when we are meant to look only at the clinical picture without any greater understanding than what the criminals in high places want us to know.

Everything Hurts

A fifty-five-year-old woman came to see me with her husband. Her doctor had referred her in to see whether I could fix her TMJ problem, which he believed was the cause of her pain. Her symptoms were numerous and confusing and completely debilitating for her. She had constant facial neuralgia, worse on the left side of her face, with pain radiating up the left jaw and into her head. The skin on her face was so sensitive that the lightest touch was interpreted as severe pain. She had serious clicking in her jaws. She had been deaf in her left ear for several years. She had very limited mobility in her neck and could turn only slightly to the right. It was an effort for her to move, as she had to be careful not to make any jarring movements. Cold winds had to be avoided, as she crumbled with the pain they caused in many parts of her body and especially in her face and neck.

Dental examination revealed missing teeth in the lower left quadrant and a few teeth intermittently missing in the upper arch. There was amalgam, root canals, crowns, bridges, and an ill-fitting partial chrome-cobalt denture. I had no idea where to start, and after about an hour of exploring possibilities I was about to give up and join the other good company who could not work out her problem. A last look at the X-ray revealed a metal speck in the left lower jaw. As the radiologist had left the denture in her mouth when taking the X-ray, the metal frame of the denture was clearly visible. The speck was about two millimetres back from this framework. Examination of the denture clearly showed that the metal speck was not there. A closer examination of the mouth revealed that there was an amalgam tattoo (mercury and silver are released and focus in the gum, as a tattoo) in the gum in exactly the spot that the metal showed on the X-ray. Unthinkingly, I touched this spot with my finger, and the patient screamed in agony. The husband was on his feet and getting angrily concerned. I don't blame him.

The reaction was so intense that I was able to convince her to let me touch it again very gently, but this time I wanted her to tell me where the pain radiated to. The pain went straight into her left ear. With her permission, but without telling her why, I placed a few drops of local anaesthetic around this area where the amalgam speck was. The reaction was the perfect Heuneke lightening reaction. She went pale and a little shocked and insisted on sitting up. By this stage the husband, who was on her left side, demanded to know what I was doing to his wife, and he shook his clenched fists at me. What happened next surprised all of us.

The patient told her husband to sit down, as she could hear him speaking through her deaf left ear. In fact, she was suddenly hearing again fully. She then proceeded to gingerly turn her head from side to side without any effort or pain. The pain in her face had completely dissipated, and the radiating pains had also vanished. She told me that she no longer felt cold (something that she had forgotten in the medical history), and I could now touch her face rather firmly without causing pain.

It took ten minutes to remove the piece of amalgam from below her gum- it was resting between the bone and the gum. All discoloured bone was removed, and a couple of sutures were placed. This little piece of amalgam measured only about two millimetres in diameter but acted like the thorn in the elephant's foot. Every time she bit down, her denture would bump against it, acting as a constant irritant to a powerful neural interference.

She rang me a few months later to say that she and her husband were having a wonderful time walking on the beach in the cold winter wind and that she was completely pain free. Ten years later, she is still well.

MS Again

I have included another MS-related case simply to stress how common this condition is. This lady was in her mid-fifties when she was diagnosed. The only treatment offered was palliative, as is so often the case. The X-ray showed two root-canalled teeth on the lower right, and the condensing osteitis around these teeth was so dense that the extractions were rather difficult. The bone was as hard as a rock. The immune system was wrecked. Her symptoms included muscle weakness, difficulty walking, and constant flu-like symptoms. Sinusitis was constant. It was a matter of removing all metal from her mouth, both root-canalled teeth and one other dead tooth from the other side of her mouth. Almost all symptoms had gone within six months, and a year later she was declared free of MS by her doctor. This claim is adhered to despite the remarkable research by people like Ratner and Stortebecker. The dental profession refuses to acknowledge a relationship between dead teeth, cavitations, and Trigeminal Neuralgia. I showed earlier that the Trigeminal Nerve is, in fact, severely affected by all toxins coming from dead teeth. In Sydney we have a major pain clinic staffed by expert dentists who treat facial pain all the time. These great dentists routinely recommend antidepressants for their Trigeminal Neuralgia patients. If this does not work, they recommend a psychiatrist. The only other treatment that is offered is brain surgery to separate the trigeminal nerve at the base of the brain. This produces complete numbness of the side of the face and neck but often does not stop the pain.

After treating ten patients with Trigeminal Neuralgia, I can happily affirm that all of them are pain free after I removed the dead teeth or, in two cases, cleaned out the cavitations.

How many people must keep suffering because of the egoistic ignorance of the dental profession? How many antidepressants have to be administered to maintain the status quo? I have never met a person who is suffering pain and is not depressed. Of course, such a person is depressed both emotionally and physically, and often financially. In fact, when the pain is of such long-standing nature, the whole of his or her central nervous system, the Vagus and other cranial nerves, and the rest of the autonomic nervous system are depressed. I would suggest that referral to psychiatry is a poor excuse for misdiagnosis and neglect by the dental experts in the pain clinics. Apart from dentists, I have never met another human being who would opt for brain surgery rather than take out a dead tooth!

This information has been in the published literature for over sixty years. It has been repeated over and over for this period. It is a sad reflection of our specialists, professors, and deans that this attitude of denial is promoted in our universities to this day, when the very literature they deny is published in their own journals! It's simply criminal to suggest brain surgery instead of acknowledging the published science. It is a dedication to ignorance!

All facial pain, and especially Trigeminal Neuralgia, must be diagnosed carefully to explore the relationships that are often found in the mouth.

Mary was sixty-eight when she first started to see me for her general dentistry. She had many missing teeth, gold crowns, amalgam, and root fillings. All this was combined with badly fitting Chrome Cobalt dentures. I was not surprised after looking in her mouth to learn that she was living on Serepax to control her pains. As far as she was concerned, it was not ideal to keep taking such long-term medications, but at least they stopped the pains in her head even though they made her feel foggy. She also knew that if she missed a day of painkillers, she would be immobilized. It turned out that she was suffering from Trigeminal Neuralgia.

She was fascinated to learn that the pains could be coming from her dead teeth, as she remembered that the last root therapy was performed some eight years earlier and that most of her pains started about six months after this was completed.

The three root therapies were removed in one go, and that was literally the end of her Trigeminal Neuralgia. About a month later, she came back a little disappointed, as some of the pains had returned in the left part of her face just below the eye. Although they were not as intense as previously, she was worried that it was all starting again.

We are taught that referred pain cannot cross the midline. Although it does not happen often, I have seen it occur in a number of patients. It is thus very difficult to diagnose. What's interesting about Mary's pain is that it did not respond to any local anaesthetic injections on the left side of her mouth. Instead, injecting local anaesthetic around the upper right lateral incisor area (second from the front—this had been part of the initial extraction sites) knocked out the pain completely. There was still some residual neural interference around this area and the local anaesthetic completely and permanently stopped it.

Mary has not had a Serepax for the past three years and is back to her work as a seamstress.

A Case of the Shakes

I was presented before lunch one day with a very sad patient. He was thirty-eight years old. He needed help just to walk from the waiting room to the surgery. He had for many years held two jobs, one as the foreman of a mine and the other as a trainer of racehorses. He had been a jockey when younger. He was also halfway through an engineering degree which he had been passing with honours. Years earlier, he had a root therapy placed in the upper right central and lateral incisors—two front teeth. The teeth had been damaged in a fall. Although the root therapies had been considered to have been done properly, they still developed abscesses and, according to his dentist, needed retreatment.

He was referred to an oral surgeon for an apicectomy on both teeth. This is a surgical procedure which attempts to remove the abscess from the bone, and then a seal is placed at the end of the root. This treatment is notoriously unsuccessful. Halfway through, he asked the surgeon *not* to put amalgam into the ends of the root, as he was concerned about mercury coming out of the material. The response of the surgeon was that he did this all of the time and that amalgam was what would be put in the end of the root no matter what the patient thought or asked for. (If ever you want to see the effects of mercury in the creation of mad hatters, all you have to do is visit the local dentist.)

I saw this patient just seven weeks after this abusive treatment was done. He had given up his studies, had dropped his horse training job, and was about to resign from his position as foreman of the mine. He had full-body tremors similar to those seen in advanced Parkinson's disease. He had great difficulty comprehending and remembering. I had to repeat everything slowly and several times for him to grasp what had happened to him. Needless to say, my lunchtime was spent

314

taking these two teeth out of his head. He immediately started on a full mercury detox.

I saw him a week later for suture removal. His tremors had eased by about 70 per cent, and he was feeling stronger. It took a few more months for them to disappear completely. Eleven years later, he is an engineer and is back into his passion of training horses.

Mercury amalgam has been the traditional material of choice to fill the end of the canal of a root. The reality is that it is an implant of amalgam into the bone and, more realistically, an implant of mercury directly into the brain. There is absolutely no excuse for using amalgam in this way, as the dental literature clearly demonstrates that amalgam has the worst leakage problems of all root-filling materials. As well, its use as a retrograde filling was contraindicated by the manufacturers in 1997. Surprisingly, this patient did not want to follow my suggestion of taking legal action against the oral surgeon, who was, after all, a Macquarie Street specialist.

The Neural Spider Bite

This is the case of a twenty-nine-year-old lady who herself, is a naturopath and is related to one of the leading Neural Therapy specialists in the world. Her uncle, the specialist, diagnosed that her lower left molars were the cause of her fatigue, itching, and kidney disorders.

On examination, I was presented with two teeth that were supposedly a problem but did not even have a filling. At her insistence, I tested the teeth; and to my surprise, I found that they were both dead. How could this be? There were no fillings or decay in these teeth. To confirm the diagnosis, I drilled through the teeth, without any local anaesthetic, to the pulp chamber, to try to elicit pain. The pulp chambers of both teeth were empty, and the teeth were certainly dead. The extractions were uneventful, and she left happy that they were removed.

The suture removal appointment a week later was incredible. All of her symptoms had already gone. What came instead was mind blowing. She stood up from the dental chair, undid her jeans, and lowered them to reveal a huge abscessed area on her right buttock. This abscess developed within a day of the extractions and was precisely the location that she had been bitten ten years earlier by a spider. It appears that the spider venom the factor responsible for killing the teeth, and when this interference was removed, the original bite became active again. Three weeks later, there was a complete resolution of this area on her buttock and all other symptoms.

A word of warning to dentists: if you decide to take up the information presented in this book, I must warn you to become accepting of the most bizarre health changes that any practitioner could ever see. People are not shy, and the really interesting ones will include you in the story. They are our real teachers. These are the people who are living the paradigm, which is different from the one the dental associations would like you to believe. I am sure that most of the changes I heard about occurred only a week after my intervention. When I worked in Sydney, I used mainly silk sutures for my surgical cases. These do not dissolve but must be removed a week after placement. This was the opportunity to start a good follow-up programme with the patients. When I worked in rural NSW, this was not always feasible, because people would travel many hours to come to the surgery.

Pain in the Neck

A forty-six-year-old lady who, after having root canal procedure on the lower left first molar two years earlier, had suffered from intense neck and shoulder pain. She felt weakened and generally unwell. By accident she came across my website and read my version of root therapies. She returned to her dentist and insisted that the tooth be removed. This was done as a regular extraction using forceps and no curettage of the bone. For a couple of days, her neck pain disappeared, but it then returned with a vengeance. At this stage, she contacted me and attended for a consultation.

I injected local anaesthetic into the area of the extraction, which immediately and totally removed all her pain. This relief lasted for about two days; she then returned in pain. Another injection like the first had the same dramatic results. We decided to immediately go back into this area and surgically clean out the infected tissue and dead bone. The wound was washed with local anaesthetic, as this helps to remove the neural interference.

She returned a week later to have the sutures removed and has had no pain for the past 1½ years since this surgery.

This case highlights the need to remove teeth surgically and completely clean out the sockets. The neural interference is often retained in the bone around the tooth, which is also infected. It is imperative that this area be taken back to healthy bone. As dentists, we must look beyond the teeth and understand that the bone surrounding them is just as important, if not more so. It's not good enough to just remove a tooth with forceps, place a piece of gauze over the socket, and send the patient home. Teeth really are an integral part of the body.

Bladders

Joe came to the surgery with what can only be described as a mouthful of rotten teeth. He was quite happy to be told that he needed to remove most of them, as he also felt that they were making him sick. Within one week of the extractions, Joe realized that from the day of the extractions, he did not have to go to the toilet six times per night. Instead he went before going to bed, and that was it. He had lost years of sleep and rest from this condition, which has not returned for nine months.

Everything Wrong

Ruth was referred to me by her local GP as she had everything wrong and no one had yet helped her. Several years ago, she had a fairly serious car accident, which caused several broken ribs, severe facial injuries, dental injuries, and several other minor injuries, such as scraped legs. She had excellent medical and dental treatment to rebuild her battered body, and she came out of it looking pretty good. She had a great smile of crowns and bridges. She had lost several teeth in the accident. The crowns and bridges were supported on root-therapied teeth. The remaining teeth were all heavily filled with amalgam. Her medical history was voluminous, and she had many main complaints, including fatigue, ear pain, ringing in her head, shooting pain and weakness in her right arm and hand, difficulty focusing her right eye, and the inability to read. But most of all, she was scared that she was going insane. She just could not maintain her attention, and she felt she was really losing her grasp on reality. Ruth was a high-profile international professional. This is not the way she was before the car accident. She'd had to stop working for two years because of her illness.

She did not want to hear about dead teeth at first but was happy to have the visible amalgams removed. We had removed three quarters of the amalgam fillings when she turned up unexpectedly at the surgery complaining about pain in the upper right canine (eye-tooth). This tooth had been root-therapied after the car accident and had remained asymptomatic all this time. She felt sure that this tooth was a large part of her problems and begged to have it removed. I was not sure, so I injected some local anaesthetic over the root of this canine, and instantly all her head pain vanished. I extracted the tooth three days later. Till then, her pain relief lasted only a day and a half, but this was a very encouraging sign. Anaesthetizing the tooth for the extraction produced the same immediate reaction. When she came in a week later to have her sutures removed and to have a post-operative consultation, she made the following report. Firstly, the feeling of impending madness had completely vanished and had not returned.

The noises in her head had disappeared from the time of the injection and had not returned. The ear pain was gone, and she felt that she had a 70 per cent improvement in the strength of her right arm and hand. The pain in her arm was also greatly reduced but not completely gone. By the way, the tooth had been root-therapied by an endodontist, and it looked perfect on the X-ray.

I have often seen that during the amalgam removal phase of their treatment, the asymptomatic root-canalled teeth would suddenly become painful. They either become painful or there is a "knowing" by the patient that there is something wrong with the tooth. I have no explanation for this and have not seen it in any of the published literature, but I have seen it many times with my patients. My way of explaining it is that when one layer of stress is removed, the next stressor shows up. It's a bit like peeling the layers off an onion. I know that this is an unsatisfactory and unscientific explanation, but I'm afraid it is the best I can do for now. The rest of Ruth's story supports it.

A couple of weeks after the extraction, she came back to have her last remaining amalgams removed. These were three very large fillings in the lower right second and first molars and the second premolar. Still, all of the health improvements were holding, and she was starting to feel positive instead of hopeless. As usual, I administered a "block" injection to make everything numb. A block injection is a local anaesthetic injection which is positioned to block the whole of the nerve trunk as it emerges from the jawbone. One knows that it has worked when the lip goes numb. Ruth's lip went very numb. We placed the rubber dam and started drilling. She jumped in pain on each tooth as soon as I drilled through the amalgam. I knew that the local anaesthetic had worked, but had I to stop, as the drilling was causing too much pain. I therefore did an injection technique called an intra-ligamentous injection, in which case the local anaesthetic is placed into the periodontal ligament between the tooth and the bone at each root. The rubber dam went back on, the drilling continued, and again there was pain.

By this stage, most of the amalgam was out and there remained only a couple of stainless-steel pins, one in each of the molars. Ruth was very brave and allowed me to continue. When I removed the first pin, she gave a reasonable scream, as the pain was sharp and intense. I then removed the pin from the next molar, at which point she sat bolt upright. She was hurt and shocked, but she then softened and said, "That's the one; that's it. That's the one that has caused all the problems." By this stage, I was seriously concerned about the type of patient I had in my chair. I knew that there was still some drilling to do to tidy up the teeth and warned Ruth that it may hurt. To my total astonishment, she sat there completely pain free. The local anaesthetic started to have its full effect as soon as that last pin came out. This was the first time that I had seen a galvanic (electrical) interference causing a local anaesthetic not to work.

Ruth came in the next day just to tell us how wonderful she felt. Her teeth did not hurt, and she was completely free of her neck and shoulder pain. She felt also that she had now regained 100 per cent of the strength in her right arm and hand. Any remaining fuzziness in her head was also gone.

Ruth's case is a wonderful demonstration of the complexity that we face in treating and diagnosing illness. This is particularly so when the establishment totally disregards possibilities which are outside of the accepted belief systems. Galvanic or electrical interferences are real and happen far more commonly than is recognized. I have seen this sort of interference cause neck muscle spasms, conjunctivitis, and severe period cramps. It's a reminder that we, as dentists, do not have the right to place multiple different metals permanently in people's mouths. Dentistry ignores this as a problem and keeps dumping any metal in the mouth, purely based on mechanical properties.

Electrical interferences simply are not an issue in modern dentistry. After all, the textbook for dental students states, "**... but the efforts which would be necessary to resolve this issue seem *not to be*** *worthy of the time and energy required.*"[702] Clearly with this sort of teaching we are all back to the Wild West, where anything goes.

Lower Back Pain

Collin was an active forty-two-year-old until three years before he contacted me. During that time, he had severe knee pains and equally severe pains in the buttock and lumbar vertebrae. (L3,4,5). I removed the lower right first molar, which had been root-therapied and on the X-ray looked perfect. All of Collin's pains disappeared the day after the extraction and have not returned. Sometimes the briefest stories might be the most dramatic in healing after extraction.

Hands and Arms

Karen had an accident as a child and bumped her front tooth. The tooth died, and her dentist at the time tried a root canal therapy to save it. After several years, the tooth became dark, and her dentist did a post and core crown. This means that a post is cemented into the top of the root canal and a crown made to go over it. A few years later, the crown fell out, and a dentist re-cemented it.

Karen came to me about nine months after this event, as the post and crown had come out yet again. On examination I found that the root of the tooth had cracked vertically and that there was nothing left mechanically that I could do except extract the root. This tooth was removed in September of 1997. After the tooth was removed, Karen noted that the pains she had been experiencing in her hands and halfway up her inner forearm and feet had disappeared completely from the time of the extraction. This pain had started only after the crown was re-cemented the first time and the tooth sealed in August the previous year. The pain was accompanied with loss of power in both hands.

Endometriosis

Kim came to see me in 1993, wondering whether her teeth might be contributing to her chronic ill health. Until six years earlier, she was a healthy and fit sport enthusiast. At thirty-one years of age when I met her, she was barely able to hold her job and spent most of the evenings recovering. She had only a couple of amalgam fillings that were visible, but it was obvious that her upper left lateral incisor (second tooth from the front) had in the past had root therapy. An X-ray revealed an enormous abscess in the bone around this root and a retrograde amalgam filling in the end of it.

Within one month of the fillings and this tooth coming out, she reported the following health changes: no endometriosis pain, no hormone-related cramps, acne almost disappeared completely, no fatigue, blood pressure normalized, jaw pain and muscle spasms completely gone.

Five years later, Kim has improved to the point that she is now a triathlete competitor and works a demanding full-time job and is back on the road with a steady and fulfilling relationship.

Thick-Headed

Not all the cases are as dramatic as the previous one. Heather was a forty-five-year-old executive businesswoman who was finding work and living difficult after she had a root therapy in the upper right first molar. She came to the surgery wondering whether the tooth could be the problem. After the extraction, she reported that the foggy, disoriented feeling in her head had gone within a day. Within a month, her candida problem had disappeared, and within a year her food intolerance had completely gone. She was now able to eat whatever she wished and was again living a busy work life.

Liverish Dentist

The patient was a forty-six-year-old male dentist. He had been in relatively excellent health and had no great problems except that the lower right second premolar was dying, and he knew that he was faced with a decision. As a dentist, you really do not want to go through the things that you put your patients through, no matter how much you know about what is going on. As a human being, you have a natural fear of losing a part of your body. The tooth became so painful, and the dentist became so tired of it, that an extraction was organized.

After the tooth came out and the wound was being curetted and cleaned out, this dentist placed his hands over the area of his stomach and liver and immediately noted that the sensitivity in the liver was gone. In 1981, he was doing a lot of yoga and inadvertently overstretched and caused a tear in the muscle over the area of the liver. Although this did not cause any great inconvenience to him, it nonetheless meant that he was for years (about once a week) readjusting the tissue that popped through the hernia. This was the first time that he noticed this part of his body feeling normal again. For the past nine months since the extraction, he has had *no* pain in the liver area, the hernia has healed by itself, there is greater mobility in his back, and the traces of lower back pain—which were present for years—have completely dissipated. I can speak confidently about the reality of this case, as the dentist being discussed is me! At seventy this is still true.

Migraine

This is a short story but is none the less important, as it demonstrates how possible it is to treat cases which are considered not important by medicine. Julia was a thirty-five-year-old woman who ran two businesses and had very high-profile management skills. She suffered for about three and a half years from persistent headaches and migraines (medically diagnosed), sinusitis, and increasing numbers of allergies. She came to have her amalgams removed and decided that she did not want to know about removing any teeth. Within a few months of the amalgam removal, she had improved, but only slightly. By this time, the upper left first molar was beginning to become tender, and she accepted that perhaps it should be removed. From that day on, the headaches and sinusitis were completely eliminated and have not returned.

Hypoglycaemia

Bill was a fifty-three-year-old man who had for years been diagnosed as hypoglycaemic. He had candida, nervous disorders, high blood pressure, and irritable bowel syndrome, and he was understandably depressed most of the time. He also had three root-therapied teeth.

Within four months of removing these teeth, all of the above symptoms disappeared. The irritable bowel took a little longer but also improved dramatically. Even Weston Price reported how dead teeth can easily affect our ability to metabolize sugars. I have seen many diabetics either get better or at least reduce their insulin intake after the dead teeth are removed.

Overwhelm

Barry was a patient of mine in a previous practise many years ago. In his late thirties, his wife passed away, and he was left with three young children and a business to look after. Over the course of a few years, his health was deteriorating. Being a sole parent was completely distressing for him, as he needed to be there for his children. His symptoms were so varied that medical practitioners could not understand what was going wrong. By the time I saw him, he had lost an enormous amount of weight and was thin and frail. His symptoms were like a "who's who" of any pathology book, all put together. He was losing his hearing, had ringing in his ears, had a metallic taste in his mouth, and had a range of psychosomatic disorders, kidney problems, and great difficulty digesting his food.

Over the past ten years he had spent a small fortune trying to save his teeth with root therapies and crowns. He was utterly depressed at the thought of losing at least ten teeth and getting a full upper denture and partial lower denture. He was even more depressed about it, as I was the one who did three of these root therapies so many years ago and was now telling him that they could have been the cause of his illness. This was a huge decision for Barry, and eventually he decided to remove all the dead and infected teeth.

Within one month, and with new and uncomfortable dentures, he had already begun to gain weight. Within six months, almost all of his health problems had gone and he was well on the way to recovery and long-term parenting.

Everything and a Bit More

Harry was fifty-one and starting to feel more than his age. He suffered from constant headaches, and neck and shoulder pain. He had dry, itchy eyes and ringing in the ears. He suffered from severe shortness of breath, and the lightest exertion found him gasping for air. His emotional life was on the edge, as he found great difficulty maintaining a sexual relationship. Harry was also losing wait rapidly. He was getting worried. After countless medical consultations, he decided to try out dentistry as a last resort. He had a mouthful of amalgam fillings and two root-therapied teeth—the two front ones. He did not smoke, and he did take immaculate care of his oral hygiene.

The treatment plan was complex, but he decided to get rid of the amalgams first, as he could not bear to lose his two front teeth. This was completed over the next two months. He remained on a detox programme for eleven months, which included IV chelation therapy.

After a couple of months, his neck pain had gone and his headaches had been reduced to about one per week and were less intense. All other symptoms remained, except for slightly improved digestion. After a great deal of time and reading and discussing the possibilities of the root therapies being a potential cause, he decided to have them out.

Within a couple of days, Harry was starting to feel positive about his health. He was already feeling stronger and noticed that he was not puffing as much. When he came in for his six-monthly check-up, he was almost unrecognizable. He had put on about ten kilograms in weight; his strength had returned, as witnessed by his handshake; and he reported that he felt normal again for the first time in years. To Harry, normal meant a little more than to most of us. All of his head and neck pains were gone. The ringing in his ears was gone. His eyes felt normal. He had a new girlfriend. Most importantly, Harry was no longer short of breath and was jogging two to three kilometres per day. He also pointed to his head and showed me how his hair had grown back. (In the references to Focal infection, there are reports of alopecia in relation to oral infections.) His libido and function had returned, and he felt like a new man. As he said, getting rid of the two dead front teeth was the cheapest treatment he had ever had.

Back Pain

Bill was a masseur. He was thirty-six and fighting fit. He meditated daily and was in prime health. One day he awoke from sleep unable to move very much owing to excruciating back pain. Knowing many people in the healing industry, he started doing the rounds to fix his back. He finally found a doctor who diagnosed a short leg and several other injuries. The leg length discrepancy was adjusted for in his shoes, and after several months he was able to get out of the house for more than an hour at a time.

I saw Bill two and a half years later, and he was still able to stand for only about twenty minutes at a time, before needing to lie down. He came in for a routine check-up and told me his story. I noted that the lower right first molar had a root therapy and a gold and porcelain crown over pins, and what looked like an amalgam filling. On the X-ray, the root therapy looked perfect. The bone around the tooth appeared healthy, and the filling looked complete. By any dental standards, it was a perfect root therapy. After discussing the possibility of a relationship to his pain, he allowed me to inject local anaesthetic into the gum next to the tooth. Within minutes, his back pain had reduced by about 50 per cent, and this lasted for the duration of the injection. He returned for another local anaesthetic two days later. This time the pain went immediately and stayed away for half a day. Two days later, we repeated the local anaesthetic, and this time the pain was gone for a day.

Within a day of removing this tooth, the back pain disappeared completely. Six months later, Bill was back at work—helping other people with back pain.

Although on the X-ray the bone looked good, it was obvious at surgery that there was quite a large amount of soft infected tissue at the ends of the roots. This is a common finding on many of the root-therapied teeth I have extracted. I have learnt not to trust an X-ray to the extent that I used to. Most, if not all, radiographically perfect root-canalled teeth have apical abscesses. This is a critically important point to remember when your dentist assures you that the tooth is perfect by looking at the X-ray. They usually declare the tooth to be free of infection, which is, of course, nonsense.

Eczema and Gut Problems

Peta, a forty-one-year-old woman, was referred to me by her GP, who had been trying to track down the cause of her rapidly declining health. Her symptoms seemed to go on forever. She suffered from the following: low blood pressure, eczema over most of her body, a constant bloated feeling, diarrhoea, and excessive body weight. She had an underactive thyroid gland, chronic fatigue, and commonly felt nauseated. She was sensitive to bright light and often wore sunglasses in the surgery. She also had liver problems, colon toxicity, and an ever increasing number of food allergies, and she was irritable most of the time. This list is not made up. It is real.

Her mouth contained almost everything that dentistry could offer. She had nine teeth which were covered with metal and porcelain crowns. All of these teeth had amalgam under the crowns. No amalgam was visible in any of the other teeth. There were five teeth that had root therapies. One of these in the front also had a retrograde amalgam filling. There were two other teeth which were dead and not yet root filled.

Peta's treatment continued for several months. I believe the health benefits which accrued from this approach were only in part due to the removal of the dead teeth. I think it was one of the bigger parts but still just a part. The first phase of the treatment was to remove all of the dead teeth. This was accomplished over two appointments. Although this was a huge physical and emotional assault, she noticed immediate benefits. Within one week, the eczema reduced dramatically and had almost completely gone within another week. Diarrhoea, nausea, and feelings of bloating were dramatically reduced.

The next phase was to remove all of the crowns and clean out all of the amalgam that we found under each of them. In effect this was a complex form of amalgam removal. After all the amalgams were removed, the irritability vanished almost as quickly. Eventually all the crowns were replaced with compatible materials.

Within a year, the rest of her symptoms virtually disappeared completely, and they have not returned for the past four years. Other professionals were also referred to, as for many people there are a number of things going on at the same time. Biomechanical support was achieved with podiatry orthotics, and massage and osteopathic adjustments were needed at times. The medical doctor who first referred her to me specializes in environmental and nutritional medicine, and is one of the finest in Sydney for chelation therapy. He was treating her the whole time. At one stage, she had a series of colonic irrigation treatments.

To bring a person back to good health requires a multidisciplinary approach and a patient who is willing to make every effort possible to get healthy.

Chronic Fatigue and Retrograde Amalgams

Jill had a great deal of difficulty getting to my surgery. For the previous couple of years, her chronic fatigue had kept her mainly at home. To come into the city was a major expedition, and she came a half hour early to have time to recover before talking to me. Jill had a few amalgam fillings and three root-therapied teeth. She had severe menstrual problems and constant body pains that seemed to shift around all of the time. Occasionally she would have a day without headaches, and she generally had no energy even to walk around the house. She had stopped working years earlier, as she just could not do it. The OPG X-ray revealed not only the presence of root-canalled teeth but also that two of them had apical retrograde amalgam fillings. Jill's X-rays were a shock to her as well, because she remembered telling the dentist who was going to do the retrogrades that she did not want amalgam placed in her bone. She never understood what the dark stains in her gum were.

You might recall this happening in a previous case study. I mention it again because these are only two of the hundreds of times I've heard a similar story. I don't comprehend the arrogance of a dentist to blatantly go against the patient's expressed wishes. I repeat it because I want you, the patient, to know that you have a right to choose what is done to you and that you don't have to put up with treatment like this.

Not only did Jill have retrograde root fillings, but as you can see from the picture, she had bits of amalgam spread from one side of her jaw to the other. It was like the spread of a shotgun. When I cleaned out all of the bits, I was literally working on her jawbone down as far as the tip of her chin.

I'm sometimes accused of being angry about what I see. This is the type of dentistry which I find appalling, and yes, it does make me angry. That a dentist can do this to someone and then pretend that he or she is doing the patient a favour is plain ugly!

Jill now has a couple of partial dentures to replace the missing teeth. Within one week of the last surgical procedure, all of her headaches finished, and they have not returned for the past six months. Her chronic fatigue lifted gradually, and she is now back in full-time employment as a landscape gardener, putting in day after day of physical labour. She is no longer sick and is once again in a fulfilling relationship.

I was telling a colleague about Jill's case, and he accused me of creating a patient-load of TMJ problems and said that I was making "dental cripples." Although accused of creating dental cripples, I am delighted that I did not do his sort of dentistry, which creates medical cripples.

Canadian Eczema

Pat found my website and sent me a couple of photos with the following story. Four months prior, she'd had a root canal done on an upper molar tooth. About a month later, her chest broke into an eczema nightmare. There were no creams, lotions, or potions that helped her. In desperation, she wrote to me as the eczema was spreading and becoming more intense. "Is it possibly related to the dead tooth? Is it really possible? What should I do next?" The advice was simple: Have the tooth removed and socket cleaned and see what happens. Then you'll know for sure.

I received more photos a couple of weeks after the tooth came out. They speak for themselves. It took just under two weeks for the eczema to clear completely, but the improvement was noticeable in terms of symptoms and itchiness after only twenty-four hours. Sometimes the Internet can provide magic. This condition is so commonly associated with dead teeth, whether root-canalled or not, that I have seen this on many patients. If you are a doctor treating eczema, then you need to see whether there is a cause in the mouth.

Implant on Abscess

Hillary was twenty-nine years old and was having pains radiating down her right arm and the right side of her body. She felt unwell all the time and had been having terrible menstrual cramps for the previous eight months. This period is marked by the placement of a titanium implant into the bone, where her upper right second incisor used to live. It had a very bad abscess on it, and the dentist decided that extraction and replacement with the implant would be a better way to go than a root treatment. She was referred to me by a friend when the area of the gum above the implant began to swell. An X-ray of the area revealed a huge hole in the bone where the abscess had remained. I suggested that she return to the oral surgeon (in fact the most respected in Sydney at the time, of course with rooms in Macquarie Street) to have the implant removed.

To the surprise of both of us, the oral surgeon wrote that he could not see the abscess on the X-ray and refused to remove his wonderful work. Perhaps he could not see the abscess when he placed the implant into it? The abscess was so clear that it would be like looking at the Sydney Opera House and saying that it doesn't exist. This case is, of course, one that resolved completely when the implant and infection were removed—and one that serves as another window into the dental profession.

The original oral surgeon who did the job was regarded back then with such high esteem (and fear) that it was almost impossible to find an oral surgeon who would remove god's work. When I finally did find someone, I had to give him a written pledge that no lawsuits would follow. This was signed by the patient and me, and then he grudgingly agreed to take out the implant. Nothing was ever said about placing a titanium implant directly into infected bone and abscess! Nothing was ever said about his complete lack of responsibility or his lack of professionalism. The dental boards are very flexible when it comes to positioning the goalposts of professional misconduct. It is far more related to who you are than what you did. His blatant denial was all that was needed to shut the case up completely. Remarkably, this great oral surgeon was still in practice by the time I retired. Is there any wonder that God has no interest in being an oral surgeon?

Bell's Palsy

A sixty-year-old lady searched us out to remove her amalgams. She presented with severe Bell's Palsy and thought that removing the amalgams might improve the half of her face that did not move. I immediately referred her to my partner, who was a gifted acupuncturist as well as a great dentist. Within a few weeks, we saw about a 50 per cent improvement in her condition. During the amalgam removal, we were able to maintain her. Then came the time to remove a dead tooth. Another close look at the OPG X-ray revealed what looked like a very small area of Osteitis (a cavitation) in the upper wisdom tooth area. Local anaesthetic deposited in the area brought immediate and almost total relief from the Bell's palsy. Immediately she was able to close her eye completely—something she had not done for months. We decided to treat with neural therapy for at least a couple of weeks, till surgery could be scheduled. Each week I injected, and each week she would improve. When we got into the surgery, we found a huge hole in the bone—cavitation, which was carefully cleaned and irrigated with Procaine LA.

There was a 95 per cent improvement of the Bell's palsy. She still has a slight slowness in some of the muscles around her face, but she claims that she feels like a new woman, with much improved energy levels and clarity of thought. She is now a happy person with a great sense of humour and joy for life. Neural interferences must be sought out and treated; many diseases start in the mouth!

A Big Toe

An elderly female patient who had had a tooth removed some months earlier was sent to me by a podiatrist. She had presented to him with severe lancing pain to the big toe. This particular podiatrist was someone I had worked closely with for many years, and he was fully aware of the dental relationships. Finding nothing wrong with her feet, he pulled out the EAV chart. The upper premolar which had been extracted had not healed properly, and an area of interference existed. This was demonstrated when a local anaesthetic injection was placed next to the socket. Within one minute of the local being injected, the pain in the toe went. A trial was performed. We waited till the pain returned a couple of days later, when she limped back into my surgery. Another local anaesthetic into the same area provided immediate relief of the pain. This was enough to convince her that the area needed treatment. After cleaning, she has remained completely pain free.

Point That Finger

Harry was a sixty-year-old man who had come to have his amalgams removed. He was aware of the problems associated with dead teeth and asked me to take out the two that he had. For the next six months, his health improved to the point that physically he was feeling about ten years younger. At his six-monthly check-up, he told me how great he felt except for the arthritis which had set in recently in one of his fingers. The second finger on the left hand (same side as the extractions) had become severely swollen, and any slight movement caused severe pain. Out of interest, I injected local anaesthetic next to the old extraction site. Within ten minutes, the finger was returned to almost full mobility without any pain. This was again repeated a number of times, till we were both satisfied that there was a neural interference. Since we cleaned this area surgically, he has had no sign of pain in any joints, including the original finger.

Sinusitis and Headaches

Forty-seven-year-old female Georgia presented with a number of complaints ranging from chronic head and neck pain to gut disorders. She had been on Serepax for the past three years. The upper right first and second premolars and the upper left second molar had been root-therapied many years earlier. Georgia had noticed some improvement after the amalgam fillings were removed two years earlier, but she had continued with the headaches and migraines, which were accompanied by chronic sinusitis. Within a couple of days of removing the dead teeth, all pains disappeared. She no longer had a sinus problem. From clinical observation, it is clear that there are very few people who have root-therapied upper teeth that do not have sinus problems.

Electric Heart Attack

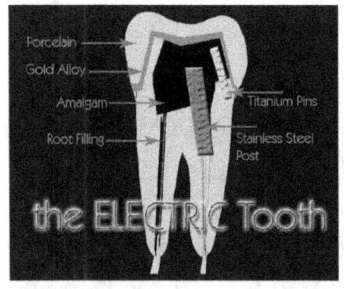

This case is not one about root canals, except that the extraction was that of a root-canalled tooth. It was an upper premolar which had developed an abscess and was causing severe acute pain. My colleague at the time looked at the X-ray, and clearly, the only rational treatment was to remove the tooth. There was other metal in the mouth, including amalgam and gold crowns.

The tooth was removed uneventfully, and the patient was grateful to be out of pain. That night, however, he found himself in hospital with a heart attack. In the particular business that he was in, he knew many cardiologists worldwide. He rang one who was a friend in the United States, who told him that there was nothing wrong with his heart but lots wrong with his teeth.

After his time in hospital, he came and saw me, and we started the process of removing the metal from his mouth, this time taking out one filling at a time according to the electrical currents that we measured at each appointment. He was able to monitor his progress each time with an Electrocardiogram and was able to report that every filling that came out led to a visible improvement in the ECG. The last thing to do was remove the only root-canalled tooth that was left—the lower first premolar. From that night on, his ECG was perfect, and it has remained so till this day.

The reason for including this here is to demonstrate the need to understand electrical interferences in the head. We are measuring currents in the range of microamps, which are a thousand times higher than the nanoamp currents found in the nervous system. They can act as powerful interferences.

The Point Is Silver

Jack was a fifty-nine-year-old naturopath who had developed kidney cancer some time earlier. He had been able to keep it under control with natural medicines but was now getting to the stage where he was considering using chemotherapy. A friend told him about the work we were doing, so he decided to pay us a visit. The lower left first molar had not only a root canal but also a metal crown and a massive infection in the bone at the back of the tooth. He had seen a periodontist (gum specialist) who had tried to treat this area without treating the cause—the dead tooth.

The extraction was both simple and exciting. The tooth had a vertical split down the crown, and both roots came out in two pieces with abscess attached. Neither I nor my colleague, who removed the tooth, had seen anything like it. This tooth had been filled with both gutta percha and silver points (a fairly old and forgotten technique, which is of course useless, as it does not seal anything). The corrosion of the silver points was such that all that remained was the black staining on the inside of the tooth.

The kidney tumour was completely resolved within two months of this disaster coming out of his mouth.

Appendix 1

Material Safety Data Sheet Information RCP

Ask your dentist what materials he or she plans to use for the root canal procedure to clean, disinfect, and seal into your tooth as a filling. Then go and look at what's in these materials and their effects on your health. Most are listed here. If they're not listed here, simply search "MSDS + Product Name."

~~~~~~~~~~~~~~~~~~~~~~~~~~~~~~~~~~~~~

Medical and dental students, in their second year of university, had to study anatomy. In the 1970s and 1980s, this included weekly dissections of cadavers. These bodies were preserved in formaldehyde. The students who were made sick from being in the dissecting rooms were given no exemption or support. They were just written off as being "squeamish"! For the dental students, the exposure was compounded by exposure to mercury in the clinics of the dental hospitals. None of us were told!

~~~~~~~~~~~~~~~~~~~~~~~~~~~~~~~~~~~~~

Papers published in dental journals will often conclude that these materials are "Biocompatible". Their use is promoted by *all* dental schools. Dentists rarely read the MSDSs for these materials and blindly do as they are told by their professors. The professors and deans rarely read or pay attention to the MSDSs for these materials. Only the manufacturers set the warnings on these materials.

To dentists who are still doing root canals, it's time to think about what you're implanting into people's bodies!

Buckley's Formocresol—A Very Special Material: Formalin and Cresol

Buckley's formocresol was created in the early 1920s by the past president of the American Dental Association, Dr Buckley—the very same person who tried to rubbish the work of Dr Weston Price. This poison is placed into baby teeth (i.e., the teeth of young children) in the procedure called pulpotomy and is sealed in permanently! It will leak into the child's body 24/7.

From the MSDS:

> Contains: Cresol, Formaldehyde Carc. Harmful by inhalation. Toxic in contact with skin and if swallowed. Causes burns. Limited evidence of a carcinogenic effect. May cause sensitization by skin contact. Keep locked up and out of the reach of children.
>
> **Potential Health Effects:**
>
> **Eyes:** Causes burns to eyes with redness, pain and tearing. Eye damage is possible.
>
> **Skin:** If spilled on skin, numbness is followed promptly by pain and reddening. Chemical burns are possible.

Toxic when absorbed through skin with symptoms similar to ingestion. May cause an allergic skin reaction.

Ingestion: Swallowing causes intense burning of mouth and throat. Cause epigastric pain, muscular weakness, headache,

dizziness, nausea, vomiting, collapse, shock, CNS depression, and death. May cause injury to the kidneys, liver, heart,

pancreas, and spleen. Symptoms may be delayed.

Inhalation: Inhalation of mists may cause mucous membrane and upper respiratory tract irritation. Toxic when inhaled with symptoms similar to ingestion. May cause an allergic reaction.

Chronic Health Effects: May cause injury to the kidneys, liver, heart, pancreas, lungs, and spleen.

Carcinogenicity: Formaldehyde is listed by IARC as "Carcinogenic to Humans," (Group 1), by NTP a "Known to be a Human Carcinogen," by ACGIH as a "Suspected Human Carcinogen" (A2), by the European Union as a Carcinogen

Category 3. Cresol Isomers- Possible human carcinogen. Based on an increased incidence of skin papillomas in mice in an initiation-promotion study. The three cresol isomers produced positive results in genetic toxicity studies both alone and in combination. None of the components are listed as a carcinogen by IARC, NTP, OSHA, ACGIH or the EU Substances Directive.

Mutagenicity: No data available

Medical Conditions Aggravated by Exposure:
Employees with pre-existing eye, skin, kidneys, liver, heart, pancreas, lungs, and spleen disorders may be at increased risk from exposure.

Reproductive Toxicity Data: No data available for mixture. In a reproductive study, rats were exposed to 0-40 ppm formaldehyde for 6 hr/days on days 6-20 of gestation. At 40 ppm, maternal toxicity was observed. Formaldehyde is slightly fetotoxic at 20 ppm. Neither embryolethal nor teratogenic effects were observed following inhalation exposure at levels up to 40 ppm.

Specific Target Organ Toxicity (STOT):

Single Exposure: Exposure to high doses of formaldehyde (>100 ppm) showed salivation, acute dyspnea, vomiting, cramps and death in laboratory animals. Mice treated with formaldehyde on skin developed severe liver damage.

Repeated Exposure: Animal data revealed a qualitative relationship between formaldehyde absorption and hepatotoxicity.

These data indicate that exposure to formaldehyde at 3 ppm or less for periods up to 6 months causes adverse effects upon the liver; higher exposure concentrations for shorter time periods produce similar effects upon the liver

~~~~~~

Cresol

Potential Health Effects

Eye: Causes eye burns. May result in corneal injury. Contact with liquid is corrosive to the eyes and causes severe burns. May cause conjunctivitis and keratitis.

Skin: May be absorbed through the skin in harmful amounts. May cause skin sensitization, an allergic reaction, which becomes evident upon re-exposure to this material. Causes severe skin irritation and burns.

Ingestion: May cause severe and permanent damage to the digestive tract. May cause vascular collapse and damage.

Causes severe digestive tract burns with abdominal pain, vomiting, and possible death. May cause kidney, liver and spleen damage. Rapidly absorbed from the gastrointestinal tract. Cresols may cause abnormalities of the central nervous system, respiratory system, spleen and pancreas.

Inhalation: May be fatal if inhaled. Irritation may lead to chemical pneumonitis and pulmonary edema. May cause liver and kidney damage. Causes severe irritation of upper respiratory tract with coughing, burns, breathing difficulty, and possible coma. Causes chemical burns to the respiratory tract. May cause headache. May cause nausea and possible vomiting.

Chronic: May cause liver and kidney damage. Repeated exposure may cause sensitization dermatitis.

May cause appetite loss, diarrhea, skin abnormalities, and digestive tract disturbances.

~~~~~~~~~~~~~~~~~~~~~~~~~~~~~~~~~~~~~~~

Formaldehyde

Formaldehyde is the main constituent in the root filling material called N2. It, too, is permanently sealed into the tooth, and it, too, will leak 24-7 into the body.

> **WARNING:** POISON! DANGER! SUSPECT CANCER HAZARD. MAY CAUSE CANCER. Risk of cancer depends on level and duration of exposure. VAPOR HARMFUL. HARMFUL IF INHALED OR ABSORBED THROUGH SKIN. CAUSES IRRITATION TO SKIN, EYES AND RESPIRATORY TRACT. STRONG SENSITIZER. MAY BE FATAL OR CAUSE BLINDNESS IF SWALLOWED. CANNOT BE MADE NONPOISONOUS. FLAMMABLE LIQUID AND VAPOR.
>
> Tumorigen, mutagen, reproductive effector;
>
> Causes burns. Very toxic by inhalation, ingestion and through skin absorption. Readily absorbed through skin. Probable human carcinogen. Mutagen. May cause damage to kidneys. May cause allergic reactions. May cause sensitisation. May cause heritable genetic damage. Lachrymator at levels from less than 20 ppm upwards. Very destructive of mucous membranes and upper respiratory tract, eyes and skin.
>
> **Acute Exposure;** Death if inhaled or absorbed; severe eye irritation and burns. Allergic dermatitis, skin burns;

bronchitis pulmonary oedema; headache dizziness nausea vomiting, abdominal pain; blindness.

Chronic Exposure: Nasal Cancer, respiratory tract irritation, reproductive disorders, asthma, dermatitis, multiple organ damage. Carcinogen Toxic fumes of: carbon monoxide, carbon dioxide Effects may be delayed Most formulations of formaldehyde also contain Methanol; Repeated or prolonged exposure to methanol could result in visual impairment and central nervous system effects.

KNOWN TO THE STATE OF CALIFORNIA TO CAUSE CANCER.

~~~~~~~~~~~~~~~~~~~~~~~~~~~~~~~~~~~~~

Materials Used to Wash and Clean the Root Canal

The materials listed below are often forced through the end of the root and into the surrounding bone, with devastating consequences.

Hydrogen Peroxide

Vapors, mists, or aerosols of hydrogen peroxide can cause upper airway irritation, inflammation of the nose, hoarseness, shortness of breath, and a sensation of burning or tightness in the chest. Prolonged exposure to concentrated vapor or to dilute solutions can cause irritation and temporary bleaching of skin and hair. Exposure to vapor, mist, or aerosol can cause stinging pain and tearing of eyes.

Confirmed Animal Carcinogen with Unknown Relevance to Humans' (A3)

Causes burns by all exposure routes

Inhalation of vapour may result in mucous membrane irritation of the nose and throat with coughing. At high levels nausea, dizziness and chemical burns to the respiratory tract.

Skin Corrosive. Prolonged or repeated contact may result in drying the skin, rash, dermatitis and chemical burns.

Ingestion Highly corrosive. Ingestion will cause severe chemical burns to the mouth and throat. The rapid releasing of oxygen can cause distension and bleeding of the mucosa in the stomach and lead to severe damage of the internal organs.

Sodium Hypochlorite

Ingestion: May be harmful if swallowed. Will cause severe irritation and corrosion (chemical burns) of the mucous membranes of the mouth, throat and gastrointestinal tract with nausea, vomiting, abdominal pain and inflammation. Systemic effects include fall of blood pressure, delirium and coma.

Eye: A severe eye irritant will cause stinging, blurring, tearing, severe pain. Causes serious eye damage. Corrosive to eyes, contact can cause corneal burns. Can result in permanent injury.

Skin: Corrosive to skin. May cause skin burns. Contact with skin will cause redness, itching, irritation, severe pain and chemical burns with resultant tissue destruction.

Inhalation: Inhalation of mists or vapours will result in respiratory irritation, cough, shortness of breath and possible harmful corrosive effects including lesions of the nasal septum, pulmonary oedema, pneumonitis and emphysema.

Inhalation causes slight to severe respiratory tract irritation and delayed pulmonary edema. Prolonged or repeated inhalation may cause allergic respiratory reaction (asthma)

~~~~~~~~~~~~~~~~~~~~~~~~~~~~~~~~~~~~~

Biocides

Biocides are chemicals placed into the dead teeth between appointments. They are intended to kill the microorganisms in dead teeth. They are sealed in with a temporary filling. They remain in the tooth for usually a week or two and sometimes up to months. They are washed out with water, sodium hypochlorite, and hydrogen peroxide. They include but are not limited to those listed below.

Chlorhexidine

Chronic Effects: The substance is toxic to lungs, mucous membrane (human)

Routes of Entry: Eye contact, inhalation, ingestion.

Health Effects – Acute

Swallowed Very hazardous in case of ingestion. May be harmful if swallowed. Accidental ingestion may cause human health damage. It is likely to result in irritation of the gastrointestinal tract.

Eye Severe irritant to the eye. This material is considered to represent risk of serious damage to eyes.

Skin Hazardous in case of skin contact (irritant). It is not expected to cause significant or prolonged irritation by skin contact. Repeated exposure may cause dermal disturbances. It is not expected to cause systemic harmful effects after skin contact. Product is a photosensitiser. This material showed low primary skin irritation potential to rabbit skin. Eczema and leg ulcer patients patch tested with 1% Chlorhexidine Digluconate solutions developed contact dermatitis. Topical applications of solutions in patients have caused urticaria, dyspnea and anaphylactic shock.

Inhaled Hazardous in case of inhalation. The substance is toxic to lungs, mucous membrane (human).

Do NOT let product reach waterways, drains and sewers. Very toxic to aquatic organisms.

Calcium Hydroxide

Potential Acute Health Effects: Very hazardous in case of eye contact (irritant). Hazardous in case of skin contact (irritant), of eye contact (corrosive), of ingestion, of inhalation. Corrosive to eyes and skin. The amount of tissue damage depends on length of contact. Eye contact can result in corneal damage or blindness. Skin contact can produce inflammation and blistering. Inhalation of dust will produce irritation to gastro-intestinal or respiratory tract, characterized by burning, sneezing and coughing. Severe overexposure can produce lung damage, choking, unconsciousness or death. Inflammation of the eye is characterized by redness, watering, and itching.

Potential Chronic Health Effects: Hazardous in case of skin contact (irritant). Repeated exposure of the eyes to a low level of dust can produce eye irritation. Repeated skin exposure can produce local skin destruction, or dermatitis. Repeated inhalation of dust can produce varying degree of respiratory irritation or lung damage.

Phenol

Note: formaldehyde and cresol are both phenolic agents.

Material is extremely destructive to tissue of the mucous membranes and upper respiratory tract, eyes, and skin., spasm, inflammation and edema of the larynx, spasm, inflammation and edema of the bronchi, pneumonitis, pulmonary edema, burning sensation, Cough, wheezing, laryngitis, Shortness of breath, Headache, Nausea, Vomiting, Circulatory collapse, tachypnea, paralysis, Convulsions, Coma., necrosis of mouth and G.I. Tract, Jaundice, respiratory failure, cardiac arrest To the best of our knowledge, the chemical, physical, and toxicological properties have not been thoroughly investigated.

Passes through the placental barrier. May cause adverse reproductive effects and birth defects (teratogenic) Embryotoxic and/or foetotoxic in animal. May affect genetic material (mutagenic)

Target Organs: Pancreas, Respiratory system, Central nervous system (CNS), Central Vascular System (CVS), Eyes, Kidney, Liver, Skin, Eyes, Kidney, Liver, Respiratory system, Skin.

Toxic to aquatic life with long lasting effects.

Para-chlorphenol

Warning! Harmful if swallowed, inhaled, or absorbed through the skin. Toxic to aquatic organisms, may cause long-term adverse effects in the aquatic environment. May cause methemoglobinemia. May cause liver and kidney damage. May cause adverse reproductive effects based upon animal studies.

Target Organs: Blood, kidneys, liver, respiratory system, gastrointestinal system, blood forming organs, skin.

Potential Health Effects

Eye: May cause eye irritation. Exposure to solid may cause pain and redness.

Skin: Causes severe skin irritation. Harmful if absorbed through the skin. May cause blistering of the skin.

Ingestion: Harmful if swallowed. May cause gastrointestinal irritation with nausea, vomiting and diarrhea.

Inhalation: May cause respiratory tract irritation. Harmful if inhaled.

Chronic: May cause liver and kidney damage. May cause methemoglobinemia, which is characterized by chocolate-brown colored blood, headache, weakness, dizziness, breath shortness, cyanosis (bluish skin due to deficient oxygenation of blood), rapid heart rate, unconsciousness and possible death. Adverse reproductive effects have been reported in animals. Toxic to aquatic organisms.

Camphorated Para-chlorphenol

Effect of overexposure: ingestion of even small amounts may cause naruea, vomiting, circulatory collapse, tachypnea, paralysis, convulsions, coma, greenish or smokey brown urine, necrosis of mouth and gastrointestinal tract, icterus, death from respiratory failure, sometimes form cardiac arrest. Average fatal dose is 15 g but death form as little as one gram has been reported. Fatal poisoning may also occur by skin absorption following application to large areas.

Antibiotics

Many antibiotics have been tried in root canals either as dressings or as the main filling inside the tooth. They kill bacteria only if they can reach the bacteria in suitable concentrations. This dosage is unachievable in the dentine tubules and accessory canals. Consequently, the low dosage applied to the bacteria stimulates a *resistance in the bacteria to the antibiotic.* This increases the already tragic number of bacteria that are resistant to antibiotics. The medical world struggles with this daily.

Exposure of bacteria to mercury produces both mercury and antibiotic resistance in many bacteria.

Antibiotics administered orally may be helpful to reduce infection that has spread form the tooth. They will not, however, be able to do anything to the bugs inside your tooth, as the blood supply has been removed and there is no way for antibiotics or the cells of your immune system to enter the tooth.

~~~~~~

A Word on Trigeminal Neuralgia

All materials placed in the tooth will travel throughout the body. Some are transported along nerve fibres directly back to the brain (Retrograde Axonal Transport). The nerves that innervate the teeth, jaws, gums, and lips derive form one cranial nerve. This is called the

Trigeminal Nerve. It arises from a major structure in the brain called the Trigeminal Ganglion. All materials placed in the tooth will easily travel to this major area of the brain.

Is it a wonder that the Trigeminal Nerve is often affected by these toxins? Irritation of this nerve may produce paraesthesia, neuralgia, and severe pains, including Trigeminal Neuralgia.

Trigeminal Neuralgia is not just a big name; it represents pain which is so intense that people have been known to commit suicide.[i], [ii]

The accepted treatment of Trigeminal Neuralgia totally ignores the wealth of published literature which associates this disaster with both dead root-treated teeth and cavitations in the jawbone. The dental profession simply denies this relationship, and thus both the diagnosis and treatment are wrong. Most patients diagnosed with this condition are placed on antidepressants. If this does not work (is it really a surprise?), they are advised to have brain surgery to section the trigeminal nerve from the base of the brain. When this still does not work, the patient is referred to a psychiatrist. These days the pain clinics in some of Sydney's largest hospitals will not see a patient unless they first have a consultation with a psychologist!

With just a little integrity and acceptance of the published literature, many patients could be spared this outrageous abuse. Would you prefer to have a dead tooth removed, a hole in the jawbone cleaned, or to undergo brain surgery? There is a wealth of literature, much of it published in the dental journals, which supports the position that dead teeth and cavitations are the main causes of trigeminal neuralgia. [iii],[iv],[v],[vi],[vii],[viii],[ix],[x],[xi],[xii],[xiii],[xiv],[xv],[xvi],[xvii],[xviii],[xix],[xx],[xxi],[xxii],[xxiii],[xxiv],[xxv]

Root-Filling Materials

Root-filling materials are permanently implanted into the tooth. They are used to try to seal the canal and maintain the sterility that was not there in the first place. They are placed in the tooth after it has stopped hurting, it no longer smells, and the dentist has run out of time and money worthiness. Dentistry still does not have any means by which to test the sterility of such a tooth, and in other material presented here, it is clear that such a dead tooth cannot be sterilised.

The American Association of Endodontists claims that teeth should be "sealed with a sterile, **biocompatible** material."[i]

A quick reminder on the technique is that once the tooth is considered ready to fill, a cement is spun down the root canal to within one millimetre of the end of the root. This cement forms a sort of mortar that holds the bricks in place and supposedly seals any gaps between the bricks. The bricks are made of rubbery points called gutta percha. Often patients are told that the tooth is filled with a "natural" material made from rubber—this same gutta percha.

Unfortunately, these little bricks are neither pure gutta percha nor safe. GP points may contain Gutta Percha, Zinc Oxide, Barium Sulphate, Titanium Oxide, Antioxidant, Iron Oxide (Colour agent), and Mastication Agents (a trade secret and not disclosed).

Dentistry has used gutta percha and no other material to try to seal the canal in teeth for over one hundred years. Any of the metals now included in GP points may cause severe autoimmune reactions.[ii] If you happen to be one of those people who are sensitive or allergic to latex, then you should know that you may also be sensitive to gutta percha, as it is derived from latex. I guess it is just too bad if you *are* sensitive; you will get it implanted into your body anyway, because that is what dentistry teaches. I have seen many patients in this situation. Their health was fine till the root filling was completed. They were even able to tolerate the sterilizing medicaments, but their latex sensitivity finally got them when the GP points were sealed into the tooth. How is this possible if, as the dental profession claims, all of the implanted materials stay sealed in a tooth? The answer is obvious! All GP points show high levels of toxicity, which is attributed to the leakage of Zinc ions (ZnO) into fluids.[iii] Everything that is placed in a tooth will leak into the surrounding tissues and then the rest of the body. This has been made patently clear by the American Association of Endodontists. "Moreover, scientific evidence has demonstrated that the damage from paraformaldehyde-containing filling materials and sealers is not necessarily confined to tissues near the root canal. The active ingredients of these filling materials and sealers have been found to travel throughout the body and have been shown to infiltrate the blood, lymph nodes, adrenal glands, kidney, spleen, liver, and brain."[iv]

Many cements have been used by dentistry to try to seal the canal. None work. Many are on the market, and it is the decision of the dentist as to which material will be used, like the decision as to which material to use to try to sterilise the tooth. This decision also has *nothing* to do with any scientific support for its efficacy. It is a decision based on supposition, cost, and ease of use, as well as how pretty the dental sales representative is (no joke).

Zinc Oxide and Euginol (a derivative of the oil of cloves) is the traditional root-filling cement. It has been around for decades. The extended use of this material is not an indication that it is safe. Zinc Oxide root-filling cements release zinc, high levels of which are found in distant organs: the liver, kidney, uterus, and brain. AH26 induced changes in calcium levels in these organs.[v]

All root-filling cements are cytotoxic; they kill cells.[vi],[vii],[viii],[ix],[x],[xi],[xii], [xiii],[xiv],[xv],[xvi],[xvii],[xviii],[xix],[xx],[xxi],[xxii],[xxiii]

Many root-filling cements are Mutagenic—they cause cancer—as published in the *Journal of Endodontics* in 2000. They cause changes in DNA which "could lead to birth defects or malignant transformation of the tissue"[xxiv ii]

> Many root filling cements are also neurotoxic. This means that they damage nerve tissue. In several studies the materials tested blocked nerve transmission either

partially or totally and in some cases the effect was irreversible.[xxv],[xxviii]

"The neurotoxic effects of the root canal filling materials- Endomethasone, N2 Universal, Traitment SPAD, Sealapex, and Calciobiotic root canal Sealer (CRCS)-were investigated on isolated rat sciatic nerves after local application."

"Inhibitory effects of root filling materials on the conduction of action potentials evoked in rat phrenic nerves were evaluated in vitro. **Endomethasone and N2 Normal completely and irreversibly inhibited conductance; ProcoSol caused complete but reversible inhibition; Kloroperka N-O caused total inhibition which was sometimes reversed; and AH26 and Diaket showed partial inhibition which was partially reversible."**

From the Manufacturers

Most products which are to be used inside or on the body are usually accompanied by a written description which must be lodged with the Food and Drug Administration in America and the Therapeutic Goods Administration in Australia. They must be publicly available on demand. They are called "material safety data sheets". (If you search the net for "MSDS + product name" you will find the full articles.) These materials are placed inside the tooth and left there. These compounds are supposedly "sealed" into the tooth. The problem is that they do not stay there. Everything that is placed in a tooth will spread throughout the body. In fact, dentistry has never been able to find a way to seal a root canal. They will leak from the tooth slowly all of the time, twenty-four hours a day. The same is true for their decomposition products.

All materials which are placed in a tooth will spread throughout the body via the blood and the lymph, and will be transported back to the brain along nerve fibres! Surely this information is critical to making an informed decision about the treatment to be embarked upon. I would like to know if a poison was to be placed in my body. I would expect that most people would want to know if a poison was to be placed in their bodies.

~~~~~~

AH26 Powder—Dentsply DeTrey GmBH

Dangerous Components:

Bismuth (111) Oxide, Methanamine 25%, Silver 10%, Titanium Dioxide 5%

Dangerous Decomposition Products: Formaldehyde, Nitrogen Oxides, Ammonia

Warnings: Skin Irritant, Eye Irritant, Sensitization Inhalation and Skin contact

Additional Toxicological Information: Harmful. Irritant. Do not allow undiluted product or large quantities of it to reach ground water, water course or sewage system

~~~~~~~~~~~~~~~~~~~~~~~~~~~~~

AH26 Resin—Dentsply DeTrey GmBH

Contents: Bisphenol-A-diglycidylether

Keep away from foodstuffs, beverages and feed.

Wash hands before breaks and at the end of work.

Avoid contact with eyes and skin.

Use skin protection cream for skin protection

Warnings: Skin Irritant, Eye Irritant, Sensitization by Skin contact

After Swallowing: Rinse mouth thoroughly and then drink plenty of water. Call a doctor immediately.

Ecological Information: Do not allow product or large quantities of it to reach ground water, water course or sewage system

~~~~~~~~~~~~~~~~~~~~

Pro Root MTA (Mineral Trioxide Aggregate)—Dentsply

Note: This material is used to seal the end of a root canal at its apex in the procedure known as *Retrograde Root Filling*. In other words, it is placed in the bone within a couple inches of your brain. It is a wet area of the body!

All versions of Portland Cement / MTA contain measurable levels of *Arsenic*, the most toxic substance known to science, followed by lead in second place and then mercury in third. These findings are published in dental journals!

- GonÃ§alves, J. L., Viapiana, R., Miranda, C. E., Borges, A. H., and Cruz, Filho, "Evaluation of physico-chemical properties of Portland cements and MTA", *Braz Oral Res*, 24/3 (2010 Jul–Sep), 277–83.
- Chang, S. W., Baek, S. H., Yang, H. C., Seo, D. G., Hong, S. T., Han, S. H., Lee, Y., Gu, Y., Kwon, H. B., Lee, W. Bae, and Kum, K. S., "Heavy metal analysis of ortho MTA and ProRoot MTA", *J Endod,* 37/12 (2011 Dec),1673–6.
- Chang, S. W. Shon, W, J., Lee, W. Kum, K. Y., Baek, S. H., and Bae, K. S, "Analysis of heavy metal contents in gray and white MTA

and 2 kinds of Portland cement: a preliminary study", *Oral Surg Oral Med Oral Pathol Oral Radiol Endod*, 109/4 (2010 Apr), 642–6.

- Monteiro Bramante, C., Demarchi, A. C., de Moraes, I. G., Bernadineli, N., Garcia, R. B., Spangberg, L. S., and Duarte, M. A., "Presence of arsenic in different types of MTA and white and gray Portland cement", *Oral Surg Oral Med Oral Pathol Oral Radiol Endod*, 106/6 (2008 Dec), 909–13.
- Duarte, M. A., De Oliveira Demarchi, A. C., Yamashita, J. C., Kuga, M. C., and De Campos, Fraga S., "Arsenic release provided by MTA and Portland cement. *Oral Surg Oral Med Oral Pathol Oral Radiol Endod*, 99/5 (2005 May), 648–50.

The following is from the MSDS (my emphasis):

Dangerous Components: Portland Cement Clinker 75%, Gypsum 5%, Bismuth Oxide 20%

Impurities may include **Crystaline Silica (Carcinogen)**, calcium oxide, magnesium oxide, potassium and sodium sulphate compounds

This product contains chemicals (trace metals) known to the state of California to cause cancer, birth defects or other reproductive harm.

The major components of Pro Root (calcium silicate compounds, and calcium compounds containing aluminium oxide and gypsum) are considered **Hazardous**.

Warnings

Exposure to wet substance may cause irreversible skin or eye destruction in the form of chemical third degree burns.

May cause blindness.

Prolonged exposure can cause severe skin damage in the form of caustic chemical burns.

Exposure **to moisture** will produce **caustic calcium Hydroxide.**

Pro Root MTA ... chemically reacts with water, and some of the intermediate products of this reaction pose a far more severe hazard than does the material itself.

~~~~~~~~~~~~~~~~~~~~~

Ferric Sulphate

Note: This material is now used as the material of choice to seal treat baby teeth, in a procedure called "pulpotomy". It is placed daily in children's teeth and bodies. No consideration is given to the systemic effects.

WARNING! HARMFUL IF SWALLOWED OR INHALED. CAUSES IRRITATION TO SKIN, EYES AND RESPIRATORY TRACT. AFFECTS THE LIVER.

Skin Protection: Wear impervious protective clothing, including boots, gloves, lab coat, apron or coveralls, as appropriate, to prevent skin contact.

First Aid Measures;

Inhalation: Remove to fresh air. If not breathing, give artificial respiration. If breathing is difficult, give oxygen. Get medical attention.

Ingestion: Induce vomiting immediately as directed by medical personnel. Never give anything by mouth to an unconscious person. Get medical attention.

Skin Contact: Immediately flush skin with plenty of soap and water for at least 15 minutes. Remove contaminated clothing and shoes. Get medical attention. Wash clothing before reuse. Thoroughly clean shoes before reuse.

Eye Contact: Immediately flush eyes with plenty of water for at least 15 minutes, lifting lower and upper eyelids occasionally. Get medical attention immediately.

Warnings:

Inhalation: Causes irritation to the respiratory tract. Symptoms may include coughing, shortness of breath.

Ingestion: Low toxicity in small quantities but larger dosages may cause nausea, vomiting, diarrhea, and black stool. Pink urine discoloration is a strong indicator of iron poisoning. Liver damage, coma, and death from iron poisoning has been recorded.

Skin Contact: Causes irritation to skin. Symptoms include redness, itching, and pain. May cause skin discoloration with irritation.

Eye Contact: Causes irritation, redness, and pain.

Chronic Exposure: Prolonged exposure of the eyes may cause discoloration. Repeated high exposure could cause too much iron to build up in the body. Symptoms of upset stomach, nausea, constipation and black bowel movements may occur. Chronic exposure may cause liver effects.

Aggravation of Pre-existing Conditions: Persons with pre-existing skin disorders or eye problems, or impaired liver, kidney or respiratory function may be more susceptible to the effects of the substance.

~~~~~~~~~~~~~~~~~~~~~~

AH Plus Paste A—Dentsply DeTrey GmBH

Eye & Skin irritation, Sensitization by Skin

Warning: contains epoxy resins or amines which may cause Sensitisation in susceptible persons

Ecological Information: Do not allow product to reach ground water, water course or sewage

~~~~~~~~~~~~~~~~~~~~~~

AH Plus Paste B—Dentsply DeTrey GmBH

Dangerous Components; 113506-22-2 N, N-Dibenzyle-5-oxanoandiamin-1,9 Xn; R 22-36-37-38, 768-94-5 10% amantadine Xn; R 20-21-22-36-37-38 5%Amines, Calcium Tungstate, Zirconium Oxide, Silica, Silicone Oil

Irritant Gases / vapours.

Irritating to eyes, respiratory system and skin.

Sensitization by Skin

Local and systemic allergic reaction have been reported

Do not allow to enter sewers/surface or ground water. Water Hazard class 2 (German regulation) (Self assessment): hazardous for water.

~~~~~~~~~~~~~~~~~~~~~~

Tubli-Seal Base—Kerr Corporation

Mineral oil-not disclosed, Zinc Oxide, Cornstarch, Barium Sulphate, Lecithin

May cause allergic dermatitis. Latex gloves to avoid skin contact recommended

Inhalation: Prolonged exposure may cause drowsiness

~~~~~~~~~~~~~~~~~~~~~~~

Tubli-Seal Accelerator—Kerr Corporation

4-allyl-2-methoxyphenol (Euginol oil of cloves), Thimol, Iodide, Dimeric acid resin

Skin and Eye irritant. May cause allergic dermatitis

~~~~~~~~~~~~~~~~~~~~~~~

Pulp Canal Sealer Powder—Kerr Corporation

Silver Powder, Zinc Oxide, Thymol Iodide

Eye and Skin Irritant

Allergic Dermatitis

May cause Drowsiness

~~~~~~~~~~~~~~~~~~~~~~~

Pulp Canal Sealer Liquid—Kerr Corporation

4-allyl-2-methoxyphenol (Euginol oil of cloves), Balsam Resin,

Eye and Skin Irritant

Allergic Dermatitis

May cause Drowsiness

~~~~~~~~~~~~~~~~~~~~~~

Ketac-Endo Aplicap—ESPE

Glass Ionomer

Eye irritation

~~~~~~~~~~~~~~~~~~~~~~

Roeko Seal Automix—Roeko Dental

Polydimethylpolymethylhydrogensiloxane, Silicone oil, Paraffin Oil, Zirconium Dioxide, Hexachoroplatinic acid.

Procosol—Dentalez Inc.

Zinc Oxide, Bismuth Subcarbonaate, Hydrogenated Resin, Sodium Borate, Barium Sulphate, Euginol Liquid,

Decomposes to: **Toxic Sodium Oxide**, **Carbon Monoxide**, Carbon Dioxide

Eye and skin irritation

Dermatitis

~~~~~~~~~~~~~~~~~~~~~~

Gutta Percha Points

A little note from me: gutta percha points are the "bricks" that are placed in the canal to try to seal it. They are inserted after the cement is spun into the canal.

Patients are usually *not* informed that they are latex-based. If you have a latex allergy, you may have serious consequences to your health from having these inserted into your tooth.

~~~~~~~~~~~~~

Natural GP tm Septodont

> Dexamethasone, Hydrocortisone acetate, Thymol Iodide, Paraformaldehyde, Barium Sulphate, Radio-opaque excipient (not known), Euginol, Peppermint Oil, Anise Oil, Zinc Oxide

~~~~~~~~~~~~~~~~~~~~~~

N2

This material is a disaster of unequalled proportion. There is a lot to get your head around with this one.

~~~~~~~~~~~~

> **WARNING: ... ... contains therapeutic agents known to be potentially Neurotoxic.**
>
> Therefore due to the known toxicity of Paraformaldehyde in particular, the paste should be confined to the root canal and should not penetrate nor be extruded beyond the apex.

"N2" is a short name for the most dangerous of all root-filling cements. This material is used widely in the UK, most poorer countries, and those with national dental health schemes, as well as the United States.

~~~~~~~~~~~~~~~~~~~~

Zinc Oxide, Euginol, Formaldehyde, Peanut Oil

Formaldehyde is a potent carcinogen.

Many people are seriously allergic to peanut oil

~~~~~~~~~~~~~~~~~~~~

Sealapex (Base and Catalyst)—Kerr Corporation

Isobutyl Salycilate Resin

Silicon Dioxide

Barium Sulphate

Titanium Dioxide Pigment

N-ethyl Toluene solfanamide resin

Zinc Oxide

~~~~~~~~~~~~

Endomethasone

Contains: Dexamethasone, Hydrocortisone acetate, Paraformaldehyde, Thymol Iodide, Barium Sulphate, Radio-opaque excipient, Euginol, Peppermint Oil, Anise Oil, Zinc Oxide

"WARNING: ... ... contains therapeutic agents known to be potentially Neurotoxic." "Therefore due to the known toxicity of Paraformaldehyde in particular, the paste should be confined to the root canal and should not penetrate nor be extruded beyond the apex." Can cause allergy.

Dexamethasone—A Component of Endomethasone, Above

Experimental teratogen. Signs of overdose include retinal toxicity, glaucoma, subcapsular cataract, gastrointestinal bleeding, pancreatitis, aseptic bone necrosis, osteoporosis, myopathies, obesity, edemas, hypertension, proteinuria, diabetes, sleep disturbances, psychiatric syndromes, delayed wound healing, atrophy and fragility of the skin, ecchymosis, and pseudotumor cerebri.

Glossary

Term	Description
abutment	a supporting structure on either side of a space
aerobic	requiring oxygen to reproduce and live
aerobic action	the need for oxygen for cells to function properly
alveolar bone	the bone that supports the teeth
anaerobic	not requiring oxygen to reproduce or live
anecdotal	based on casual observations or indications rather than rigorous or scientific analysis
Apicectomy	the procedure of cutting off the end of the root of a tooth, in an attempt to get rid of infection (usually accompanied by a retrograde root filling)
bacteraemia	the spread of bacteria throughout the blood and body which may or may not localize in different organs/tissues.
bone resorption	the loss of bone usually around an implant or dead tooth
Carcinogenic	able to cause cancer
cardiotoxic	damaging or destructive to heart cells
caries	another word for tooth decay, the process of demineralization of tooth structure producing a hole in the tooth
Cavitations	also called NICO - Neuralgia- Inducing Cavitational Osteonecrosis

clinical observation	anecdotal observation by a specialist which supports the status quo
commensal	living on or within another organism and deriving benefit without harming or benefiting the host individual
Compression Necrosis	the death of bone which has had too much pressure applied to it.
condensing osteitis	condensation of the bone around the end of the root, which looks white and dense on an X-ray—an indication that the immune system is wrecked
coronectomy	removal of the crown of the tooth, which leaves the dead and decaying root in the bone, so the dentist does not have to get blood on his or her hands by doing surgery
cortical bone	bone on the surface, as compared to the cancellous bone on the inside of bones
crown of the tooth	the part of the tooth that is in the mouth above the gum line
cumulative toxin	a toxin, such as mercury, which is excreted very slowly and is therefore stored in the body long term as it.
cytotoxic	damaging or destructive to cells
decoronation	a relatively new term in dentistry English which suggests removing the crown of the tooth and leaving the root in place (the lazy dentist's excuse for doing lousy work)
dental caries	decay in a tooth
devitalized	no longer alive; killed
EAV	Electro Acupuncture after Voll
edentulous	without teeth—one or all
Electrodermal	studying the electrical transmission of the skin
electrolyte	a salt solution capable of conducting electricity and mobilizing the atoms of the salts and other substances involved
embryogenic	relating to the development of an embryo

EMF	Electro Magnetic Frequency
EMR	Electro Magnetic Radiation
ENT	ear, nose, and throat specialist
FDA	Federal Drug Administration
galvanic cell	battery
histotype	any of a range of tissue types that arise during the growth of a tumour
intraradicular	inside the dentine tubules
ischemic	lacking blood supply
leukoplakia	precancerous changes in the tissue lining the mouth
lingual surface	the part of the tooth facing the tongue
liquefaction necrosis	death and liquifying destruction of the bone, usually around the end of a root that has been overfilled, as is commonly done
maxillary sinus	The sinus spaces in the cheekbones
neoplasms	cancerous changes in tissues
neurotoxic	damaging or destructive to nerve cells
obturation	sealing of the root canal with toxic materials to try to seal the canal from the rest of the body
odontogenous toxins	toxins from teeth
oseointegration	the supposed desired reaction of titanium implants integrating with bone—nonsense
OSHA	Occupational Safety and Health Authority
palatal surface	the part of the tooth facing the palate
periapical	the area around the the apex of the root
periapical radiolucency	around the apex of the root - ' radiolucency' an area of the Xray which is darker than it should be. Usually indicating that there is an abscess there.
periapical X-ray	an X-ray taken on film that you hold with a finger in your mouth, usually in a very uncomfortable position; contrast with a Bite Wing X-ray, which is one where you bite down on a tag that is attached to the film in your mouth

Peri-implantitis	a destructive inflammatory process affecting the soft and hard tissues surrounding dental implants, the name of which was invented to describe a situation that dentistry has no way of controlling
periodontitis	inflammation and infection of the periodontal ligament which holds the tooth to the bone
physiologic balance	a fantasy term invented by the dental profession to describe the inability of any procedure to sterilize a tooth
Procaine	The first synthetic local anaesthetic developed after cocaine
Proposition 65	The proposition that protects California's drinking water sources from being contaminated with chemicals known to cause cancer, birth defects, or other reproductive harm, and requires businesses to inform Californians about exposures to such chemicals
PTO	Private Trade Organisation - all dental and medical associations
pulp chamber	the part of the root canal that is in the crown of the tooth
pulpless	having no dental pulp, which is made of connective tissue, body fluid, veins, arteries, and nerve fibres (A pulpless tooth is a dead tooth.)
Radiograph	X-ray
radiolucent area	a dark area on an X-ray that represents bone loss— usually an abscess (As there is less bone for the X-rays to pass through, the X-ray becomes darker in this area.)
RCP	root canal procedure.
RCT	root canal treatment (or "therapy")—this is a misnomer
retrograde root filling	a filling placed at the end of the root after the apex has been removed. All materials used to fill this end of the root are highly toxic.

RFR	Radio Frequency Radiation
roentgenograph	an alternative term for an X-ray
scintograph	a technique in which a scintillation counter or similar detector is used with a radioactive tracer to obtain an image of a bodily organ or a record of its functioning
somatotopic projection	the projection of the body surface onto a brain area that is responsible for our sense of touch and that is called the somatosensory cortex
spontaneous remission	the disappearance of a disease that medicos don't understand
synapses	a junction between two nerve cells, consisting of a minute gap across which impulses pass by diffusion of a neurotransmitter.
teratogenic	able to cause developmental malformations
TGA	Therapeutic Goods Administration (Australia)
TMJ	Temporo Mandibular Joint (i.e., the jaw joint.)
Trigeminal Neuralgia (TN)	neuralgia or pain along the Trigeminal Nerve
vasoconstrictor	a substance included with a local anaesthetic which will constrict the local blood vessels in order to extend the anaesthetic affect.
WHO	World Health Organization
X-ray negative	not showing any abcessed area at the end of the root; showing what looks like normal bone, which the dental profession claims as a good outcome of RCPs
X-ray positive	showing a well-defined abscess at the end of a root on an Xray

Endnotes

[1] Alice In Wonderland – Louis Carrol – the people who made hats, used mercuric nitrate to cure the felt for the hats. Many went mad from the mercury exposure. Hence the phrase "as 'mad as a hatter'.

[2] Dr Joseph Issels 'Cancer a Second Opinion' http://issels.com

[3] "The Changing Face Of Dentistry - Endodontics" by Dr Paul V. Abbott Australian Dental Association News Bulletin April 1996

[4] Australian Dental Journal Endodontic Supplement Volume 52, Number 1, March 2007

[5] Endodontics and implants, a catalogue of therapeutic contrasts. White SN, Miklus VG, Potter Ks, Cho J, Ngan AYW,. J Evid Based Dent Pract. 2006;6:101-109

[6] Australian Dental Association Endodontic Supplement Vol 52 No 1 March 2007

[7] Yuval Noah Harari, 21 Lessons for the 21st Century

[8] Focal Infection - The endodontic point of view Ehrmann *Oral Surgery* Vol 44 No 4 October 1977

[9] The American Association of Endodontists (http://www.aae.org): "Facts About Root Canal Treatment and Endodontists

[10] Gary Hunter, "How much does a Root Canal cost in Australia?", finder, last updated 8 April, 2021, https://www.finder.com.au/root-canal-therapy.

[11] The Canadian Academy of Endodontics claims that; Endodontic Retreatment treatment is extremely successful, but occasionally the tooth will fail to heal or will develop new problems. In this case, a second endodontic procedure may be recommended to save the tooth.

[12] "The Changing Face Of Dentistry - Endodontics" by Dr Paul V. Abbott BDSc, MDS, FRACDS(Endo). Australian Dental Association News Bulletin April 1996

13   https://www.aae.org/specialty/wp-content/uploads/sites/2/2017/06/rootcanalsafetytalkingpoints.pdf

14 Summary report on the joint commission on Neurology. Yahr MD Neurology 25: 497-501 1975

15 https://www.aae.org/specialty/about-aae/aae-history/

16 Laura Lee. Interview with George Meinig, DDS & Dr. M. LaMarche Cavitations & Root Canals http://www.tldp.com/issue/157-8/157rootc.htm

17 https://www.nationallibertyalliance.org/files/NaturalHealing/Rife/History%20of%20Dr%20Rife.pdf

18 https://www.quantumbalancing.com/rife-historyifhtm

19   https://www.aae.org/specialty/wp-content/uploads/sites/2/2017/06/rootcanalsafety.pdf

20 Shakman, S. Hale (2010-06-16). MEDICINE'S GRANDEST FRAUD PHD

21 Curtis, A. Focal infection. American Textbook of operative Dentistry Ed 7, M. L. Ward, ed., Lea & Febiger, philadelphia, 1840

22 Billings, E: Focal infection. The Lane medical Lectures. D. Appleton & Co., New York, 1916.

23 Shuster, M. Relationship of arthritis to oral diagnosis, defocalization, and streptococcus vaccine therapy. Am. J. ortodont."& oral Surg. (oral Surg. Sect.), .27: 149 (March), l941

24 Journal of the American Dental Association Vol 42 June 1951(619-633)

25 S.H. Shakman, Fraud and Root Canals – medicines greatest fraud – dentistry, deception, quackery 1998 Institute of Science www.instituteofscience.com

26 Grossman, Louis (1940), "Pulpless teeth and focal infection", Root Canal Therapy, Philadelphia: Lea & Febiger, pp. 16–17

27 https://www.medicinenet.com/script/main/art.asp?articlekey=12923

28 Gilman, A.G., T.W. Rall, A.S. Nies and P. Taylor (eds.). Goodman and Gilman's The Pharmacological Basis of Therapeutics. 8th ed. New York, NY. Pergamon Press, 1990., 1001

29 Risk factors for dental caries in small rural and regional Australian communities. Zander A1, Sivaneswaran S, Skinner J, Byun R, Jalaludin B. Rural Remote Health. 2013;13(3):2492. Epub 2013 Aug 13.

30 http://www.ada.org/public/topics/root_canal.asp

[31] IARC Working Group on the Evaluation of Carcinogenic Risks to Humans (2006);.

[32]

[33] Patterns of dental caries following the cessation of water fluoridation. Maupomé G, Clark DC, Levy SM, Berkowitz J. Community Dent Oral Epidemiol. 2001 Feb;29(1):37-47Decline of caries prevalence after the cessation of water fluoridation in the former East Germany. Künzel W, Fischer T, Lorenz R, Brühmann S. Community Dent Oral Epidemiol. 2000 Oct;28(5):382-9

[34]

[35] Caries trends 1992-1998 in two low-fluoride Finnish towns formerly with and without fluoridation. Seppä L, Kärkkäinen S, Hausen H. Caries Res. 2000 Nov-Dec;34(6):462-8.

[36] The decline of caries in New Zealand over the past 40 years. de Liefde B. N Z Dent J. 1998 Sep;94(417):109-13.

[37] Caries prevalence after cessation of water fluoridation in La Salud, Cuba. Künzel W, Fischer T. Caries Res. 2000 Jan-Feb;34(1):20-5.

[38] Journal of the American Dental Association, Editorial, October 1, 1944

[39] R.Steinman J Dent Res St. Louis, Vol 37 #5 1958

[40] R.Steinman J Dent Res St. Louis, Vol 37 #4 1958

[41] R.Steinman Indiana State Dental Journal Vol 39 1960

[42] R.Steinman J Southern California State Dental Assoc. Vol 28, No11 November 1960

[43] R.Steinman J of Southern California State Dental Association Vol 29 1961

[44] R.Steinman J of Southern California State Dental Association Vol 30 1962

[45] R.Steinman J of Southern California State Dental Association Vol 31 1963

[46] R.Steinman J of Southern California State Dental Association Vol 32 1964

[47] R.Steinman Caries and Cellular Nutrition, Dental Progress Vol.2; #3 April 1962

[48] R.Steinman J Southern California State Dental Assoc. Vol 35 No 4 April 1967

[49] R. Steinman J. Dent Res. Vol 47, No5, Sept 1968

[50] R. Steinman J. Dent Res. Vol 50, No6, Part 2. Nov-Dec 1971

[51] R. Steinman J. Dent Res. Vol 50, No6, Part 2. Nov-Dec 1971

[52] Aars H Gazelius B Edwall L Olgart L Effects of autonomic reflexes on tooth pulp blood flow in man. Acta Physiol Scand (1992 Dec) 146(4)

[53] R Steinman Dental Progress Vol 2 1962 Abstracts of Steinman p42 International Academy of Microendocrinology

[54] Edwall L Gazelius B Involvement of afferent nerves in pulpal blood-flow reactions in response to clinical and experimental procedures in the cat. In: Arch Oral Biol (1991) 36(8):575-81

[55] Aars H Gazelius B Edwall L Olgart L Effects of autonomic reflexes on tooth pulp blood flow in man. In: Acta Physiol Scand (1992 Dec) 146(4):423-9

[56] Desiderio DM Kai M Tanzer FS Trimble J Wakelyn C Measurement of enkephalin peptides in canine brain regions, teeth, and cerebrospinal fluid with high-performance liquid chromatography and mass spectrometry. In: J Chromatogr (1984 Aug 3) 297:245-60

[57] Olgart L Gazelius B Effects of adrenaline and felypressin (octapressin) on blood flow and sensory nerve activity in the tooth. In: Acta Odontol Scand (1977 May) 35(2):69-75

[58] Heyeraas KJ Kim S Raab WH Byers MR Liu M Effect of electrical tooth stimulation on blood flow, interstitial fluid pressure and substance P and CGRP-immunoreactive nerve fibers in the low compliant cat dental pulp. In: Microvasc Res (1994 May) 47(3):329-43

[59] Matthews B, Vongsavan N. Interactions between neural and hydrodynamic mechanisms in dentine and pulp. Arch Oral Biol 1994;39 Suppl:S87-S95.

[60] S. Vongsavan N, Matthews B. Fluid flow through cat dentine in vivo. Arch Oral Biol 1992;37:175–85.

[61] An overview of the dental pulp: its functions and responses to injury C Yu, PV Abbott from (2)

[62] Stanley H "Pulpal responses to ionomer cements" JADA 1990

[63] Samulson H., Sieraski S "diseases of the dental histopathology and pulp" ed/ Franklin S weine endodontic therapy 1989

[64] U. Schellenberg et al J. Endo 18:3 1992

[65] D. Pashley Clinical Considerations of Microleakage J. Endo 16:2 1990

[66] Buck, R. A. DMD; Eleazer, P. D. DDS, MS; Staat, R. H. PhD; Scheetz, J. P. PhD Effectiveness of Three Endodontic Irrigants at Various Tubular Depths in Human Dentin Journal of Endodontics: Volume 27(3) March 2001 pp 206-208

[67] J. Guttman et al J. Endo 13:12 1987

[68] Yusuf H The significance of the presence of foreign material periapically as a cause of failure of root treatment. Oral Surg Oral Med Oral Pathol 1982:54;566-574

[69] The principles of techniques for cleaning root canals GR Young, P Parashos, HH Messer Aust Dent J. 2007 Mar;52(1 Suppl):S52-63.

[70] Kakehashi S et al. The effect of surgical exposure of dental pulps in germ-free and conventional laboratory rats. Oral Surg oral mMed Oral Pathol 1965:20:340-349

[71] A survey of sodium hypochlorite use by general dental practitioners and endodontists in Australia. Clarkson RM, Podlich HM, Savage NW, Moule AJ. Aust Dent J. 2003 Mar;48(1):20-6.

[72] Treatment Planning the endodontic case' by T. Yeng, HH Messer, p. Parashos as part of (2)

[73] Australian Dental Journal Endodontic Supplement Volume 52, Number 1, March 2007 **(My emphasis)**

[74] https://f3f142zs0k2w1kg84k5p9i1o-wpengine.netdna-ssl.com/specialty/wp-content/uploads/sites/2/2017/06/rootcanalsafety.pdf

[75] Easlick K: An Evaluation of the Effect of Dental Foci of Infection on Health. JADA 42:615-686, 694-697, June 1951

[76] Stortebecker P "Dental Infectious Foci and diseases of the nervous system - spread of microorganisms and their products from dental infectious foci along direct cranial venous pathways eliciting a toxic - infectious encephalopathy" Acta. Psych Neural Scand 36 Suppl. 157 (1961) 62; Stortebecker P "Dental significance of pathways for dissemination from infectious foci." J Can Dent Assoc 33:6 1967 301–11; Stortebecker P "Chronic dental infections in the etiology of Glioblastomas. 8th int congress" Neuropathy. Washington D.C. Sept 1978 J Neuropth. Exp. Neurology 37(s) 1978; Shklar, Person, Ratner. Oral pathology and Trigeminal Neuralgia III J Dent Res. 1976;55(B):299; Ratner E., Langer., Evins M., alveolar Cavitational Osteopathosis manifestations of an infectious process and its implications in the causation of chronic pain. J Periodoontal 1986;57:593–603.

[77]

[78]

[79]

[80]

[81]

[82] Cell wall deficient bacterial variants from man in experimental cardiopathy. Merline JR, Golden A, Mattman LH Am J Clin Pathol (1971 Feb) 55(2):212–20;

[83] Cell wall-deficient forms of mycobacteria. Mattman LH Ann N Y Acad Sci (1970 Oct 30) 174(2):852-61

[84] Structures suggesting cell-wall-deficient forms detected in circulating erythrocytes by fluorochrome staining. Mattman LH, et al Appl Microbiol (1972 Feb) 23(2):262-7

[85] More Cures for Cancer Translation form the German by Dr Josef Issels Helfer Publishing E. Schwabe, Bad Homburg FRG.

[86] Cancer; a second opinion. Dr Joseph Issels. Published 2005 by Square One Publishers ISBN13: 9780757002793

[87] I. Bender J. Endo 23:1 1997

[88] Kesel RG a critique of methods in filling root canals. In Grossman LI editor. Transactions of the international conference on endodontics, Philadelphia 1958

[89] http://www.bbc.co.uk/history/historic_figures/nelson_horatio.shtml

[90] Kesel RG a critique of methods in filling root canals. In Grossman LI editor. Transactions of the international conference on endodontics, Philadelphia 1958;

[91] Malcolm Davis. Periapical and Intracanal Healing following incomplete root canal fillings in dogs. Oral surgery May 1971 vol. 31 no 5

[92] "Teeth decay because of an initial alteration in the internal metabolism." R. Steinman J. Dent Res. Vol 50, No6, Part 2. Nov-Dec 1971

[93] Actinomycotic Oral Infection (Modern Dental Implants and Root Canals) R.S. Carlson, DDS May 2017 Biological Dentistry Journal

[94] Implant Failures Associated With Asymptomatic Endodontically Treated Teeth David L. Brisman, D.M.D.; Adam S. Brisman, D.M.D.; Mark S. Moses, D.D.S. JADA February 2001, page 191

[95] Weston Price. *Dental Infections Oral and Systemic* Vols 1 & 2

[96] http://journal.iabdm.org/wp-content/uploads/2014/07/Endo-Pathology-Carlson.pdf

[97] Australian Dental Association handout December 1996

[98] E. Mandel Scanning Electron Microscope Observation of Canal Cleanliness. J. Endo. 16:6 1990

[99] 'Journal of the Australian Dental Association Endodontic Supplement' Vol 52 No 1 March 2007

[100] Schafer E., Lohman D Eficiency of rotary nickel-titanium Flexmaster instruments compared with stainless steel hand K-Flexofile – part 2. Cleaning effectiveness and instrumentation results in severely curved root canals of extracted teeth. Int Endod J 2002;33:297–310

[101] Schafer E., Schlingemann R Eficiency of rotary nickel-titanium K3 instruments compared with stainless steel hand K-Flexofile – part 2. Cleaning effectiveness and instrumentation results in severely curved root canals of extracted teeth. Int Endod J 2003;36:2208-217

[102] Peters OA et al.; Effects of four NiTi preparation techniques on root canal geometry assessed by microcumputed tomography. Int Endod J 2001;34:221-230

[103] Sim TP, Knowles JC, Ng YL, et al. Effect of sodium hypochlorite on mechanical properties of dentine and tooth surface strain. Int Endod J 2001;34:120–32.

[104] Marending M, Luder HU, Brunner TJ, et al. Effect of sodium hypochlorite on human root dentine–mechanical, chemical and structural evaluation. Int Endod J 2007;40:786–93.

[105] Effect of final irrigation protocols on microhardness reduction and erosion of root canal dentin Oral Research 31 · May 2017 Flávia Emi Razera BALDASSO et al

[106] Intracanal Irrigating Solutions Prior to Calcium Hydroxide Medication and Its Effects on Root Dentin Strength Leila Clarisse Hillesheim Brazilian Dental Journal (2017) 28(1): 46-50

[107] Intracanal Irrigating Solutions Prior to Calcium Hydroxide Medication and Its Effects on Root Dentin Strength Leila Clarisse Hillesheim et al Brazilian Dental Journal (2017) 28(1): 46-50

[108] Evaluation of the Effect of Endodontic Irrigation Solutions on the Microhardness and the Roughness of Root Canal Dentin Journal of Endodontics 30(11):792-5· December 2004

[109] Yusuf H The significance of the presence of foreign material periapically as a cause of failure of root treatment. Oral Surg Oral Med Oral Pathol 1982:54;566–74

[110] Anaerobic bacteremia and fungemia in patients undergoing endodontic therapy: an overview. Debelian J1, Olsen I, Tronstad L. Ann Periodontol. 1998 Jul;3(1):281–87.

[111] http://www.smile-mag.com/?pid=artd&artid=10&magid=4

[112] "The Changing Face Of Dentistry - Endodontics" by Dr Paul V. Abbott BDSc, MDS, FRACDS(Endo). Australian Dental Association News Bulletin April 1996

[113] Interim and temporary restoration of teeth during endodontic treatment AL Jensen, PV Abbott J Castro Salgado

[114] Kakehashi S et al The effects of surgical exposure of dental pulpsin germ-free and conventional laboratory rats. Oral Surg Oral med Oral Pathol 1965;20:340–49; Moller A Microbilogical examination of root canals and periapical tissues of human teeth. Methodological studies.Odont Tidskr 1966; 74:Suppl:1–380; Sundqvist G Bacteriological studies of necrotic dental pulpsUmea University Odontological dissertations No 7 Umea:Umea University Sweden 1976; Moller A, Fabricius L, Dahlen G, Ohman A, Heyden G. Influence on periapical tissues of indigenous oral bacteria and necrotic pulp tissue in monkeys. Scand J Dent Res 1981;89:475–84; Bergenholtz G. Micro-organisms from necrotic pulp of traumatized teeth, Odom Rev 1974;25:347–58; Fabricius L, Dab len G, Holm S, Moller Influence of combinations of oral bacteria on periapical tissues of monkeys. Scand J Dent Res 1982;90:200–206; Sundqvist Eckerbom M. Larsson A, Sjogren U. Capacity of anaerobic bacteria from necrotic dental pulps to induct purulent infections. Infect Immunol 1979;25:685–93; Seltzer S, Farber P. Microbiologic factors in endodontology. Oral Surg Oral Med Oral Pathol Oral Radio] Endod 1994;78:634- 645.

115

116

117

118

119

120

121

[122] The principles of techniques for cleaning root canals GR Young, P Parashos, HH Messer from Journal of the Australian Dental Association Endodontic Supplement' Vol 52 No 1 March 2007; Peters LB et al Viable bacteria in root dentinal tubules of teeth with apical periodontitis J Endod 2001;27:76–81; Love RM

[123] Peters LB et al Viable bacteria in root dentinal tubules of teeth with apical periodontitis J Endod 2001;27:76-81

[124] Love RM Regional variation in root dentinal tubule infection by Streptococus gordonii. J Endod 1996;22;290-293

[125] U. Schellenberg et al J. Endo 18:3 1992

[126] Stanley H "Pulpal responses to ionomer cements" JADA 1990;.

[127] Samulson H., Sieraski S "diseases of the dental histopathology and pulp" ed/ Franklin S weine endodontic therapy 1989

[128] A Athanassiadis, PV Abbott, LJ Walsh The use of calcium hydroxide, antibiotics and biocides as antimicrobial medicaments in endodontics. As part of the Special Supplement on Endodontics by the Journal of the Australian Dental Association March 2007

[129] Love MR Enterococous Faecalsi a mechanism for its role in endodontic failure Int Endod J 2001;34:399-405

[130] Peters OA Current challenges and concepts in the preparation of root canal systems: a review J Endod 2004;30:559-567

[131] Wu MK et al., Consequences of and strategies to deal with residual post-treatment root canal infections. Int Endod J 2006;39:343-356

[132] Nair PNR et al., Microbial status of apical root canal system of human mandibular first molars with primary apical periodontitis after 'one-visit' endodontic treatment. Oral Surg Oral Med Oral Pathol Oral Radiol Endod 2005;99:231-252

[133] A big role for the very small — understanding the endodontic microbial flora D Figdor, G Sundqvist

[134] Rants WE. Henry CA. Isolation and classification of anaerobic bacteria from intact pulp chambers of non-vital teeth in man. Ardis Oral Biol 1974;19:91-96. Sundqvist G. Taxonomy, ecology, and pathogenicity of the root canal flora. Oral Surg Oral Med Oral Pathol 1994:78:522-530.

[135] Wittgow WC, Jr., Sabiston CB, Jr. Microorganisms from pulpal chambers of intact teeth with necrotic pulps. J En do d 1975:1:168-171.

[136] Sundqvist G. Bacteriological studies of necrotic dental pulps. Umea University Odontological Dissertations No 7.Umea Umea University, Sweden, 1976.

[137] Sundqvist G. Taxonomy, ecology, and pathogenicity of the root canal flora. Oral Surg Oral Med Oral Pathol 1994:78:522-530.

[138] Mims C. Dimmock N, Nash A, Stephen Mims pathogenesis of infectious disease. 4th edn. London: Academic Press, 1995.

[139] Nair PN, Sjogren U, Krey G, Kahnberg KE, Sundqvist G J Endod 1990 Dec;16(12):580-588 Intraradicular bacteria and fungi in root-filled, asymptomatic human teeth with therapy-resistant periapical lesions: a long-term light and electron microscopic follow-up study

[140] J. Baumgartner J. Endo. 17:8 August 1991

[141] Kobayashi T, Hayashi A, Yoshikawa R, Okuda K, Hara K Niigata Int Endod J 1990 Mar;23(2):100-106 The microbial flora from root canals and periodontal pockets of non-vital teeth associated with advanced periodontitis

[142] Kobayashi T, Hayashi A, Yoshikawa R, Okuda K, Hara K Niigata Ando N, Hoshino E Int Endod J 1990 Jan;23(1):20-27 Predominant obligate anaerobes invading the deep layers of root canal dentin. Ando N, Hoshino E

[143] Sundqvist G, Figdor D, Persson S, Sjogren U Oral Surg Oral Med Oral Pathol Oral Radiol Endod 1998 Jan;85(1):86-93 Microbiologic analysis of teeth with failed endodontic treatment and the outcome of conservative re-treatment

[144] Sundqvist G, Figdor D, Persson S, Sjogren U B Wayman et a. J. Endo 18:4 1992

[145] Asikainen S, Alaluusua S Eur Heart J 1993 Dec;14 Suppl K:43-50 Bacteriology of dental infections.

[146] M.K. Wu, Moorer Wesselink Int. Endodontic Journal (1989) 22, 269-277

[147] The use of Calcium Hydroxide, antibiotics and biocides as antimicrobial medicaments in endodontics B Athanassiadis, PV Abott LJ Walsh from 'Journal of the Australian Dental Association Endodontic Supplement' Vol 52 No 1 March 2007

[148] Sundqvist, in 1976, isolated 88 species of bacteria from32 root canals with periapical disease.

[149] Wu, Moorer, Wesselink. Capacity of anaerobic bacteria enclosed in a simulated root canal to induce inflammation. Int. Endodontic Journal (1989) 22, 269-277

[150] Molecular analysis of bacteria in asymptomatic and symptomatic endodontic infections. Sakamoto M, Rôças IN, Siqueira JF, Benno Y. Oral Microbiol Immunol. 2006 Apr;21(2):112-22

[151] Charlton BR Channing-Santiago SE Bickford AA Cardona CJ Chin RP Cooper GL Droual R Jeffrey JS Meteyer CU Shivaprasad HL et al Preliminary

[152] characterization of a pleomorphic gram-negative rod associated with avian respiratory disease. J Vet Diagn Invest (1993 Jan) 5(1):47-51

[153] Cantwell AR Variably acid-fast pleomorphic bacteria as a possible cause of mycosis fungoides. A report of a necropsied case and two living patients J Dermatol Surg Oncol (1982) 8(3):203-213

[154] Cantwell AR Lawson JW Necroscopic Findings Of Pleomorphic, Variably Acid-Fast Bacteria In A Fatal Case Of Kaposi's Sarcoma J Dermatol Surg Oncol (1981) 7(11):923-930

[155] Eisenberg RJ Montgomery PC Characterization of an antibody directed against a surface component of normal and pleomorphic cells of Streptococcus sanguis. Infect Immun (1975 Sep) 12(3):668-78

[156] Maeda N Anaerobic, gram-positive, pleomorphic rods in human gingival crevice. Bull Tokyo Med Dent Univ (1980 Mar) 27(1):63-70

[157] Ishikawa O Aerobic gram-positive pleomorphic rods isolated from dental plaque and gingival crevice. Bull Tokyo Med Dent Univ (1980 Mar) 27(1):71-7

[158] Bauld J Marshall KC Quantitative description of morphological changes during growth of a pleomorphic budding bacterium. Antonie Van Leeuwenhoek (1971) 37(4):401-7

[159] Wainwright M Highly pleomorphic staphylococci as a cause of cancer. Med Hypotheses (2000 Jan) 54(1):91-4

[160] The persecution and trial of Gaston Naessens by Christopher Bird isbn 0-915811-30-8

[161] Townsend Letter for Doctors & Patients Feb/March 1999 Cell Wall Deficient Forms and Their Association with Root Canaled Teeth and Cavitational Osteonecrosis

[162] Dr Weston A Price, Dental Infections – Oral and Systemic 1923

[163] Philip Delivanis Oral Surgery 1981 Vol 52 No 4

[164] Nagaoka S, Miyazaki Y, Liu Hj, Iwamoto Kitano M, Kawagoe M. Bacterial invasion into dentinal tubules of human vital and nonvital teeth. j Endod 1995;21:70-73.

[165] Linden LA, Kallskog 0, Wolgast M. Human dentine as a hydrogel. Arch Oral Biol 1995;40:991-1004.

[166] Vongsavan N, Matthews B. The permeability of cat dentine in vivo and in vitro. Arch Oral Biol 1991;36:641-646.

[167] Matthews B, Vongsavan N. Interactions between neural and hydrodynamic mechanisms in dentine and pulp. Arch Oral Biol 1994;39 Suppl:887-895.

[168] S. Vongsavan N, Matthews B. Fluid flow through cat dentine in vivo. Arch Oral Biol 1992;37:175-185

[169] This story has been adapted from a news release issued by University of California - Berkeley.

[170] British Dental Association, 64 Wimpole Street, London, W1M 8AL 1996

[171] "Irrigation in Endodontics," https://bda.org/dentists/education/sgh/Documents/Irrigation%20in%20endodontics%202.pdf.

381

[172] Recent Advances in Root Canal Disinfection: A Review Zahed Mohammadi, et al Iran Endod J. 2017 Fall; 12(4): 402–406.

[173] Jha D Guerrero A Ngo T Helfer A Hasselgren G Inability of laser and rotary instrumentation to eliminate root canal infection. J Am Dent Assoc (2006 Jan) 137(1):67-70

[174] Kreisler M, Kohnen W, Beck M, Al Haj H, Christoffers AB, Gotz H, et al. Efficacy of NaOCl/H2O2 irrigation and GaAlAs laser in decontamination of root canals in vitro. Lasers Surg Med 2003;32:189-96

[175] Bergmans L, Moisiadis P, Teughels W, Van Meerbeek B, Quirynen M, Lambrechts P. Bactericidal effect of Nd:YAG laser irradiation on some endodontic pathogens ex vivo. Int Endod J 2006;39:547-57.

[176] Klinke T, Klimm W, Gutknecht N. Antibacterial effects of Nd:YAG laser irradiation within root canal dentin. J Clin Laser Med Surg 1997;15(1):29-31.

[177] The Use of Lasers in Disinfection and Cleanliness of Root Canals: a Review Ivona Bago Jurič and Ivica Anić Acta Stomatol Croat. 2014 Mar; 48(1): 6–15.

[178] The Disinfecting Efficacy of Root Canals with Laser Photodynamic Therapy Aliu Xhevdet, et al J Lasers Med Sci. 2014 Winter; 5(1): 19–26.

[179] Piccolomini R, D›Arcangelo C, D›Ercole S, Catamo G, Schiafino G, De Fazio P. Bacteriologic evaluation of the effect of Nd:YAG laser irradiation in experimental infected root canals. J Endod 2002;28(4):276-8.

[180] Meire MA, De Prijck K, Coenye T, Nelis HJ, De Moor RJ. Effectiveness of different laser systems to kill Enterococcus faecalis in aqueous suspension and in an infected tooth model. Int Endod J 2009;42,351-9.

[181] Kangarloo A, Fekrazad R, Salar O. Antibacterial effect of Er, Cr: YSGG laser and 2%chlorhexidine solution on dental tubules infected by E. faecalis. Thesis No:2519-2004.

[182] Moritz A, Jakolitsch S, Goharkhay K, Schoop U, Kluger W, Mallinger R, et al. Morphologic changes correlating to different sensitivities of Escherichia coli and Entrococcus faecalis to Nd:YAG laser irradiation through dentin. Lasers Surg Med 2000;26:250-61.

[183] Le Goff A, Dautel-Morazin A, Guigand M, Vulcain JM, Canal Disinfection by Laser during Root Canal Therapy 16 Journal of Lasers in Medical Sciences Volume 4 Number 1 Winter 2013 Bonnaure-Mallet M. An evaluation of the CO2 laser for endodontic disinfection. J Endod 25(2):105-8.

[184] Gutknecht N, Van Gogswaardt D, Conrads G, Apel C, Schubert C, Lampert F. Diode laser radiation and its bactericidal effect in root canal wall dentin. J Clin Laser Med Surg 2000;18(2):57-60.

[185] De Sauza EB, Cai S, Simionato MR, Lage-Marques JL. High power diode laser in the disinfection in depth of the root canal dentin

[186] Vezzani MS, Pietro R, Silva-Sousa YT, Brugnera-Junior A, Sousa-Neto MD. Disinfection of root canals using Er: YAG laser at different frequencies. Photomed Laser Surg 2006; 24(4):499-502.

[187] Godon W, Atabakhsh VA, Meza F, Doms A, Nissan R, Rizoiu I, et al. The antimicrobial efficacy of the erbium, chromium:yttrium-scandium-gallium-garnet laser with radial emitting tips on root canal dentin walls infected with Enterococcus faecalis. J Am Dent Assoc; 138(7):992-1002.

[188] Moritz A, Schoop U, Goharkhay K, Jakolitsch S, Kluger W, Wernisch J, et al. The bactericidal effect of Nd:YAG, Ho:YAG, and Er:YAG laser irradiation in the root canal

[189] Foschi F, Fontana CR, Ruggiero K, Riahi R, Vera A, Doukas AG, et al. Photodynamic inactivation of Enterococcus faecalis in dental root canals in vitro. Lasers Surg Med 2007;39(10):782-7.

[190] Fimple JL, Fontana CR, Foschi F, Ruggiero K, Song X, Pagonis TC, et al. Photodynamic treatment of endodontic polymicrobial infection in vitro. J Endod 2008;34(6):728- 34.

[191] Lasers in Dentistry: Is It Really Safe? Hamed Mortazavi 2016 Volume: 7 Issue: 4 Page: 123-127

[192] C. Budd J.Endo 17:6 1991

[193] Murazabal M Erausquin J Devoto FH A study of periapical overfilling root canal treatment in the molar of the rat. Arch Oral Biol (1966 Apr) 11(4):373-83

[194] Russell DI Ryan WJ Towers JF Complications of automated root canal treatment. Apical perforation and overfilling. Br Dent J (1982 Dec 7) 153(11):393-8

[195] Bruno E Gagliani M Fantoni A Di Gianvittorio A Canal overfilling: clinico-therapeutic considerations Dent Cadmos (1987 Jul 15) 55(12):77-8

[196] A comparison of short-term periapical responses to hand and ultrasonic file overextension during root canal instrumentation in the Macaca fascicularis monkey. J Endod (1987 Aug) 13(8):388-91

[197] Nitzan DW Stabholz A Azaz B Concepts of accidental overfilling and overinstrumentation in the mandibular canal during root canal treatment. J Endod (1983 Feb) 9(2):81-5

[198] Bergenholtz G Lekholm U Milthon R Engstrom B Influence of apical overinstrumentation and overfilling on re-treated root canals. J Endod (1979 Oct) 5(10):310-4

[199] Garcia JR Loianno F [Accidental overfilling with medicated cement] Rev Soc Odontol La Plata (1990 Oct) 3(5):7-10

[200] Kockapan C [Overfilling into the mandibular canal as an endodontic complication. A review] Schweiz Monatsschr Zahnmed (1993) 103(1):20-8

[201] Buser D Hotz P [Complications in overfilling of the root canals] Schweiz Monatsschr Zahnmed (1990) 100(10):1184-93

[202] Nikolic T Pathology and treatment in overfilling of the root canal Stomatol Glas Srb (1974 May-Jul) 21(3):175-8

[203] Liston PN Walters RF Foreign bodies in the maxillary antrum: a case report. Aust Dent J (2002 Dec) 47(4):344-6

[204] Gutierrez JH Brizuela C Villota E Human teeth with periapical pathosis after overinstrumentation and overfilling of the root canals: a scanning electron microscopic study. Int Endod J (1999 Jan) 32(1):40-8

[205] Barkhordar RA Nguyen NT Paresthesia of the mental nerve after overextension with AH26 and gutta-percha: report of case. J Am Dent Assoc (1985 Feb) 110(2):202-3

[206] Tamse A Kaffe I Littner MM Kozlovsky A Paresthesia following overextension of AH-26: report of two cases and review of the literature. J Endod (1982 Feb) 8(2):88-90

[207] Koseoglu BG Tanrikulu S Subay RK Sencer S Anesthesia following overfilling of a root canal sealer into the mandibular canal: a case report. Oral Surg Oral Med Oral Pathol Oral Radiol Endod (2006 Jun) 101(6):803-6

[208] Blanas N Kienle F Sandor GK Inferior alveolar nerve injury caused by thermoplastic gutta-percha overextension. J Can Dent Assoc (2004 Jun) 70(6):384-7

[209] Giardino L Pontieri F Savoldi E Tallarigo F Aspergillus mycetoma of the maxillary sinus secondary to overfilling of a root canal. J Endod (2006 Jul) 32(7):692-4

[210] Khongkhunthian P Reichart PA Aspergillosis of the maxillary sinus as a complication of overfilling root canal material into the sinus: report of two cases. J Endod (2001 Jul) 27(7):476-8

[211] Neaverth EJ Disabling complications following inadvertent overextension of a root canal filling material. J Endod (1989 Mar) 15(3):135-9

[212] Manisali Y Yucel T Erisen R Overfilling of the root. A case report. Oral Surg Oral Med Oral Pathol (1989 Dec) 68(6):773-5

[213] Gatot A Tovi F Prednisone treatment for injury and compression of inferior alveolar nerve: report of a case of anesthesia following endodontic overfilling. Oral Surg Oral Med Oral Pathol (1986 Dec) 2(6):704-6

[214] Spielman A Gutman D Laufer D Anesthesia following endodontic overfilling with AH26. Report of a case. Oral Surg Oral Med Oral Pathol (1981 Nov) 52(5):554-6

[215] Holland R Nery MJ de Mello W de Souza V Bernabe PF Otoboni Filho JA Root canal treatment with calcium hydroxide. I. Effect of overfilling and refilling. Oral Surg Oral Med Oral Pathol (1979 Jan) 47(1):87-92

[216] Yaltirik M Ozbas H Erisen R Surgical management of overfilling of the root canal: a case report. Quintessence Int (2002 Oct) 33(9):670-2

[217] Journal of Endodontics: Volume 26(1) January 2000 pp 29-31

[218] Saliva penetration of filled root canals was considered to be clinically significant M. Magura J. Endo 17:7 1991

[219] Leakage of Amalgam, Composite, and Super-EBA, Compared with a New Retrofill Material: Bone Cement Holt, Gary Matthew BS; Dumsha, Thom C. DDS, MS

[220] Chong BS Pitt Ford TR Watson TF Wilson RF Sealing ability of potential retrograde root filling materials. Endod Dent Traumatol (1995 Dec) 11(6):264-9

[221] Adamo HL Buruiana R Schertzer L Boylan RJ A comparison of MTA, Super-EBA, composite and amalgam as root-end filling materials using a bacterial microleakage model. Int Endod J (1999 May) 32(3):197-203

[222] Higa RK Torabinejad M McKendry DJ McMillan PJ The effect of storage time on the degree of dye leakage of root-end filling materials. Int Endod J (1994 Sep) 27(5):252-6

[223] Peters LB Harrison JW A comparison of leakage of filling materials in demineralized and non-demineralized resected root ends under vacuum and non-vacuum conditions. Int Endod J (1992 Nov) 25(6):273-8

[224] Ayhan H Alacam A Olmez A Apical microleakage of primary teeth root canal filling materials by clearing technique. J Clin Pediatr Dent (1996 Winter) 20(2):113-7

225 Yatsushiro JD Baumgartner JC Tinkle JS Longitudinal study of the microleakage of two root-end filling materials using a fluid conductive system. J Endod (1998 Nov) 24(11):716-9

226 Wu MK Kontakiotis EG Wesselink PR Long-term seal provided by some root-end filling materials. J Endod (1998 Aug) 24(8):557-60

227 Torabinejad M Hong CU Pitt Ford TR Kettering JD Cytotoxicity of four root end filling materials. J Endod (1995 Oct) 21(10):489-92

228 Fogel BB A comparative study of five materials for use in filling root canal spaces. Oral Surg Oral Med Oral Pathol (1977 Feb) 43(2):284-99

229 Tollens H [Root canal filling materials (electron scanning microscope comparison of root canal adaptation to 3 endodontic filling products) Rev Belge Med Dent (1979) 34(4):351-84

230 Bacterial leakage in root canals filled with conventional and MTA-based sealers A. C. M. Oliveira International Endodontic Journal 28 January 2011

231 Oliver CM Abbott PV An in vitro study of apical and coronal microleakage of laterally condensed gutta percha with Ketac-Endo and AH-26. Aust Dent J (1998 Aug) 43(4):262-8

232 Malcolm Davis. Periapical and Intracanal Healing following incomplete root canal fillings in dogs. Oral surgery May 1971 vol. 31 no 5

233 C. Budd J.Endo 17:6 1991

234 F. Goldberg et al J. Endo 21:1 1995

235 J. Simons et al J. Endo 17:3 1991

236 Prevalence of apical periodontitis and the quality of endodontic treatment in an adult Belarusian population. Int Endod J. 2005 Apr;38(4):238-45 Kabak Y, Abbott PV

237 Yatsushiro JD Baumgartner JC Tinkle JS Longitudinal study of the microleakage of two root-end filling materials using a fluid conductive system. J Endod (1998 Nov) 24(11):716-9

238 Fogel BB A comparative study of five materials for use in filling root canal spaces. Oral Surg Oral Med Oral Pathol (1977 Feb) 43(2):284-99

239 Tollens H [Root canal filling materials (electron scanning microscope comparison of root canal adaptation to 3 endodontic filling products) Rev Belge Med Dent (1979) 34(4):351-84

240 Outcome of primary root canal treatment: Systematic review of the literature – Part 2. Influence of clinical factors Y.-L. Ng et al Int Endo J 11 October 2007

[241] Stortebecker P "Dental Infectious Foci and diseases of the nervous system - spread of microorganisms and their products from dental infectious foci along direct cranial venous pathways eliciting a toxic - infectious encephalopathy" Acta. Psych Neural Scand 36 Suppl. 157 (1961) 62

[242] Stortebecker P "The cranial venous system filled from pulp of a tooth - Proceedings" 3rd Int. Congress of Nero Surg. Copenhagen Aug 1965

[243] Stortebecker P "Dental significance of pathways for dissemination from infectious foci." J Can Dent Assoc 33:6 1967 pp301-311

[244] Stortebecker P "Chronic dental infections in the etiology of Glioblastomas. 8th int congress" Neuropathy. Washington D.C. Sept 1978 J Neuropth. Exp. Neurology 37(s) 1978

[245] Capra N. Andersopn KV. Pride JB. Jones TE simultaneous "Demonstration of Neuronal Somata that innovate the tooth pulp and adjacent periodontal tissues using two retrogradely transported anatomic markers." Exp. Neurol 86(1984) 1670

[246] Marfurt C. Turner D Uptake and transneuronal transport of Horseradish Peroxidase - Wheat Germ aglutinin by Tooth Pulp Primary Afferent Neurons' Brain Res. 452(1988) 381-387

[247] Marfurt C. Turner D 'The central Projections of tooth pulp afferent neurons in the rat as determined by the Transganglionic transport of Horseradish Peroxidase" J. of Comp.Neuro 223 (1984) 535-547.

[248] Arvidson J. Gobel S. "An HRP study of the Central Projections of Primary Trigeminal Neurons which innovate tooth pulps in the cat." Brain Res. 210 (1981) 1-16

[249] Implant Failures Associated With Asymptomatic Endodontically Treated Teeth David L. Brisman, D.M.D.; Adam S. Brisman, D.M.D.; Mark S. Moses, D.D.S. JADA February 2001, page 191

[250] Management of endodontic failures: case selection and treatment modalities. Aqrabawi J Gen Dent (2005 Jan-Feb) 53(1):63-5

[251] Implants failures related to endodontic treatment. An observational retrospective study. Eduardo Jaramillo D Clin Oral Implants Res (2015 Sep) 26(9):992-5

[252] Molecular analysis of the root canal microbiota associated with endodontic treatment failures. Sakamoto M Siqueira JF Rocas IN Benno Y Oral Microbiol Immunol (2008 Aug) 23(4):275-81

[253] Rubin et al Oral Surg 1976 Vol 41 No 1

[255] Ancestry of pink disease (infantile acrodynia) identified as a risk factor for autism spectrum disorders. Shandley K, Austin DW J Toxicol Environ Health A (2011) 74(18):1185-94

[256] International Endodontic Journal, Vol. 33 Issue 1, 2000

[257] Materials used for root canal obturation: technical, biological and clinical testing DAG ØRSTAVIK Endodontic Topics 2005, 12, 25–38

[258] Use of radioactive iodine as a tracer in the study of the physiology of teeth. BARTELSTONE HJ, MANDEL ID, et al N Y State Dent J (1947 Nov) 13(9):515-8

[259] Lewis BB Chestner SB Formaldehyde In Dentistry: A Review Of Mutagenic And Carcinogenic Potential J Am Dent Assoc (1981) 103(3):429-434

[260] https://www.aae.org/specialty/wp-content/uploads/sites/2/2017/06/paraformaldehydefillingmaterials.pdf

[261] Safavi K et al. "Tumor necrosis factor identified in periapical tissue exudates in teeth with periapical periodontitis. J. of Endo. 17 (1991) 12-13

[262] Perna E et al. "Actinomycotic Granuloma of the Gasserian Ganglion with primary site in a dental root" J of Neurosurg 54 (1981) 553-555

[263] Hata G. et al. "Systemic distribution of 14 c-labeled Formaldehyde applied in the root Canal following pulpectomy" J. of Endo 15 No11 1989 539-543

[264] Geurtsen W Leyhausen G Biological aspects of root canal filling materials--histocompatibility, cytotoxicity, and mutagenicity. Clin Oral Investig (1997 Feb) 1(1):5-11

[265] Arenholt-Bindslev D Horsted-Bindslev P A simple model for evaluating relative toxicity of root filling materials in cultures of human oral fibroblasts. Endod Dent Traumatol (1989 Oct) 5(5):219-26

[266] Chong BS Owadally ID Pitt Ford TR Wilson RF Cytotoxicity of potential retrograde root-filling materials. Endod Dent Traumatol (1994 Jun) 10(3):129-33

[267] Chong BS Ford TR Wilson RF Radiological assessment of the effects of potential root-end filling materials on healing after endodontic surgery. Endod Dent Traumatol (1997 Aug) 13(4):176-9

[268] Peltola M Salo T Oikarinen K Toxic effects of various retrograde root filling materials on gingival fibroblasts and rat sarcoma cells. Endod Dent Traumatol (1992 Jun) 8(3):120-4

[269] Chong BS Ford TR Kariyawasam SP Tissue response to potential root-end filling materials in infected root canals. Int Endod J (1997 Mar) 30(2):102-14

[270] Pascon EA Spangberg LS In vitro cytotoxicity of root canal filling materials: 1. Gutta- percha. J Endod (1990 Sep) 16(9):429-33

[271] Zhu Q Safavi KE Spangberg LS Cytotoxic evaluation of root-end filling materials in cultures of human osteoblast-like cells and periodontal ligament cells. J Endod (1999 Jun) 25(6):410-2

[272] Ersev H Schmalz G Bayirli G Schweikl H Cytotoxic and mutagenic potencies of Endod (1999 May) 25(5):359-63

[273] Brodin P Roed A Aars H Orstavik D Neurotoxic effects of root filling materials on rat phrenic nerve in vitro. J Dent Res (1982 Aug) 61(8):1020-3

[274] Serper A Ucer O Onur R Etikan I Comparative neurotoxic effects of root canal filling materials on rat sciatic nerve. J Endod (1998 Sep) 24(9):592-4

[275] Maseki T Yasumura K Nanba I Kobayashi F Nakamura H Alterations in macrophages after exposure to root canal filling materials. J Endod (1996 Sep) 22(9):450-4

[276] Torabinejad M Ford TR Abedi HR Kariyawasam SP Tang HM Tissue reaction to implanted root-end filling materials in the tibia and mandible of guinea pigs. J Endod (1998 Jul) 24(7):468-71

[277] Lambrecht JT Panzer G [The toxicity of root-canal filling materials in primary osteoclast cell cultures (see comments)] Die Toxizitat von Wurzelfullmaterialien in primaren Osteoklasten- Zellkulturen. Schweiz Monatsschr Zahnmed (1995) 105(7):899-906

[278] Tsuzuki N A histopathological study of various root canal filling materials. Showa Shigakkai Zasshi (1990 Jun) 10(2):196-202

[279] Resorcinol-Formaldehyde Resin ?Russian Red" Endodontic Therapy. Schwandt et al Journal of Endo vol 29., No 7 July 2003

[280] Pascon EA Spangberg LS In vitro cytotoxicity of root canal filling materials: 1. Gutta- percha. In: J Endod (1990 Sep) 16(9):429-33 ISSN: 0099-2399

[281] Materials used for root canal obturation: technical, biological and clinical testing DAG ØRSTAVIK Endodontic Topics 2005, 12, 25–38

[282] Mittal M Chandra S Chandra S Comparative tissue toxicity evaluation of four endodontic sealers. Endod (1995 Dec) 21(12)

[283] Chang SW Baek SH Yang HC Seo DG Hong ST Han SH Lee Y Gu Y Kwon HB Lee W Bae KS Kum KY Heavy metal analysis of ortho MTA and ProRoot MTA. J Endod (2011 Dec) 37(12):1673–76

284 https://www.epa.gov/sites/default/files/2015-09/documents/train1-background.pdf

285 Water Quality Association https://www.wqa.org/Portals/0/Technical/Technical%20Fact%20Sheets/2014_Arsenic.pdf

286 Chang SW Baek SH Yang HC Seo DG Hong ST Han SH Lee Y Gu Y Kwon HB Lee W Bae KS Kum KY Heavy metal analysis of ortho MTA and ProRoot MTA. J Endod (2011 Dec) 37(12):1673-6

287 Duarte MA De Oliveira Demarchi AC Yamashita JC Kuga MC De Campos Fraga S Arsenic release provided by MTA and Portland cement. Oral Surg Oral Med Oral Pathol Oral Radiol Endod (2005 May) 99(5):648-50

288 Monteiro Bramante C Demarchi AC de Moraes IG Bernadineli N Garcia RB Spangberg LS Duarte MA Presence of arsenic in different types of MTA and white and gray Portland cement. Oral Surg Oral Med Oral Pathol Oral Radiol Endod (2008 Dec) 106(6):909-13

289 GonÃ§alves JL Viapiana R Miranda CE Borges AH Cruz Filho AM Evaluation of physico-chemical properties of Portland cements and MTA. Braz Oral Res (2010 Jul-Sep) 24(3):277-83

290 Journal of Endodontics: Volume 29(11) November 2003 pp 743-746 In Vitro Neurotoxic Evaluation of Root-end-filling Materials

291 Nylander et al. Fourth international symposium: Epidemiology in Occupational Health., Como Italy Sept 1985

292 Periapical tissue response to two calcium hydroxide-containing endodontic sealers IlsonSoaresDDS1et al Journal of Endodontics Volume 16, Issue 4, April 1990, Pages 166-169

293 Evaluation of pH and Calcium Ion Release of Root-end Filling Materials Containing Calcium Hydroxide or Mineral Trioxide Aggregate MárioTanomaru-Filho et al Journal of Endodontics Volume 35, Issue 10, October 2009, Pages 1418-1421

294 The hemolytic and cytotoxic properties of a zeolite-containing root filling material in vitro David C.ThomBSc, DMD, MSc (Endodontics) et al Oral Surgery, Oral Medicine, Oral Pathology, Oral Radiology, and Endodontology Volume 95, Issue 1, January 2003, Pages 101-108

295 Toxicity of endodontic filling materials JON E. DAHL Endodontic Topics 05 April 2006

296 Alveolodental ankylosis induced by root canal treatment in rat molars JorgeErausquinD.D.S.(Dr. Odont.)*Francisco C.H.DevotoD.D.S., M.D.(Dr. Odont.) Volume 30, Issue 1, July 1970, Pages 105-116

[297] N. Tani et al J. Endo 18:2 1992 "A wide range of pathobiological properties are attributed to the most frequently isolated endodontic pathogens".

[298] http://www.ada.org Jan 2005

[299] British Dental Association, 64 Wimpole Street, London, W1M 8AL 1996

[300] California's Proposition 65.

[301] https://www.mayoclinic.org/diseases-conditions/endocarditis/symptoms-causes/syc-20352576

[302] Boyd ND Benediktsson H Vimy MJ Hooper DE Lorscheider FL Am J Physiol (1991 Oct) 261(4 Pt 2):R1010-4

[303] "Silver" Dental Fillings Provoke An Increase in Mercury and Antibiotic Resistant Bacteria in the Mouth and Intestines of Primates. Anne 0. Summers, Murray Vimy and Fritz Lorscheider, The Alliance for the Prudent Use of Antibiotics (APUA) Newsletter, Fall 1991, Vol.9, No.3, pp.4-5.

[304] "Resistance of the Normal Human Microflora to mercury and antimicrobials", Clin Infect Dis 22(6):944-950, 1996.

[305] Richards H Mullany P Wilson M Prevalence and antibiotic resistance profile of mercury-resistant oral bacteria from children with and without mercury amalgam fillings. J Antimicrob Chemother (2002 May) 49(5):777- 83

[306] Debelian GJ, Olsen I, Tronstad L Electrophoresis of whole-cell soluble proteins of microorganisms isolated from bacteremias in endodontic therapy. Eur J Oral Sci (1996 Oct-Dec) 104(5-6): 540-6

[307]

[308] N. Tani et al J. Endo 18:2 1992 A wide range of pathobiological properties are attributed to the most frequently isolated endodontic pathogens

[309] Siskin M Oral Surg. 1977 Vol 43 No 3 Various immunologic diseases may be associated with Pulpal-Periapical Disease

[310] Rubin et al Oral Surg 1976 Vol 41 No 1 Three cases of infection of total hip replacements following Root Canal Therapy in 2 cases and Periodontal Surgery in 1 case.

[311] J Am Dent Assoc 1995 Apr;126(4):469-72; quiz 499-500 Abscess involving the left eye that originated as a dental abscess

[312] J Oral Maxillofac Surg 1995 Feb;53(2):203-8 1995 Feb Cervical cellulitis and mediastinitis caused by odontogenic infections

[313] Rapoport Y et al Oral Surg Oral Med Oral Pathol 1991 Jul;72(1):15-8 Cervical necrotizing fasciitis of odontogenic origin

[314] Mattila KJ et al Atherosclerosis 1993 Nov;103(2):205-11 Dental infections and coronary atherosclerosis

[315] J Am Dent Assoc (1989 Sep) 119(3):397-8, 401-2 Infection of pulpally involved teeth near the maxillary sinus sometimes spreads into the sinus and causes serious complications

[316] Steiner G J Neuropath. 1952;11:343-72 Support for the Oral Spirochaetes theory relating MS to oral infections

[317] Eliezer et al Oral Surg June 1978 Vol 45 No 6 Brain Abscess following Dental Infection

[318] Valachovic R Hargreaves JA Oral Surg Oral Med Oral Pathol (1979 Dec) 48(6):495-500

[319] Perna E et al. "Actinomycotic Granuloma of the Gasserian Ganglion with primary site in a dental root" J of Neurosurg 54 (1981) 553-555 Some brain cancers can be caused by infection in a tooth

[320] Black R., laboratory model for Trigeminal Neuralgia. Adv. Neuro.1974; 4:651-8 there is now evidence of demyelenation of the Gasserian Ganglion after damage as far away as a tooth pulp

[321] Westrum LE., Canfield RC., Black R., Transganglionic Degeneration in the spinal trigeminal nucleus following the removal of tooth pulps in adult cats. Brain Res 1976; 6:100:137-40

[322] Westrum LE., Canfield RC., Electron microscopy of degenerating axons and terminals in the spinal trigeminal nucleus after tooth pulp exterpation. Am J Anat. 1977; 149:591-6

[323] Gobel S., Bink J., degenerative changes in primary trigeminal axons and in neurons in nucleus caudalis following tooth pulp extirpation in the cat., Brain Res. 1977;132:347-54

[324] Mucke L Clinical management of neuropathic pain Neurol clin 1987;5:649-63 Peripheral nerve damage in human beings can result in central nervous system damage or hyperexcitability in the trigeminal ganglion and nuclei with subsequent development of Trigeminal Neuralgia

[325] Fromm G., et al Trigeminal Neuralgia. Current concepts regarding etiology and pathogenisis Arch Neurol 1984;41: 1204-7

[326] Bayer D. et al Trigeminal Neuralgia an overview. Oral Surg. Oral Med. Oral Pathol. 1979:48:393-9

[327] Selby G., Diseases of the fifth cranial nerve. In Dyke PJ., Thomas PK.,

[328] Peripheral Neuropathy. Philadelphia. W.B. Saunders 1984;1224-65

[329] King R. Interaction of noxious and nonnoxious stimuli in primary sensory nuclei Adv Neurol 1974; 4:659-63

[330] The changing face of dentistry Endodontics Paul V. Abbott BDSc, MDS, FRACDS(Endo) Insert in April 1996 Australian Dental Association News Bulletin

[331] Serious complications of endodontic infections: Some cautionary tales L. J. Walsh Australian Dental Journal 1997;42:(3):156-9

[332] Meurman JH Dental infections and general health. Quintessence Int (1997 Dec) 28(12):807-11

[333] Karow, J. Taken to Heart; Scientific American, May 2001, page 20

[334] Stortebecker 3rd Int Cong of Neurological Surgery Copenhagen 1965

[335] Stortebecker P "Dental significance of pathways for dissemination from infectious foci." J Can Dent Assoc 33:6 1967 pp301-311

[336] Stortebecker P Chronic dental infections in the etiology of Glioblastomas. 8th int congress" Neuropathy. Washington D.C. J Neuropth. Exp. Neurology 37(s) 1978

[337] Kristensson K., Olssan Y., Diffusion Pathways and Retrograde Transport in peripheral nerves" Prog. In Neurobio. 1 (1973)

[338] Price DL., Griffin J., Neurons and ensheathing cells as targets of disease processes. Ed. P.S. Spencer. Experimental and Clinical Neurotoxicology (Schaumburg: Wilkens and Wilkens 1980

[339] Stortebecker P "Dental Infectious Foci and diseases of the nervous system - spread of microorganisms and their products from dental infectious foci along direct cranial venous pathways eliciting a toxic - infectious encephalopathy" Acta. Psych Neural Scand 36 Suppl. 157 (1961) 62

[340] Stortebecker P "The cranial venous system filled from pulp of a tooth - Proceedings 3rd Int. Congress of Nero Surg. Copenhagen Aug 1965

[341] Horiba et al. Oral Surg. Oral Med. Oral Path. 1991 Vol 71 R. Nissan et al J. Endo 21:2 1995

[342] Alves J.A., Barrieshi K, Walton R. E., Wertz P. Wilcox L., Drake D. J Dent Res 1996; 75 (special issue):373 abstract 2847).

[343] Schein B J. of Endodontics 1975 Vol 1 No 1

[344] Penner A et al. J Exp Med 1960;111:145-53

[345] Palmiro C J Exp Med 1962; 115:609-12

[346] Alper M Proc Soc Exp Biol Med 1967;124:537-8 Parnas I Science 1971;171:1153-5

[347] Dr. Boyd Haley and Dr. Curt Pendergrass; [Affinity Labeling Technologies, Inc., USA] Bio-Probe journal (Vol 14-5); 1998

[348] Systemic Diseases Caused by Oral Infection XIAOJING LI,1* kristin m. Kolltveit,1 leif tronstad,2 and ingar olsen1 clinical microbiology reviews, Oct. 2000, p. 547–558

[349] Yiping Han et al. Transmission of an uncultivated Bergeyella strain from the oral cavity to amniotic fluid in a case of preterm birth. Journal of Clinical Microbiology 2006; 44:1475–83;.

[350] Maternal oral origin of Fusobacterium nucleatum in adverse pregnancy outcomes as determined using the 16S-23S rRNA gene intergenic transcribed spacer region. Gonzales-Marin C, Spratt DA, Allaker RP J Med Microbiol. 2013 Jan;62(Pt 1):133-44

[351] 16-year remission of rheumatoid arthritis after unusually vigorous treatment of closed dental foci. Breebaart AC1, Bijlsma JW, van Eden W. Clin Exp Rheumatol. 2002 Jul-Aug;20(4):555–57

[352] AAP November 13, 2006 01:36pm

[353] Radiology 2006;239:187-194.

[354] J Am Dent Assoc 1995 Apr;126(4):469-72; quiz 499-500

[355] Abscess of the orbit arising 48 h after root canal treatment of a maxillary first molar. Int Endod J. 2006 Aug;39(8):657-64 Koch F, Breil P, Marroquín BB, Gawehn J, Kunkel M.

[356] J Dent Res. 2006 Aug;85(8):761-5.Treponema denticola in disseminating endodontic infections.

[357] M. E. Vianna, G. Conrads, B. P. F. A. Gomes, H. P. Horz. 2006. Identification and quantification of Archaea involved in primary endodontic infections. Journal of Clinical Microbiology, 44. 4: 1274-1282

[358] Microbiol Immunol. 2005;49(5):399-405. Experimental abscess formation caused by human dental plaque.

[359]

[360] Okayama H, Nagata E, Ito HO, Oho T, Inoue M.

[359] Journal of Clinical Microbiology, July 2006, p. 2601-2604, Vol. 44, No. 7

[360] Periodontal, Cervical and Vaginal Microbiota in Pregnancy S.C. LU, A. Dasanayake, H. Saito, M. TAM, J. M. Theva

[361] http://www.asm.org/

[362] Infection and Immunity, April 2004, p. 2272-2279, Vol. 72, No. 4

[363] Journal of Clinical Microbiology, April 2006, p. 1475-1483, Vol. 44, No. 4

[364] Yiping Han et al. Transmission of an uncultivated Bergeyella strain from the oral cavity to amniotic fluid in a case of preterm birth. Journal of Clinical Microbiology 2006; 44:1475-1483.

[365] ZWR. 1989 Oct;98(10):850, 852, 854

[366] J Am Dent Assoc (1989 Sep) 119(3):397-8, 401-2

[367] Eliezer et al Oral Surg June 1978 Vol 45 No 6

[368] Valachovic R Hargreaves JA Oral Surg Oral Med Oral Pathol (1979 Dec) 48(6):495-500

[369] Perna E et al. "Actinomycotic Granuloma of the Gasserian Ganglion with primary site in a dental root" J of Neurosurg 54 (1981) 553-555

[370] Black R., laboratory model for Trigeminal Neuralgia. Adv. Neuro.1974; 4:651-8

[371] Westrum LE., Canfield RC., Black R., Transganglionic Degeneration in the spinal trigeminal nucleus following the removal of tooth pulps in adult cats. Brain Res 1976; 6:100:137-40

[372] Westrum LE., Canfield RC., Electron microscopy of degenerating axons and terminals in the spinal trigeminal nucleus after tooth pulp exterpation. Am J Anat. 1977; 149:591-6

[373] Gobel S., Bink J., degenerative changes in primary trigeminal axons and in neurons in nucleus caudalis following tooth pulp extirpation in the cat.,: Brain Res. 1977;132:347-54

[374] Evidence of Periopathogenic Microorganisms in Placentas of Women With Preeclampsia Shlomi Barak, Orit Oettinger-Barak, Eli E. Machtei, Hannah Sprecher, Gonen Ohel Journal of Periodontology 2007, Vol. 78, No. 4, Pages 670-676

[375] Case report: brain and liver abscesses caused by oral infection with Streptococcus intermedius. Oral Surg Oral Med Oral Pathol Oral Radiol Endod. 2006 Oct;102(4):e21-3. Epub 2006 Aug 10. Wagner KW, Schön R, Schumacher M, Schmelzeisen R, Schulze D

[376] Are dental infections a cause of brain abscess? Case report and review of the literature. Oral Dis. 2001 Jan;7(1):61-5 Corson MA, Postlethwaite KP, Seymour RA.

[377] Dtsch Z Mund Kiefer Gesichtschir. 1990 Jul-Aug;14(4):297-300 [Odontogenic brain abscess. 2 case reports] Feldges A, Heesen J, Nau HE, Schettler D.

[378] Intracranial complications of sinusitis in children. A sequela of periapical abscess. Ann Otol Rhinol Laryngol. 1982 Jan-Feb;91(1 Pt 1):41-3 Brook I, Friedman EM.

[379] Microbiology of intracranial abscesses and their associated sinusitis. Arch Otolaryngol Head Neck Surg. 2005 Nov;131(11):1017-9 Brook I.

[380] Oral Surg Oral Med Oral Pathol Oral Radiol Endod. 2006 Oct;102(4):e21-3.

[381] Oral Microbiology and Immunology Volume 17 Issue 2 Page 113 - April 2002

[382] Rubin et al Oral Surg 1976 Vol 41 No 1

[383] Professor P Miossec Clinical Immunology Unit, Departments of Immunology and Rheumatology, Hôpital Edouard Hérriot, 69437 Lyon Cedex 03, France

[384] American Journal of Obstetrics and Gynecology Volume 195, Issue 4, October 2006, Pages 1086-1089

[385] Published online January 24, 2007 Diabetes Care 30:842-847, 2007

[386] J Med Microbiol 55 (2006), 1285-1289

[387] Sinusitis of odontogenic origin Itzhak Brook MD, MSc Available online 1 September 2006.

[388] J Clin Microbiol. 2006 Sep;44(9):3313-7. Detection of cariogenic Streptococcus mutans in extirpated heart valve and atheromatous plaque specimens. Nakano K, et al

[389] J Periodontal Res. 2006 Aug;41(4):350-3. Periodontal pathogens in atheromatous plaques isolated from patients with chronic periodontitis. Padilla C, Lobos O, Hubert E, Gonzalez C, Matus S, Pereira M, Hasbun S, Descouvieres C.

[390] International Endodontic Journal Volume 39 Issue 5 Page 343 - May 2006

[391] American Chemical Society Date: September 29, 2006

[392] Arteriosclerosis, Thrombosis, and Vascular Biology. 2005;25:1446.)

[393] J Med Microbiol 55 (2006), 1135-1140

[394] Oral Microbiology and Immunology Volume 21 Issue 4 Page 206 - August 2006

[395] Journal of Periodontal Research Volume 41 Issue 4 Page 350 - August 2006

[396] Bacterial Signatures in Thrombus Aspirates of Patients With Myocardial Infarction Tanja Pessi et al Circulation March 19, 2013

[397] J Dent Res 85(1):74-78, 2006

[398] Arteriosclerosis, Thrombosis, and Vascular Biology. 2005;25:e17.)

[399] Evaluation of the Incidence of Periodontitis-Associated Bacteria in the Atherosclerotic Plaque of Coronary Blood Vessels Journal of Periodontology2007, Vol. 78, No. 2, Pages 322-327 Maciej Zaremba, Renata Górska, Piotr Suwalski, and Jan Kowalski

[400] Correlation Between Atherosclerosis and Periodontal Putative Pathogenic Bacterial Infections in Coronary and Internal Mammary Arteries Journal of Periodontology 2007, Vol. 78, No. 4, Pages 677-682 Ana Pucar, Jelena Milasin, Vojislav Lekovic, Miroslav Vukadinovic, Miljko Ristic, Svetozar Putnik,§ and E. Barrie Kenney

[401] April 2007 Journal of Bacteriology, published by the American Society of Microbiology.

[402] Mattila KJ et al Atherosclerosis 1993 Nov;103(2):205-11

[403] Bacterial diversity in aortic aneurysms determined by 16S ribosomal RNA gene analysis Marques da Silva R, Caugant DA, Eribe ER, Aas JA, Lingaas PS, Geiran O, Tronstad L, Olsen I. J Vasc Surg. 2006 Nov;44(5):1055-60.

[404] Quintessence Int 2006;37:11–18

[405] Journal of Periodontology 2006, Vol. 77, No. 7, Pages 1110-1119

[406] Arch Intern Med. 2006;166:554-559.

[407] Sedgley CM, Lennan SL, Appelbe OK. Survival of Enterococcus faecalis in root canals ex vivo. International Endodontic Journal, 38, 735–742, 2005.

[408] International Endodontic Journal, Volume 38, Number 10, October 2005, pp. 697-704(8)

[409] http://www.medicalnewstoday.com/sections/stroke/

[410] http://iadr.confex.com/iadr/2006Brisb/techprogram/session_16556.htm

[411] International Journal of Dermatology, Volume 46, Number 4, April 2007, pp. 376-379(4)

[412] J Oral Maxillofac Surg 1995 Feb;53(2):203-8 1995 Feb

[413] Rapoport Y et al Oral Surg Oral Med Oral Pathol 1991 Jul;72(1):15-8

[414] Siskin M Oral Surg. 1977 Vol 43 No 3

[415] Consequences of and strategies to deal with residual post-treatment root canal infection M.K. Wu1, P. M. H. Dummer & P. R. Wesselink 2006 International Endodontic Journal

[416] Price DL., Griffin J., Neurons and ensheathing cells as targets of diseasse processes. Ed. P.S. Spencer. Experimental and Clinical Neurotoxicology (Schaumburg: Wilkens and Wilkens 1980

[417] Marfurt C. Turner D Uptake and transneuronal transport of Horseradish Peroxidase - Wheat Germ aglutinin by Tooth Pulp Primary Afferent Neurons' Brain Res. 452(1988) 381-387

[418] Marfurt C. Turner D 'The central Projections of tooth pulp afferent neurons in the rat as determined by the Transganglionic transport of Horseradish Peroxidase" J. of Comp.Neuro 223 (1984) 535-547.

[419] Retrograde Axonal Transport of Mercury in Primary Sensory Neurons Innervating the Tooth Pulp in the Rat. Neurosci Lett. 115(1):29-32. Jul 17, 1990

[420] Arvidson B. Retrograde Axonal Transport of Mercury. Exp Neurol 1987;98

[421] BARUAH, J.K., RASOOL, C.G. BRADLEY, W.G. and MUNSAT, 7.L: Retrograde Transport of Lead in Rat Sciatic Nerve, Neurol, 31, 612, 1981

[422] Kristensson K., Olssan Y., Diffusion Pathways and Retrograde Transport in Peripheral nerves" Prog. In Neurobio. 1 (1973)

[423] Stortebecker P "Dental Infectious Foci and diseases of the nervous system - spread of microorganisms and their products from dental infectious foci along direct cranial venous pathways eliciting a toxic - infectious encephalopathy" Acta. Psych Neural Scand 36 Suppl. 157 (1961) 62

[424] Stortebecker P "Dental significance of pathways for dissemination from infectious foci. J Can Dent Assoc 33:6 1967 pp301-311

[425] Stortebecker P "The cranial venous system filled from pulp of a tooth - Proceedings" 3rd Int. Congress of Nero Surg. Copenhagen Aug 1965

[426] Mechanisms of Blood Brain Barrier Disruption by Different Types of Bacteria, and Bacterial-Host Interactions Facilitate the Bacterial Pathogen Invading the Brain Mazen M Jamil Al-Obaidi https://pubmed.ncbi.nlm.nih.gov/30117097/ - affiliation-1, Mohd Nasir Mohd Desa Epub 2018 Aug 16.

[427] J of Endodontics Vol3 No 5 May 1976

[428] Hubert Newman Focal infection Dent Res 75 (12) 1996 t Newman Focal infection Dent Res 75 (12) 1996 edited by Irwin Mandel (Assoc. Dean for Research School of Dental and Oral Surgery Colombia University New York)

[429] Excerpt from 'Facts about Neural Therapy according to Huneke' by Peter Dosch MD 20th edition 1984 Haug Publishers ISBN 3-7760-0851-2

[430] Professor Otto Neuner Biological Therapy Vol VI No2 April 1988

[431] Peter Dosch MD Facts about Neural Therapy according to Huneke 20th German edition Haug Publishers ISBN 3-7760-0851-2 1985

[432] Mathias Dosch MD Illustrated Atlas of the Techniques of Neural Therapy with Local Anesthetics Haug publishers ISBN 3-7760-0849-0 1985.

[433] Ernesto Adler MD DDS Neural Focal Dentistry 2nd Edition 1984 Multi-Discipline Research Foundation 6550 Tarnef Houston, Texas 77074

[434] Matrix and Matrix Regulation - Basis For A Holistic Theory In Medicine by A Pischinger Haug Publishers ISBN 2-8043-4000-7

[435] Professor Otto Neuner Biological Therapy Vol VI No2 April 1988

[436] Professor Otto Neuner Biological Therapy Vol VI No2 April 1988

[437] From the 'Memory of Water' Michael Schiff 1994 ISBN 0 7225 3262 8

[438] Shklar, Person, Ratner. Oral pathology and Trigeminal Neuralgia III J Dent Res. 1976;55(B):299;.

[439] Ratner E., Langer., Evins M., alveolar Cavitational Osteopathosis manifestations of an infectious process and its implications in the causation of chronic pain. J Periodoontal 1986;57:593-603

[440] The Holographic Universe by Michael Talbot 1996 (ISBN 0 586 09171 8)]

[441] Professor Otto Neuner Biological Therapy Vol VI No2 April 1988

[442] Caulk Co – MSDS contraindications 1997

[443] Stortebecker, P. Mercury poisoning from dental amalgam through a direct nose-brain transport. The Lancet, May 27, 1989.

[444] "The Changing Face Of Dentistry - Endodontics" by Dr Paul V. Abbott BDSc, MDS, FRACDS(Endo). Australian Dental Association News Bulletin April 1996

[445] AK Olson J. Endo 16:8 1990

[446] S. Dorn J. Endo 16:8 1990

[447] K. King Et Al J. Endo 16:7 1990

[448] M. Yoshimura J. Endo 16:1 1990

[449] S. Dazey et al J. Endo 16:1 1990

[450] C. Nixon et al J. Endo 17:10 1991

[451] P. Burtscher et al J. Endo 17:10 1991

[452] E. Pissiotis et al J. Endo 17:5 1991

[453] S. Inoue et al J. Endo 17:8 1991

[454] T. Coen et al J. Endo 18:3 1992

[455] D. Smith et al J. Endo 18:1 1992

[456] P. Abbott et al J. Endo 18:11 1992

[457] J. Smith et al J. Endo 18:4 1992

[458] W. Wong et al J. Endo 20:12 1994

[459] P. Randolph et al J. Endo 21:2 1995

[460] M. Torabinejad et al J. Endo 21:3 1995

[461] F. Goldberg et al J. Endo 21:10 1995

[462] J. Welch et al J. Endo 22:11 1996

[463] N Hosoya et al J. Endo 21:9 1995

[464] F Gerhards et al J. Endo 22:9 1996

[465] C. Lee et al J. Endo 23:4 1997

[466] Avram DC, Pulver F Pulpotomy medicaments for vital primary teeth. Surveys to determine use and attitudes in pediatric dental practice and in dental schools throughout the world. ASDC J Dent Child (1989 Nov-Dec) 56(6):426-34

[467] Fraud and Root Canals Medicine's Greatest Fraud Dentistry, Deception, Quackery. S.H. Shakman Phd Institute of Science 1998 Instituteofscience.com

[468] Assessment of the systemic distribution and toxicity of formaldehyde following pulpotomy treatment: Part one. Ranly DM ASDC J Dent Child (1985 Nov-Dec) 52(6):431-4

[469] Gobel S., Bink J., degenerative changes in primary trigeminal axons and in neurons in nucleus caudalis following tooth pulp extirpation in the cat.,: Brain Res. 1977;132:347-54 6:100:137–40.

[470] Westrum LE., Canfield RC., Electron microscopy of degenerating axons and terminals in the spinal trigeminal nucleus after tooth pulp exterpation. Am J Anat. 1977; 149:591-6

[471] Westrum LE., Canfield RC., Black R., Transganglionic Degeneration in the spinal trigeminal nucleus following the removal of tooth pulps in adult cats. Brain Res 1976; 6:100:137-40

472 Lewis BB Chestner SB Formaldehyde in dentistry: a review of mutagenic and carcinogenic potential. J Am Dent Assoc (1981 Sep) 103(3):429-34

473 Periapical tissue reaction in monkeys to endodontic treatment using formocresol as a disinfectant. Simon M van Mullem PJ Lamers AC J Endod (1979 Aug) 5(8):239-41

474 Embryotoxicity and teratogenicity of formocresol on developing chick embryos. Friedberg BH Gartner LP J Endod (1990 Sep) 16(9):434-7

475 Pulpal tissue reaction to formocresol vs. ferric sulfate in pulpotomized rat teeth. Cotes O Boj JR Canalda C Carreras M J Clin Pediatr Dent (1997 Spring) 21(3):247-53

476 Lahcen, Ousehal and Lazrak, Laila. "Change in nickel levels in the saliva of patients with fixed orthodontic appliances." International Orthodontics 10.2 (2012): 190–197

477 Bengleil, Mudafara S., Juma M. Orfi, and Iman Abdelgader. "Evaluation of salivary nickel level during orthodontic treatment." Int J Med Health Pharmacol Biomed Eng 7 (2013): 735-7.

478 Effect of mobile phone use on metal ion release from fixed orthodontic appliances. Saghiri MA, Orangi J, Asatourian Am J Orthod Dentofacial Orthop. 2015 Jun;147(6):719-24.

479 Black GV. A work on special dental pathology. 2nd ed. Chicago: Medico- Dental Publ Co, 1920.

480 A work on special dental pathology. 2nd ed. Chicago: Medico-Dental Publ Co, 1920.

481 Griffiths ID. Osteonecrosis. In: Scott JT (editor). Copeman's textbook of the rheumatic diseases, 6th ed. London: Churchill Livingstone, 1986: 1207-1228

482 Jones JP Jr. Osteonecrosis. In: McCarty D (editor). Arthritis and allied conditions: a textbook of rheumatology, 11th ed. Philadelphia, Lea & Febiger, 1989, pp 1545-1562. (good general review by an internationally recognized expert)

483 Arlet J, Mazieres B (editors). Bone circulation and bone necrosis. Proceedings of the Ivth International Symposium on Bone Circulation, Toulouse (France), 17th-19th September, 1987. New York: Springer-Verlag, 1990. (the definitive work to date; this book sets the standards)

484 Hungerford DS. Diagnosis and treatment of ischemic necrosis of the femoral head. In: Mc Evarts C (editor). Surgery of the musculoskeletal system, 2nd edition. New York: Churchill Livingstone, 1990: vol 3: 2757- 2794.

485 Ono K (editor). Symposium: recent advances in avascular osteonecrosis. Clin Orthopaedics Related Res 277:2-138, 1992. (summary of research papers of the Second International Symposium on Osteonecrosis)

486

487 Steinberg ME, Steinberg DR. Osteonecrosis. In: Kelly WN, Harris ED Jr, Ruddy S, Sledge CB (editors). Textbook of rheumatology, 4th ed. Philadelphia: W.B. Saunders, 1993:1628-1650.

488 Mazieres B. Osteonecrosis. In: Klippel JH, Dieppe PA (editors). Rheumatology. St. Louis: Mosby; 1994:41.1-41.8.

489 Sweet DE, Madewell JE. Osteonecrosis: pathogenesis. In: Resnick D (editor). Diagnosis of bone and joint disorders, 3rd ed. Philadelphia: W. B. Saunders, 1995: 3445-3494. (detailed review in the encyclopedic radiology text)

490 Rywlin AM. Histopathology of the bone marrow. Boston: Little, Brown & Co., 1996:153-190.

491 Jones JP Jr. Osteonecrosis. In: Koopman WJ (ed). Arthritis and allied conditions; a textbook of rheumatology, 13th edition. Baltimore: Williams & Wilkins, 1997:1923-1942. (good general review by an internationally recognized expert, one of the first to recognize potential coagulopathies in osteonecrosis)

492 Glueck CJ, McMahon R, Bouquot J, et al. A preliminary pilot study of treatment of thrombophilia and hypofibrinolysis and amelioration of the pain of osteonecrosis of the jaws. Oral Surg Oral Med Oral Pathol Oral Radiol Endod 1998; 85:64-73.

493 Gruppo R, Glueck CJ, McMahon RE, et al. The pathophysiology of osteonecrosis of the jaw: anticardiolipin antibodies, thrombophilia, and hypofibrinolysis. J Lab Clin Med 1996; 127:481-488.

494 Shankland WE. Craniofacial pain syndromes that mimic temporomandibular joint disorders. Ann Acad Med Singapore 1995; 24:104-106.

495 Bouquot JE, Christian J. Long-term effects of jawbone curettage on the pain of facial neuralgia; treatment results in neuralgia-inducing cavitational osteonecrosis. J Oral Maxillofac Surg 1995; 53:387-397.

496 Bouquot JE, Roberts AM, Person P, Christian J. NICO (neuralgia- inducing cavitational osteonecrosis): osteomyelitis in 224 jawbone samples from patients with facial neuralgias. Oral Surg Oral Med Oral Pathol 1992; 73:307-319.

[497] Bouquot JE, Roberts AM, Person P, Christian J. Neuralgia inducing cavitational osteonecrosis (NICO). Osteomyelitis in 224 jawbone samples from patients with facial neuralgia. Oral Surg Oral Med Oral Pathol. 1992;73:307–19

[498] Shklar, Person, Ratner. Oral pathology and Trigeminal Neuralgia III J Dent Res. 1976;55(B):299;

[499] Ratner. J Periodontol Oct 1968

[500] Ratner E., Langer., Evins M., alveolar Cavitational Osteopathosis manifestations of an infectious process and its implications in the causation of chronic pain. J Periodoontal 1986;57:593-603

[501] Ratner. J Periodontol Oct 1968

[502] Roberts A., Persons P., Chandran N. Hori J., Further observations on Dental Parameters of atypical facial Neuralgias. Oral Surg, Oral Med., and Oral Path 58(2) 1984

[503] Roberts A., Persons P., "Etiology and treatment of Idioathic Trigeminal and atypical facial Neuralgias. "Oral Surg, Oral Med., and Oral Path 48(4) 1979

[504] Stewart J "Microbiological findings" Manual for Residual Infection In Bone (RIIB) Indiana Univ. Medical Centre 1988

[505] Dental Extractions, Antibiotics and Curettage – First, Do no Harm. Michael J. Wahl DDS, Jean A. Wahl DMD & Margaret M. Schmitt DMD Global Journal of Medical research: J Dentistry and Otolaryngology Volume 14 Issue 1 Version 1.0 Year 2014

[506] Cavitation & Extraction protocol Thomas E. Levy, MD, FACC, Hal A. Huggins, DDS, MS Journal of Advancement in Medicine, Volume 9, Number 4, Winter 1996

[507] Endodontic treatment and general health April 1996. A recent press report (*Daily Mail*, 9 April 1996) suggested that the removal of endodontically treated teeth could alleviate various health conditions, including arthritis and kidney and heart disease.

[508] "Transatlantic Transfer of Digitized Antigen Signal by Telephone Link," J. Benveniste, P. Jurgens, W. Hsueh and J. Aissa, "Journal of Allergy & Clinical Immunology - Program and abstracts of papers to be presented during scientific sessions AAAAI/AAI.CIS Joint Meeting February 21-26, 1997"

[509] California's PROPOSITION 65:

> Warning on dental amalgam, used in many dental fillings, causes exposure to mercury, a chemical known to the state of California to cause birth defects or other reproductive harm.

Root canal treatments and restorations including fillings, crowns and bridges, use chemicals known to the state of California to cause cancer.

[510] Dental Infections – Oral and Systemic Being a contribution to the Pathology of Dental Infections, Focal infections and the Degenerative Disseases. Weston A Price DDS., MS., FACD Cleveland Ohio The Penton Press Co Cleveland 1923

[511]

[512] Alves J.A., Barrieshi K, Walton R. E., Wertz P. Wilcox L., Drake D. J Dent Res 1996; 75 (special issue):373 abstract 2847).

[513] Monitoring the effectiveness of root canal procedures on endotoxin levels found in teeth with chronic apical periodontitis Ariane Cassia Salustiano MARINHO, et al J Appl Oral Sci. 2014 Nov-Dec; 22(6): 490–95.

[514] Martinho FC, Gomes BP. Quantification of endotoxins and cultivable bacteria in root canal infection before and after chemomechanical preparation with 2.55% sodium hypochlorite. J Endod. 2008;34:268–272.

[515] Martinho FC, Chiesa WM, Leite FR, Cirelli JA, Gomes BP. Antigenic activity of bacterial endodontic contents from primary root canal infection with periapical lesions against macrophage in the release of interleukin-1beta and tumor necrosis factor alpha. J Endod. 2010;36:1467–1474.

[516] Gomes BP, Martinho FC, Vianna ME. Comparison of 25% sodium hypochlorite and 2% chlorhexidine gel on oral bacterial lipopolysaccharide reduction from primarily infected root canals. J Endod. 2009;35:1350–1353.

[517] Schein B, Schilder H. Endotoxin content in endodontically involved teeth. J Endod. 2006;32:293–295.

[518] Gomes BP, Endo MS, Martinho FC. Comparison of endotoxin levels found in primary and secondary endodontic infections. J Endod. 2012;38:1082–1086

[519] Buck RA, Cai J, Eleazer PD, Staat RH, Hurst HE. Detoxification of endotoxin by endodontic irrigants and calcium hydroxide. J Endod. 2001;27:325–327.

[520] Burton AJ, Carter HE. Purification and characterization of the lipid A component of the lipopolysaccharides from Escherichia coli. Biochemistry. 1964;3:411–418

[521] Alves J.A., Barrieshi K, Walton R. E., Wertz P. Wilcox L., Drake D. J Dent Res 1996; 75 (special issue):373 abstract 2847);

[522] R. Nissan et al J. Endo 21:2 1995

[523] Horiba N, Maekawa Y, Matsumoto T, Nakamura H J Endod 1990 Jul;16(7):331-334 A

[524] Schein B J. of Endodontics 1975 Vol 1 No 1 Measurable quantities of endotoxins are found in root filled teeth.

[525] Schein B J. of Endodontics 1975 Vol 1 No 1

[526] Alves J.A., Barrieshi K, Walton R. E., Wertz P. Wilcox L., Drake D. J Dent Res 1996; 75 (special issue):373 abstract 2847).

[527] R. Nissan et al J. Endo 21:2 1995

[528] Horiba et al. Oral Surg. Oral Med. Oral Path. 1991 Vol 71

[529] Clinical Syndromes and Cardinal Features of Infectious Diseases: Approach to Diagnosis and Initial Management Judith A. Guzman-Cottrill,... Brahm Goldstein, in Principles and Practice of Pediatric Infectious Diseases (Fourth Edition), 2012

[530] Penner A et al. J Exp Med 1960;111:145-53

[531] Parnas I Science 1971;171:1153-5

[532] Alper M Proc Soc Exp Biol Med 1967;124:537-8

[533] Palmiro C J Exp Med 1962; 115:609-12

[534] Toxicol Lett 1996 Jan;84(1):43-53 Effects of repeated exposures of hydrogen sulphide on rat hippocampal EEG. Skrajny B, Reiffenstein RJ, Sainsbury RS, Roth SH

[535] Can J Physiol Pharmacol 1992 Nov;70(11):1515-1518 Low concentrations of hydrogen sulphide alter monoamine levels in the developing rat central nervous system. Skrajny B, Hannah RS, Roth SH

[536] Penner A et al. J Exp Med 1960;111:145-53

[537] Palmiro C J Exp Med 1962; 115:609-12

[538] Alper M Proc Soc Exp Biol Med 1967;124:537-8

[539] Parnas I Science 1971;171:1153-5

[540] J Neurophysiol 1993 Jul;70(1):81–96 The actions of hydrogen sulfide on dorsal raphe serotonergic neurons in vitro. Kombian SB, Reiffenstein RJ, Colmers WF

[541] Toxicol Ind Health 1995 Mar;11(2):185-197 Hydrogen sulfide and reduced-sulfur gases adversely affect neurophysiological functions. Kilburn KH, Warshaw RH

[542] A prospective study to investigate the relationship between periodontal disease and adverse pregnancy outcome S Moore, et al British Dental Journal volume 197, 11 September 2004: 251–258(2004)

[543] Beck J, Garcia R, Heiss G, Vokonas PS, Offenbacher J Periodontol 1996 Oct;67(10 Suppl):1123-1137 Periodontal disease and cardiovascular disease

[544] Kipioti A, Nakou M, Legakis N, Mitsis F Oral Surg Oral Med Oral Pathol 1984 Aug;58(2):213-220 Microbiological findings of infected root canals and adjacent periodontal pockets in teeth with advanced periodontitis.

[545] Kerekes K, Olsen I Endod Dent Traumatol 1990 Feb;6(1):1-5 Similarities in the microfloras of root canals and deep periodontal pockets.

[546] The role of endotoxin and its receptors in allergic disease L. Keoki Williams, MD, MPH, Dennis R. Ownby, MD, Mary J. Maliarik, PhD, and Christine C. Johnson, PhD, MPH Ann Allergy Asthma Immunol. 2005 Mar; 94(3): 323–332.

[547] Asikainen S, Alaluusua S Eur Heart J 1993 Dec;14 Suppl K:43-50 Bacteriology of dental infections.

[548] M.K. Wu, Moorer Wesselink Int. Endodontic Journal (1989) 22, 269-277 Schein B J. of Endodontics 1975 Vol 1 No 1

[549] Asikainen S, Alaluusua S Eur Heart J 1993 Dec;14 Suppl K:43-50 Bacteriology of dental infections.

[550] M.K. Wu, Moorer Wesselink Int. Endodontic Journal (1989) 22, 269-277

[551] Schein B J. of Endodontics 1975 Vol 1 No 1

[552] Horiba N, Maekawa Y, Matsumoto T, Nakamura H J Endod 1990 Jul;16(7):331-334

[553] A study of the distribution of endotoxin in the dentinal wall of infected root canals. Horiba et al. Oral Surg. Oral Med. Oral Path. 1991 Vol 71

[554] J Neurophysiol 1993 Jul;70(1):81-96 The actions of hydrogen sulfide on dorsal raphe serotonergic neurons in vitro. Kombian SB, Reiffenstein RJ, Colmers WF

[555] Toxicol Ind Health 1995 Mar;11(2):185-197 Hydrogen sulfide and reduced-sulfur gases adversely affect neurophysiological functions. Kilburn KH, Warshaw RH

[556] Annu Rev Pharmacol Toxicol 1992;32:109-134 Toxicology of hydrogen sulfide. Reiffenstein RJ, Hulbert WC, Roth SH

[557] J Appl Physiol 1995 Feb;78(2):433-440 Sulfide-induced perturbations of the neuronal mechanisms controlling breathing in rats. Greer JJ, Reiffenstein RJ, Almeida AF, Carter JE

[558] Robert McMahon A.B., DDS From Dental Interference Fields and NICO Acad of Biol Dentistry 82

[559] Keele C., Armstrong D., "Mediators of Pain" Pharmacol of pain Oxford: Pergaman 1968

[560] Wannfors K Hammarstrom L "A Proliferative inflamation in the mandible caused by implantation of an infected dental root" Inter J Of Oral and Maxilofacial Surgery 18 (1989)

[561] Brodin E., Gazelius B Edvinsson L "Tachykinins in Peripheral Sensory Nerve Endings" eds. F. Sichter, et al (B.V. Elsevier Science Publishers)

[562] Fitzgerald M Woolf C., "Axon Transport and Sensory C-Fibre Function" 29th IUPS Satelite Symposium, Australia.

[563] Muramatso I., "Peripheral Transmission of Primary Sensory Nerves" Japanese J of Pharm. 43 (1987) 113-120

[564] Dahlen C., Bergenholtz G., "Endotoxic activity of teeth with necrotic pulp" J. Dent. Res. 559 (1980) 1033-40

[565] Josef Issels MD Cancer A second Opinion 1999 ISBN 0-89529-992-5: "Odontogenic toxins wherever they may have been produced, are able to diffuse and circulate within the organism."

[566] The formation of hydrogen sulfide and methyl mercaptan by oral bacteria. Persson et al., (1990). Oral Microbiol. Immunol. 5:195-201.(2082242)

[567] Desulfuration of cysteine and methionine by Fusobacterium nucleatum. Piannotti et al., (1986). J. Dent. Res.65:913-917.(3458742)

[568] On the transformation of sulfur-containing amino acids and peptides to volatile sulfur compounds (VSC) in the human mouth. Waler (1997). Eur. J. Oral Sci. 105:534-537.(9395120)

[569] Production of volatile sulfur compounds by various Fusobacterium species. Claesson et al., (1990). Oral Microbiol. Immunol. 5:137-142.(2080068)

[570] Competition for peptides and amino acids among periodontal bacteria. Tang-Larsen et. al., (1995). J. Periodont. Res. 30:390-395.(8544102)

[571] Relationship between volatile sulfur compounds, BANA-hydrolyzing bacteria and gingival health in patients with and without complaints of oral malodor. De Boever et. al., (1994). J. Clin. Dentisrty 4:114-119. (8031479)

[572] Peptostreptococcus micros has a uniquely high capacity to form hydrogen sulfide from glutatione. Carlsson et. al., (1993). Oral Microbiol. Immunol. 8:42-45.(8510983)

[573] Science Direct https://www.sciencedirect.com/topics/engineering/methyl-mercaptan

[574] Agency for Toxic Substances and Disease Registry USA https://www.atsdr.cdc.gov/MHMI/mmg139.pdf

[575]

[576] Ecomed Verlag, Landsberg 1998 isbn 3-609-71750-5

[577] www.issels.com/publicatioins

[578] https://www.burtongoldberg.com/home/burtongoldberg/contribution-of-chemotherapy-to-five-year-survival-rate-morgan.pdf

[579] S.H. Shackman Fraud and Root Canals. Institute of Science www.instituteofscience.com

[580] Joseph Issels

[581]

[582] Kristensson K., Olssan Y., "Diffusion Pathways and Retrograde Transport in Peripheral nerves" Prog. In Neurobio. 1 (1973)

[583] Price DL., Griffin J., Neurons and ensheathing cells as targets of disease processes. Ed. P.S. Spencer. Experimental and Clinical Neurotoxicology (Schaumburg: Wilkens and Wilkens 1980

[584] Westrum LE., Canfield RC., Black R., Transganglionic Degeneration in thespinal trigeminal nucleus following the removal of tooth pulps in adult cats. Brain Res 1976; 6:100:137-40

[585] Ratner EJ, Person P, Kleinman DJ. Severe arm pain associated with pathological bone cavity of maxilla. Lancet 1978:106-107.

[586] Ratner EJ, Person P, Kleinman DJ, et al. Jawbone cavities and trigeminal and atypical facial neuralgias. Oral Surg 1979; 48:3-20

[587] Ratner EJ, Langer B, Evins ML. Alveolar cavitational osteopathosis -- manifestations of an infectious process and its implication in the causation of chronic pain. J Periodontol 1986; 57:593-603

[588] Ratner EJ, Person P, Kleinman DJ. Oral pathology and trigeminal neuralgia. I. Clinical experiences. J Dent Res 1976; 55:299. (research abstract)

[589] Shankland WE. Osteocavitational lesions (Ratner bone cavities): frequently misdiagnosed as trigeminal neuralgia-a case report. J Craniomand Pract 1993; 11:232-234.

590 Socransky SS, Stone C, Ratner E. Oral pathology and trigeminal neuralgia. III. Microbiologic examination. J Dent Res 1976; 55(B):300. (research abstract)

591 Mathis B., Oatis G., Grisius R., "Jaw bone cavities associated with facial pain syndromes' Military Med. 146 (1981)

592 Shaber E., Krol A., "Trigeminal Neuralgia - a new treatment concept" Oral Surg, Oral Med., and Oral Path. 49(4)1980

593 Xiwei J. Quinrong I., the influence of pathological bone cavities of jaw bone on the etiopathology of trigeminal neuralgia. Acta Acad Med Sichuan 12(2) 1981

594 Mortang W.,. Xiwei J., et al. "A study between the relation of the various trigger zones of idiopathic trigeminal neuralgia and jaw bone cavities," Acta Acad Med Sichuan 13(3) 1982

595 Mortang W.,. Xiwei J., et al. "Localisation method in the diagnosis of the pathological jaw bone cavity" Acta Acad Med Sichuan 13(4) 1982

596 Brodin E., Gazelius B Edvinsson L "Tachykinins in Peripheral Sensory Nerve Endings" eds. F. Sichter, et al (B.V. Elsevier Science Publishers)G., "Endotoxic activity of teeth with necrotic pulp" J. Dent. Res. 559 (1980) 1033-40

597 Wannfors K Hammarstrom L "A Proliferative inflamation in the mandible caused by implantation of an infected dental root" Inter J Of Oral and Maxilofacial Surgery 18 (1989)

598 Keele C., Armstrong D., "Mediators of Pain" Pharmacol of pain Oxford: Pergaman 1968

599 Fitzgerald M Woolf C., "Axon Transport and Sensory C-Fibre Function" 29th IUPS Satelite Symposium, Australia.

600 Muramatso I., "Peripheral Transmission of Primary Sensory Nerves" Japanese J of Pharm. 43 (1987) 113-120

601 Ecomed Verlag, Landsberg 1998 isbn 3-609-71750-5

602 Stortebecker P "Dental Infectious Foci and diseases of the nervous system - spread of microorganisM.S. and their products from dental infectious foci along direct cranial venous pathways eliciting a toxic - infectious encephalopathy" Acta. Psych Neural Scand 36 Suppl. 157 (1961) 62

603 Stortebecker P "The cranial venous system filled from pulp of a tooth - Proceedings" 3rd Int. Congress of Nero Surg. Copenhagen Aug 1965

604 Stortebecker P "Dental significance of pathways for dissemination from infectious foci." J Can Dent Assoc 33:6 1967 pp301-311

605 Stortebecker P "Chronic dental infections in the etiology of Glioblastomas. 8th int congress" Neuropathy. Washington D.C. Sept 1978 J Neuropth. Exp. Neurology 37(s) 1978

606 Selden HS The endo-antral syndrome: an endodontic complication. J Am Dent Assoc (1989 Sep) 119(3):397-8, 401-2

607 Ngeow WC Orbital cellulitis as a sole symptom of odontogenic infection. Singapore Med J (1999 Feb) 40(2):101-3

608 Maloney PL Doku HC Maxillary sinusitis of odontogenic origin. J Can Dent Assoc (1968 Nov) 34(11):591-603

609 Guglani L Maxillary sinusitis due to dental infection. Newsl Int Coll Dent India Sect (1970 Sep) 7(3):15

610 Yamazaki Y Shimada K Sakuma M Kawashima Y Kobayashi H [Odontogenic maxillary sinusitis: with special reference to surgical therapy] Nippon Jibiinkoka Gakkai Kaiho (1972 Oct) 75(10):1125-6

611 Esposito S [Maxillary sinusitis of dental origin] Rass Int Clin Ter (1970 Jan 15) 50(1):39-45

612 Azimov M Ermakova FB [Role of focal odontogenic infection in the pathogenesis of maxillary sinusitis (experimental study)] Stomatologiia (Mosk) (1978 Jan-Feb) 57(1):11-4

613 Neupokoev NI Neupokoeva NV [Periapical cyst of the maxillary teeth as a cause of odontogenic maxillary sinusitis] Stomatologiia (Mosk) (1991 May-Jun) 70(3):62-3

614 Bertrand B Rombaux P Eloy P Reychler H Sinusitis of dental origin. Acta Otorhinolaryngol Belg (1997) 51(4):315-22

615 Stefaniu A Czausescu V Popescu N Romascanu G Ceausescu A [Orbito- ocular and meningoencephalic complications in odontogenic maxillary sinusitis] Rev Chir Oncol Radiol O R L Oftalmol Stomatol Otorinolaringol (1982 Jan-Mar) 27(1):59-64

616 Tarlowska W A case of chronic inflammation of the right maxillary sinus caused by the introduction of cement into its lumen during root canal treatment of the 1st molar through the palatal root canal Czas Stomatol (1968 Jan) 21(1)

617 Sato K Pathology of recent odontogenic maxillary sinusitis and the usefulness of endoscopic sinus surgery Nippon Jibiinkoka Gakkai Kaiho (2001 Jul) 104(7):715-20

618 Selden HS The interrelationship between the maxillary sinus and endodontics. Oral Surg Oral Med Oral Pathol (1974 Oct) 38(4):623-9

[619] Selden HS August DS Maxillary sinus involvement--an endodontic complication. Report of a case. Oral Surg Oral Med Oral Pathol (1970 Jul) 30(1)

[620] Thevoz F Arza A Jaques B Dental foreign body sinusitis Schweiz Med Wochenschr (2000) Suppl 125:30S-34S

[621] Bogaerts P Hanssens JF Siquet JP Healing of maxillary sinusitis of odontogenic origin following conservative endodontic retreatment: case reports. Acta Otorhinolaryngol Belg (2003) 57(1):91-7

[622] Risk of maxillary fungus ball in patients with endodontic treatment on maxillary teeth: a case-control study. Oral Surg Oral Med Oral Pathol Oral Radiol Endod. 2007 Mar;103(3):433-6. Epub 2006 Dec 4 Mensi M, Piccioni M, Marsili F, Nicolai P, Sapelli PL, Latronico N.

[623] American Association of Endodontics Position Statement Maxillary Sinusitis of Endodontic Origin. AAE website 2021

[624] Gay D Dick G Is multiple sclerosis caused by an oral spirochaete? Lancet (1986 Jul 12) 2(8498):75-7

[625] Callaghan TS Multiple sclerosis and sinusitis Lancet (1986 Jul 19) 2(8499):160-1

[626] Jones RL Crowe P Chavda SV Pahor AL The incidence of sinusitis in patients with multiple sclerosis. Rhinology (1997 Sep) 35(3):118-9 A retrospective study was performed to assess the incidence of sinus disease in patients with M.S. The MRI scans of 108 patients referred to a regional Neurosciences Unit with a diagnosis of multiple sclerosis were examined. There were 71 females and 37 males with an age range of 22 to 67 years (mean: 39.7 years). The sagittal and axial images were reviewed and the degree of sinus disease noted. This was graded as absent, minimal, polypoid and pansinus. Fifty- seven patients (53%) had disease, the most common sinus involved was the maxillary followed by the ethmoid, frontal and sphenoid. Thirty- six patients had bilateral disease affecting the ethmoid sinuses most commonly. Three patients had fluid levels and four patients had retention cysts. The incidence of sinus disease is higher than in some other studies of normal populations.

[627] Symons AL Bortolanza M Godden S Seymour G A preliminary study into the dental health status of multiple sclerosis patients. Spec Care Dentist (1993 May-Jun) 13(3):96-101

[628] Khmel'nik VM [Combined intracranial complication in chronic odontogenic maxillary sinusitis] Kombinirovannoe vnutricherepnoe oslozhnenie pri khronicheskom odontogennom gaimorite. Vestn Otorinolaringol (1981 May-Jun)(3):87-8 ISSN: 0042-4668

411

[629] Khmel'nik VM [Combined intracranial complication in chronic odontogenic maxillary sinusitis] Kombinirovannoe vnutricherepnoe oslozhnenie pri khronicheskom odontogennom gaimorite. Vestn Otorinolaringol (1981 May-Jun)(3):87-8 ISSN: 0042-4668

[630] Jones RL Crowe P Chavda SV Pahor AL The incidence of sinusitis in patients with multiple sclerosis. Rhinology (1997 Sep) 35(3):118-9 A retrospective study was performed to assess the incidence of sinus disease in patients with M.S.631 Gay D Dick G Upton G Multiple sclerosis associated with sinusitis: case-controlled study in general practice. Lancet (1986 Apr 12) 1(8485):815-9

[632] Craelius W Comparative epidemiology of multiple sclerosis and dental caries. J Epidemiol Community Health (1978 Sep) 32(3):155-65

[633] In the words of a patient who was also featured in my documentary 'ROOTED' from 2006

[634] World Health Organization Criteria 118 Environmental Mercury 1991

[635] M.S. Hughes, Amer. J. Of Obstetrics and Gynecology, vol 143, No 4:440- 443, 1982.

[636] P. Le Quesne,"Metal-induced diseases of the nervous system",1982, Br J Hosp Med,28:

[637] J.Mai et al, Biological Trace Element Research,1990;24:109-117.

[638] B.A. Weber, "Conuctivitis sicca(dry eye study)", Institute for Naturopathic Medicine, 1994;

[639] G.Sallsten et al, "Mercury in cerebrospinal fluid in subjects exposed to mercury vapor", Environmental Research, 1994; 65:195-206.

[640] Siblerud RL Kienholz E Evidence that mercury from silver dental fillings may be an etiological factor in multiple sclerosis. Sci Total Environ (1994 Mar 15) 142(3):191-205

[641] Kahrizi F Salimi A Noorbakhsh F Faizi M Mehri F Naserzadeh P Naderi N Pourahmad J Repeated Administration of Mercury Intensifies Brain Damage in

[642] Prochazkova J Sterzl I Kucerova H Bartova J Stejskal VD The beneficial effect of amalgam replacement on health in patients with autoimmunity. Neuro Endocrinol Lett (2004 Jun) 25(3):211-8

[643] Siblerud RL A comparison of mental health of multiple sclerosis patients with silver/mercury dental fillings and those with fillings removed. Psychol Rep (1992 Jun) 70(3 Pt 2):1139-51

[644] Hugins HA Levy TE Cerebrospinal fluid protein changes in multiple sclerosis after dental amalgam removal. Altern Med Rev (1998 Aug) 3(4):295-300

[645]

[646] Fluoride exposure from infant formula and child IQ in a Canadian birth cohort. Till et al Environment International 134:105315. January 2020;

[647] Li, X.S.; Zhi, J.L.; Gao, R.O. Effect of fluoride exposure on intelligence of children. Fluoride. 28(4):189-192,1995.

[648] Clin Exp Pharmacol Physiol 1995 May;22(5):379-380 Alteration of the morphology and neurochemistry of the developing mammalian nervous system by hydrogen sulphide. Roth SH, Skrajny B, Reiffenstein RJ Department of Pharmacology and Therapeutics, Faculty of Medicine, University of Calgary, Alberta, Canada.

[649] Neurosci Lett 1989 May 8;99(3):323-327 Hydrogen sulfide exposure alters the amino acid content in developing rat CNS. Hannah RS, Hayden LJ, Roth SH Department of Anatomy, University of Calgary, Alta., Canada.

[650] S H Shakman Instituteofscience.com

[651] Stortebecker P "Dental Infectious Foci and diseases of the nervous system - spread of microorganisms and their products from dental infectious foci along direct cranial venous pathways eliciting a toxic - infectious encephalopathy" Acta. Psych Neural Scand 36 Suppl. 157 (1961) 62

[652] Journal of the Indian Prosthodontic Association 2005 Vol 5 Iss 3 P126-131

[653] Meachim G, Williams DF. Changes in nonosseous tissue adjacent to titanium implants. J Biomed Mater Res 1973;7:555-72.

[654] Solar RJ, Pollack SR, Korostoff E. In vitro corrosion testing of titanium surgical implant alloys: an approach to understanding titanium release from implants. J Biomed Mater Res 1979;13:217-50.

[655] Merrit K, Brown SA. In Compatibility of Biomedical Implants, Kovacs P., Istephanous NS. Editors, Proc.-Vol.94-15, The Electrochemical Society: Pennington NJ; 1994. p. 14.

[656] Ferguson AB, Jr, Laing PG, Hodge ES. "The ionization of metal implants in living tissue". J Bone Jt Surg 1960;42:76-89.

[657] Australian Dental Journal (Aust. Dent. J.) ISSN 0045-0421 2002, vol. 47, No3, pp. 214-217 FRISKEN K. W.; DANDIE G. W.; LUGOWSKI S.; JORDAN G.;

[658] What is the impact of titanium particles and biocorrosion on implant survival and complications? A critical review. Mombelli A et al Clin Oral Implants Res. 2018 Oct;29 Suppl 18:37–53.

[659] www.melisa.org

[660] Actinomycotic Oral Infection (Modern Dental Implants and Root Canals) R. S. Carlson BioCore Oct 2017

[661] Impact of the Food Additive Titanium Dioxide (E171) on Gut Microbiota-Host Interaction Wojciech Chrzanowski et al Front. Nutr., 14 May 2019 https://doi.org/10.3389/fnut.2019.00057

[662] Food-grade TiO2 impairs intestinal and systemic immune homeostasis, initiates preneoplastic lesions and promotes aberrant crypt development in the rat colon

Sarah Bettini, et al. Scientific Reports volume 7, Article number: 40373 (2017)

[663] Ultrafine titanium dioxide particles in the absence of photoactivation can induce oxidative damage to human bronchial epithelial cells.Gurr JR, Wang AS, Chen CH, Jan KY. Toxicology. 2005 Sep 15;213(1-2):66-73.

[664] Titanium particles stimulate bone resorption by inducing differentiation of murine osteoclasts. Bi Y, Van De Motter RR, Ragab AA, Goldberg VM, Anderson JM, Greenfield EM. J Bone Joint Surg Am. 2001 Apr;83-A(4):501-8.

[665] Immunohistochemical study of the soft tissue around long-term skin-penetrating titanium implants. Holgers KM Et Al. Biomaterials. 1995 May;16(8):611-6.

[666] Corrosion of titanium and amalgam couples: effect of fluoride, area size, surface preparation and fabrication procedures. Johansson BI Bergman B Dent Mater (1995 Jan) 11(1):41-6

[667] In vitro corrosion of titanium. Strietzel R, Et Al Biomaterials. 1998 Aug;19(16):1495-9.

[668] Influence of fluoride on titanium in an acidic environment measured by polarization resistance technique. B oere, G. J Appl Biomater, 6(4):283-8, 1995.

[669] Sensitivity to titanium. A cause of implant failure? Lalor PA, Revell PA, Gray AB, Wright S, Railton GT, Freeman MA. London Hospital Medical College, England J Bone Joint Surg Br. 1991 Jan;73(1):25-8

[670] A case of allergic reaction to surgical metal clips inserted for postoperative boost irradiation in a patient undergoing breast-conserving therapy Tamai

K, Mitsumori M, Fujishiro S, Kokubo M, Ooya N, Nagata Y, Sasai K, Hiraoka M, Inamoto T. Department of Therapeutic Radiology and Oncology, Graduate School of Medicine, Kyoto University, 54 Shogoin-Kawahara-cho, Sakyo-ku, Kyoto 606-8507, Japan Breast Cancer. 2001;8(1):90-2e

[671] Effects of titanium-dental restorative alloy galvanic couples on cultured cells. Bumgardner JD Johansson BI J Biomed Mater Res (1998 Summer) 43(2):184-91

[672] Corrosion current and pH rise around titanium coupled to dental alloys. Ravnholt G Scand J Dent Res (1988 Oct) 96(5):466-72

[673] Morphological transformation of BHK-21 cells by nickel titanium shape memory alloy particles encapsulated by titanium oxide Lautenbach E Focal Process And Electro-Skin Test With Special Reference To Stomatologyzahn Mund Kieferheilkd Zentralbl (1975) 63(1):32–41; Thermography And Focus Diagnosisthermographie Und Herddiagnostik Zwr (1975 May 25)84(10):486-88; Rost A Focal Infection And Focal Diagnosis From The Viewpoint Of Thermoregulation Freie Zahnarzt (1985 Oct) 29(10):82, 84, 86; Passim Rozenfel'd Lg Timofeev Aa Borisenko On Stupko Tn Thermographic Diagnosis Of Diseases Of The Maxillofacial Area Stomatologiia (Mosk) (1989 Jan-Feb) 68(1):54-8

PLEOMORPHIC CHANGE

Charlton Br Channing-Santiago Se Bickford Aa Cardona Cj Chin Rp Cooper Gl Droual R Jeffrey Js Meteyer Cu Shivaprasad Hl Et Al Preliminary Characterization Of A Pleomorphic Gram-Negative Rod Associated With Avian Respiratory Disease. J Vet Diagn Invest (1993 Jan) 5(1):47-51Cantwell Ar Variably Acid-Fast Pleomorphic Bacteria As A Possible Cause Of Mycosis Fungoides. A Report Of A Necropsied Case And Two Living Patients J Dermatol Surg Oncol (1982) 8(3):203-213Cantwell Ar Lawson Jw Necroscopic Findings Of Pleomorphic, Variably Acid-Fast Bacteria In A Fatal Case Of Kaposi's Sarcoma J Dermatol Surg Oncol (1981) 7(11):923-930Eisenberg Rj Montgomery Pc Characterization Of An Antibody Directed Against A Surface Component Of Normal And Pleomorphic Cells Of Streptococcus Sanguis. Infect Immun (1975 Sep) 12(3):668-78Maeda N Anaerobic, Gram-Positive, Pleomorphic Rods In Human Gingival Crevice. Bull Tokyo Med Dent Univ (1980 Mar) 27(1):63-70Ishikawa O Aerobic Gram-Positive Pleomorphic Rods Isolated From Dental Plaque And Gingival Crevice. Bull Tokyo Med Dent Univ (1980 Mar) 27(1):71- 7Bauld

J Marshall Kc Quantitative Description Of Morphological Changes During Growth Of A Pleomorphic Budding Bacterium. Antonie Van Leeuwenhoek (1971) 37(4):401–7; Wainwright M Highly Pleomorphic Staphylococci As A Cause Of Cancer. Med Hypotheses (20004 Jan) 54(1):91-4

[674] On electric current creation in patients treated with osseointegrated dental bridges. Nilner K Lekholm U Swed Dent J Suppl (1985) 28:85-92

[675] In vivo corrosion behavior of gold-plated versus titanium dental retention pins. Palaghias G Eliades G Vougiouklakis G J Prosthet Dent (1992 Feb) 67(2):194-8

[676] *Vibrational Medicine* by Gerbber 1987

[677] Effect of Electro Magnetic Field (Emf) on Dental Amalgam and General Health Sundaresan Balagopal Et al Biomed Pharmacol J 2015, 8

[678] https://ehtrust.org/wireless-braces-earrings-hip-replacements-metal-can-increase-wireless-radiation-absorption-body/;

[679] A study of changes to specific absorption rates in the human eye close to perfectly conducting spectacles within the radio frequency range 1.5 to 3.0 GHz W.G. Whittow R.M. Edwards IEEE Transactions on Antennas and Propagation (Volume: 52, Issue: 12, Dec. 2004)

[680] Othman, N., et al. "Specific Absorption Rate in the human leg and testicle due to metallic coin and zip." RF and Microwave Conference (RFM), 2015. IEEE (2015).

[681] Effect of pierced metallic objects on sar distributions at 900 MHz Jose Fayos-Fernandez, Carlos Arranz-Faz, Antonio M. Martinez-Gonzalez, David Sanchez-Hernandez Volume27, Issue5 July 2006 Pages 337-353

[682] The effect of authentic metallic implants on the SAR distribution of the head exposed to 900, 1800 and 2450 MHz dipole near field. Virtanen H. Phys Med Biol. 2007 Mar 7;52(5):1221-36. Epub 2007 Jan 31

[683] Anderson, V., and K. H. Joyner. "Specific absorption rate levels measured in a phantom head exposed to radio frequency transmissions from analog hand-held mobile phones." Bioelectromagnetics 16.1 (1995): 60-9.

[684] Mobile Phone Use and The Risk of Headache: A Systematic Review and Meta-analysis of Cross-sectional Studies Jing Wang, et al Scientific Reportsvolume 7, Article number: 12595 (2017)

[685] Does radiations emitted from cell phone effects orofacial structures and dental implants? Sunil Kumar Mishra, Ramesh Chowdhary Int J Env Health Eng 2018, 7:1

[686] Fujii Y. Sensation of balance dysregulation caused/aggravated by a collection of electromagnetic waves in a dental implant. Open J Antennas Propag 2014;2:29-35.

[687] Fujii Y. Improvement of systemic symptoms after dental implant removal. Open J Stomatol2016;6:37-46

[688] Mishra SK, Chowdhary R, Kumari S, Rao SB. Effect of cell phone radiations on orofacial structures: A Systematic review. J Clin Diagn Res 2017;11:ZE01-5.

[689] https://iabdm.org/education/articles/has-the-dental-work-in-your-mouth-turned-you-into-a-walking-antenna

[690] Mobile phone use and risk for intracranial tumors and salivary gland tumors – A meta-analysis Alicja Bortkiewicz Int J Occup Med Environ Health 2017;30(1):27–43

[691] https://microwavenews.com/news-center/more-coincidence

[692] Report of final results regarding brain and heart tumors in Sprague-Dawley rats exposed from prenatal life until natural death to mobile phone radiofrequency field representative of a 1.8 GHz GSM base station environmental emission L.Falcioni et al Environmental Research Volume 165, August 2018, Pages 496-503

[693] Release of titanium ions from an implant surface and their effect on cytokine production related to alveolar bone resorption. Wachi T et al Toxicology. 2015 Jan 2;327:1-9.

[694]

[695]

[696] Ratner E., Person, Kleinman DJ "Oral Pathology and Trigeminal neuralgia I. Cloinical Experiences." J. Dent Res. Vol 55 1976

[697] Shklar G., Person., Ratner E., "Oral Pathology and Trigeminal neuralgia II Histopathologic Observations." J. Dent Res. 55 1976

[698] Socransky S., Stone C., Ratner., "Oral Pathology and Trigeminal neuralgia III. Microbilogical examination". J. Dent Res. Vol 55 1976

[699] Ratner E., Person P., Kleinman D. Shklar G., Socransky., "Jawbone Cavities and Trigeminal and Atypical facial Neuralgias"" Oral Surg, Oral Med., and Oral Path., 48(1) 1979 3-20

[700] Ratner Langan B and Evins M., "Alveolar Cavitational Osteopathies; manifestation of an infectious Proces and it's implications in the causation of chronic pain" J. of Perio. 57(10) 1986 593-603

[701] Shankland WE. Osteocavitational lesions (Ratner bone cavities): frequently misdiagnosed as trigeminal nerualgia-a case report. J Craniomand Pract 1993;

[702] Skinner & Phillips 5th edition Dec 1964 Chap 21 p349 Text book

References for the Appendix

[i] Shklar, Person, Ratner. Oral pathology and Trigeminal Neuralgia III J Dent Res. 1976;55(B):299

[ii] Ratner E., Langer., Evins M., alveolar Cavitational Osteopathosis manifestations of an infectious process and its implications in the causation of chronic pain. J Periodoontal 1986;57:593-603

[iii] Bouquot JE, Roberts AM, Person, P, et al. The histopathology of neuralgia-inducing Cavitational osteonecrosis (NICO). J Dent Res 1989; 68:952.

[iv] Bouquot JE Roberts AM Person P Christian J Neuralgia-inducing cavitational osteonecrosis (NICO). Osteomyelitis in 224 jawbone samples from patients with facial neuralgia [see comments] Oral Surg Oral Med Oral Pathol (1992 Mar) 73(3):307-19;

[v] Bouquot J, Roberts A. NICO (neuralgia-inducing cavitational osteonecrosis): radiographic appearance of the "invisible" osteomyelitis. Oral Surg Oral Med Oral Pathol 1992; 74:600.

[vi] Bouquot JE Christian J Long-term effects of jawbone curettage on the pain of facial neuralgia. J Oral Maxillofac Surg (1995 Apr) 53(4):387-97; discussion 397-9

[vii] Fracica F Brickman J LoMonaco CJ Lin LM Trigeminal neuralgia and endodontically treated teeth. J Endod (1988 Jul) 14(7):360-2

[viii] Graff-Radford SB, Simmons M, Fox L, et al. Are bony cavities exclusively associated with atypical facial pain and trigeminal neuralgia? Proceedings, Annual Meeting, Western USA Pain Society, 198

[ix] Grecko Puzin., odontogenic Trigeminal Neuralgia. Zh Nevropathol

Psikhiatr 1984;84:1655-8

[x] Jiao X., Meng Q., the influences of pathologic bone cavty of jaw bone on eatiology of Trigeminal Neuralgia. Acta Acad Med Sichaun 1982;12(3): 243-7

[xi] Mathis B., Oatis G., Grisius R., "Jaw bone cavities associated with

facial pain syndromes' Military Med. 146 (1981)

[xii] Mortang W.,. Xiwei J., et al. "A study between the relation of the

various trigger zones of idiopathic trigeminal neuralgia and jaw bone cavities," Acta Acad Med Sichuan 13(3) 1982

[xiii] Ratner EJ Person P Kleinman DJ Shklar G Socransky SS Jawbone cavities and trigeminal and atypical facial neuralgias. Oral Surg Oral Med Oral Pathol (1979 Jul) 48(1):3-20

[xiv] Ratner EJ, Langer B, Evins ML. Alveolar Cavitational osteopathosis -- manifestations of an infectious process and its implication in the causation of chronic pain. J Periodontol 1986; 57:593-603.

[xv] Rhodus: J Okla Dent Assoc (1983 Summer) 74(1):9, 11-2 Treatment of trigeminal neuralgia associated with residual bone cavities.

[xvi] Roberts AM Person P Etiology and treatment of idiopathic trigeminal and atypical facial neuralgias. Oral Surg Oral Med Oral Pathol (1979 Oct) 48(4):298-308

[xvii] Roberts: Oral Surg Oral Med Oral Pathol (1984 Aug) 58(2):121-9 Further observations on dental parameters of trigeminal and atypical facial neuralgias.

[xviii] Shankland WE. Osteocavitational lesions (Ratner bone cavities): frequently misdiagnosed as trigeminal neuralgia-a case report. J Craniomand Pract 1993; 11:232-234.

[xix] Shankland 1993 Cranio 11:232-236.(8242788) Osteocavitation lesions (Ratner bone cavities): frequently misdiagnosed as trigeminal neuralgia-a case report.

[xx] Shaber E., Krol A., "Trigeminal Neuralgia - a new treatment concept" Oral Surg, Oral Med., and Oral Path. 49(4)1980

[xxi] Shklar, Person, Ratner. Oral pathology and Trigeminal Neuralgia III J Dent Res. 1976;55(B):299

[xxii] Socransky SS, Stone C, Ratner E. Oral pathology and trigeminal

neuralgia. III. Microbiologic examination. J Dent Res 1976; 55(B):300.

[xxiii] Wang M., et al a study of the various relation between the trigger zones of idiopathic Trigeminal Neuralgia and jaw bone cavities. Acta Acad Med Sichaun 1982;13(3):233-8

[xxiv] Xiwei J. Quinrong I., the influence of pathological bone cavities of jaw bone on the etiopathology of trigeminal neuralgia. Acta Acad Med Sichuan 12(2) 1981

[xxv] Yang J Simonson TM Ruprecht A Meng D Vincent SD Yuh WT Magnetic resonance imaging used to assess patients with trigeminal neuralgia. Oral Surg Oral Med Oral Pathol Oral Radiol Endod (1996 Mar) 81(3): 343-50

[i] (http://www.aae.org)

[ii] www.melisa.org

[iii] E. Pascon In Vitro Cytotoxicity of root canal filling materials. J. Endo. Vol 16 No 9 1990

[iv] https://www.aae.org/specialty/wp-content/uploads/sites/2/2017/06/paraformaldehydefillingmaterials.pdf

[v] In 1995, Economedes[v] studied four different root filling cements. They are amongst the most popular used at present – AH-26, Roth 811, CRCS, Sealapex all caused mild to severe tissue irritation; Roth 811, CRCS induced zinc redistribution to different organs (liver, kidney, uterus, brain; AH-26 (induced changes in Ca content in some organs). Economedes showed that zinc was distributed from root canals filled with CRCS and Roth 811. High levels were found in the brain, kidney, liver and uterus.

[vi] B. Briseno J. Endo. 16:8 1990

[vii] R. Gerosa et al J. Endo 21:9 1995

[viii] Peltola M Salo T Oikarinen K Toxic effects of various retrograde root filling materials on gingival fibroblasts and rat sarcoma cells. Endod Dent Traumatol (1992 Jun) 8(3):120-4

[ix] Chong BS Ford TR Wilson RF Radiological assessment of the effects of potential root-end filling materials on healing after endodontic surgery. Endod Dent Traumatol (1997 Aug) 13(4):176-9

[x] Chong BS Owadally ID Pitt Ford TR Wilson RF Cytotoxicity of potential retrograde root-filling materials. Endod Dent Traumatol (1994 Jun) 10(3):129-33

[xi] Arenholt-Bindslev D Horsted-Bindslev P A simple model for evaluating relative toxicity of root filling materials in cultures of human oral fibroblasts. Endod Dent Traumatol (1989 Oct) 5(5):219-26

[xii] Geurtsen W Leyhausen G Biological aspects of root canal filling materials--histocompatibility, cytotoxicity, and mutagenicity. Clin Oral Investig (1997 Feb) 1(1):5-11

[xiii] Chong BS Ford TR Kariyawasam SP Tissue response to potential root-end filling materials in infected root canals. Int Endod J (1997 Mar) 30(2):102-14

[xiv] Ersev H Schmalz G Bayirli G Schweikl H Cytotoxic and mutagenic potencies of various root canal filling materials in eukaryotic and prokaryotic cells in vitro. J Endod (1999 May) 25(5):359-63

[xv] Zhu Q Safavi KE Spangberg LS Cytotoxic evaluation of root-end filling materials in cultures of human osteoblast-like cells and periodontal ligament cells. J Endod (1999 Jun) 25(6):410-2

[xvi] Pascon EA Spangberg LS In vitro cytotoxicity of root canal filling materials: 1. Gutta- percha. J Endod (1990 Sep) 16(9):429-33

[xvii] Chong BS Pitt Ford TR Kariyawasam SP Short-term tissue response to potential root-end filling materials in infected root canals. Int Endod J (1997 Jul) 30(4):240-9

[xviii] Briseno B Willershausen B Sonnabend E [The effect of root canal filling materials on gingival fibroblast cultures] Einfluss verschiedener Wurzelfullmaterialien auf Gingivafibroblastenkulturen. Schweiz Monatsschr Zahnmed (1991) 101(3):294-8

[xix] Lambrecht JT Panzer G [The toxicity of root-canal filling materials in primary osteoclast cell cultures (see comments)] Die Toxizitat von Wurzelfullmaterialien in primaren Osteoklasten- Zellkulturen. Schweiz Monatsschr Zahnmed (1995) 105(7):899-906

[xx] Tsuzuki N A histopathological study of various root canal filling materials. Showa Shigakkai Zasshi (1990 Jun) 10(2):196-202

[xxi] Torabinejad M Ford TR Abedi HR Kariyawasam SP Tang HM Tissue reaction to implanted root-end filling materials in the tibia and mandible of guinea pigs. J Endod (1998 Jul) 24(7):468-71

[xxii] Maseki T Yasumura K Nanba I Kobayashi F Nakamura H Alterations in macrophages after exposure to root canal filling materials. J Endod (1996 Sep) 22(9):450-4

[xxiii] Kundzinia RS Komnova ZD Volozhin AI [The periodontal reaction to root canal obturation with different filling materials] Reaktsiia periodonta na zapolnenie kornevogo kanala raznymi plombirovochnymi materialami. Stomatologiia (Mosk) (1993 Jan-Mar) 72(1):4-7

[xxiv] Journal of Endodontics: Volume 26(6) June 2000 pp 321-324 The Mutagenic Potential of AH+ and AH26 by Salmonella/Microsome Assay Jukiç, Silvana DDS; Miletiç, Ivana DDS; Aniç, Ivica DDS, PhD; Britviç, Smiljana PhD; Osmak, Maja PhD; Sistig, Suzana DDS;

[xxv] Neurotoxic effects of root filling materials on rat phrenic nerve in vitro. Brodin P Roed A Aars H Orstavik D [J Dent Res (1982 Aug) 61(8):1020-3]

[ix] Comparative neurotoxic effects of root canal filling materials on rat sciatic nerve. Serper A Ucer O Onur R Etikan I [J Endod (1998 Sep) 24(9):592-4]

www.ingramcontent.com/pod-product-compliance
Lightning Source LLC
Chambersburg PA
CBHW071246220526
45468CB00001B/16